RENAL AND UROLOGIC DISORDERS

COMORBIDITIES IN CHRONIC KIDNEY DISEASE

FROM DIAGNOSIS TO MANAGEMENT

RENAL AND UROLOGIC DISORDERS

Additional books in this series can be found on Nova's website under the Series tab.

Additional e-books in this series can be found on Nova's website under the eBooks tab.

RENAL AND UROLOGIC DISORDERS

COMORBIDITIES IN CHRONIC KIDNEY DISEASE

FROM DIAGNOSIS TO MANAGEMENT

LUCA DI LULLO, MD, PHD
EDITOR

New York

Library of Congress Cataloging-in-Publication Data

ISBN: 978-1-63485-070-4
Library of Congress Control Number: 2016935815

Published by Nova Science Publishers, Inc. † New York

To my father Mario, my mother Elena, my sister Simonetta,
my wife Alessia and my beautiful sons Francesco and Ilaria

CONTENTS

PREFACE

First edition of “Comorbidities in chronic kidney disease” is focused on main clinical syndromes associated with renal failure. Chronic kidney disease (CKD) and end – stage renal disease (ESRD) are characterized by wide spectrum of comorbidities potentially complicating patients’ clinical outcomes.

In this volume, both the editor and the authors, have planned complete review of main clinical syndromes associated with renal injury and failure.

The first chapter is dedicated on epidemiological aspects of chronic kidney disease, also concerning risk factors and associated comorbidities.

Arterial hypertension and cardiovascular diseases are actually accountable as major risk factors for developing renal disease and related chapter is mainly focused to latest trials in this field.

The following chapter is dedicated to pathophysiology, diagnosis and treatment of dyslipidemia and atherosclerosis in patients with declined renal function.

An exhaustive chapter is focused on secondary hyperparathyroidism clinical features and its complications on kidneys, bone, vessels and heart from early laboratory findings ‘till severe vascular and heart valvular calcifications.

The next section reflects on secondary anemia and consequent so – called cardiorenal anemia syndrome with particular attention on latest treatment schedules.

Coronary artery disease is also discussed, especially for whom concerning clinical features and laboratory diagnosis in chronic kidney disease patients with impaired clearance of coronary acute syndrome biomarkers.

Cardiorenal syndrome and sudden cardiac death are a well-established clinical aspects in CKD patients and they are discussed both on pathophsysiological and clinical features.

Book finally ends with two sections on hepato – renal syndrome and contrast – induced nephropathy (CIN); first one tries to point up actual pathophysiological views and treatment’s strategies. CIN represents daily challenge for all nephrologists because of large amounts of instrumental diagnostic tests and increasing number of chronic kidney disease patients involved.

This volume could be appreciated both by nephrologists and all clinicians involved in chronic patients’ management due to schematic and practical editing and form.

In: Comorbidities in Chronic Kidney Disease
Editor: Luca Di Lullo ISBN: 978-1-63485-070-4

Chapter 1

EPIDEMIOLOGY OF CHRONIC KIDNEY DISEASE

Antonio Gorini, MD*
Consultant Nephrologists, Rome, Italy

ABSTRACT

Chronic Kidney Disease (CKD) is among the diseases that are most frequently underdiagnosed. The patient with CKD is affected by a high number of co-morbidities; in addition, it presents an increased risk of cardiovascular and for all-cause death which is not observed in other diseases. It is important to increase the epidemiological knowledge of the disease in order to promote appropriate strategies for prevention and treatment.

Keywords: CKD, epidemiology, mortality rate

Chronic kidney disease (CKD) in recent years has become a major public health emergency.

A characteristic of the early stages of CKD is to not show obvious symptoms, which makes early diagnosis difficult. However, if well-defined screening procedures are shared and implemented by general practitioners on the general population and at-risk populations, a realistic estimate of the prevalence of this disease can be obtained.

CKD has a key role in the so-called chronic Non-Communicable Diseases (NCDs).

The NCDs, also known as chronic diseases, are characterized by not being transmittable, having a long duration and, generally, a slow progression [1].

In the last quarter of a century NCDs have been found as a major cause of death and morbidity worldwide [2].

According to the Global Status Report of the World Health Organization (WHO) of 2014, NCDs cause more deaths than all other causes combined. Furtermore, it is estimated thatwhile deaths from infectious diseases will decrease, those from NCDs will increase by 38 million in 2012 to 52 million in 2030 [3].

---

* Correspondence to: antonio.gorini.md@gmail.com.

The most important NCDs are cardiovascular diseases (CVD) (17.5 million deaths, i.e., 46.2% of NCD deaths), cancer (8.2 million, i.e., 21.7% of NCD deaths), chronic respiratory diseases, including asthma and chronic obstructive pulmonary disease (4.0 million, i.e., 10.7% of NCD deaths), and diabetes (1.5 million, i.e., 4% of NCD deaths).

All together, these four diseases account for 82% of all NCD-related deaths.

Approximately 42% of deaths occur before the seventieth year of age; 48% of deaths from NCDs are observed in low- and middle- income countries while 28% of deaths caused by NCD in high-income countries were in individuals aged under 70 years.

Tobacco use, physical inactivity, alcohol abuse and unhealthy diet increase the risk of death for NCD [4].

CKD patients experience a reduction in kidney function and are at risk for major complications such as anemia, Mineral and Bone Disorders (MBD), infections, an increased risk of Acute Kidney Injury (AKI), atherosclerosis and the increase of cardiovascular disease (CVD).

Progression toward renal disease (ESRD), a stage when Renal Replacement Treatment (RRT) is required, also increases mortality from CVD and all-causes.

While the true incidence and prevalence of CKD is not well known, we do know exactly the number of patients undergoing dialysis treatment.

This is due to the organizational and economic cost of this therapy, which requires a careful national planning. Registers of Dialysis and Transplantation exist in most Western countries, and though some are still incomplete, they still collect data.

The world dialysis population was about 1.1 million in 2002 with an annual increase of 7%, so it is estimated to exeed 2 million people today [5].

According to the Wave III of the US National Health and Nutrition Evaluation Survey, 11% of adults observed between 1988 and 1994 had a CKD [6].

A subsequent survey (1999-2004) has estimated a higher prevalence of 13% [7].

In other countries like China and Australia, the observed prevalence is similar to that of the US at 11%, indicating that prevalence of CKD is much higher than that of dialysis patients.

The National Health and Nutrition Examination Survey (NHANES) examined the prevalence of CKD in the US population, who are not hospitalized and at least 20 years old. From this observation the prevalence of CKD was higher than the prevalence of Diabetes Mellitus (DM) [8]. (Table 1)

This survey likely overestimates the data since it was based on a single test of kidney function. This survey shows a prevalence of 13.6% for CKD and 12.3% for the DM [9].

In the three observation periods of the NHANES study (1988-1994, 1999-2004, 2007-2012), the highest increase was observed in stage 3 patients, where the prevalence increased from 4.5% to 6% [8].

From this study we can conclude that age is the most important risk factor for CKD.

Other important risk factors are the DM, hypertension, obesity and metabolic syndrome, cardiovascular disease, a family history of CKD or ESRD, and a previous acute renal failure.

The Medicare database shows the prevalence of CKD at 10.4% in 2012 in the over 65 population. However, it should be noted that this data is an undeestimation of the actual incidence of CKD due to the recruitment procedure in the database [10].

Another interesting observation that can be drawn from the Medicare database is that, once the CKD diagnosis is made, 91% of the population is visited by a general practitioner within one year from diagnosis, 62% by the cardiologist, while only 31% by a nephrologist. Within the group of stage 3-5 CKD patients, the percentage of patients that are followed by a nephrologist increases to 55% [10].

These data show that there is a lack of awareness of who can give best treament for CKD, although there is evidence that the patients followed by nephrologist have a better prognosis than those visited by other specialists [11, 12].

Table 1. Prevalences (%) of CDK in NHANES population within age, sex, race /ethnicity and risk – factor categories, (a) 1988 – 1994, (b) 1999 – 2004, (c) 2007 – 2012 (modified)

	All CKD			*eGFR < 60*			*ACR ≥ 30*		
	1988 - 1994	*1999 - 2004*	*2007 - 2012*	*1988 - 1994*	*1999 - 2004*	*2007 - 2012*	*1988 - 1994*	*1999 - 2004*	*2007 - 2012*
20 – 39	5.1	5.9	5.7	0.1	0.3	0.2	5.0	5.8	5.5
40 – 59	8.4	9.8	8.9	1.3	2.0	2.3	7.5	8.4	7.2
60 +	32.2	37.5	33.2	19.1	25.1	22.7	18.0	20.1	17.7
Male	10.2	12.3	12.1	4.1	5.0	5.4	7.4	9.2	8.7
Female	14.2	15.7	15.1	5.6	7.2	7.6	10.2	10.3	9.6
Non – Hispanic White	12.3	14.0	13.9	5.5	7.0	7.6	8.2	8.9	8.4
Non – Hispanic Black / Af Am	14.5	14.9	15.9	4.1	5.0	6.2	12.7	12.4	12.3
Other	10.5	13.5	11.7	2.2	3.4	3.1	9.2	11.7	10.1
Diabetes	43.1	42.0	39.2	15.6	17.0	19.6	36.3	33.3	28.6
SR Diabetes	42.7	42.2	40.4	16.4	18.5	21.1	35.9	32.6	29.3
Hypertension	33.3	32.7	31.0	15.3	17.1	17.1	23.4	21.3	19.8
SR Hypertension	25.3	27.2	26.0	12.9	15.8	15.2	17.1	16.4	16.2
SR Cardiovasc. disease	25.4	40.0	39.5	14.5	27.3	26.8	16.6	23.0	23.8
Obesity (BMI ≥30)	16.6	16.8	16.6	6.2	6.4	7.3	12.3	12.6	11.5
All	12.0	14.0	13.6	4.9	6.2	6.5	8.8	9.8	9.2

Data source: National Health and Nutrition Examination Survey (NHANES), 1988 – 1994, 1999 – 2004, 2007 – 2012. Participants age 20 and older. Single – sample estimates of e GFR and ACR; eGFR calculated using the CKD – EPI equation. Diabetes defined as HbA1c > 7 percent, self – reported (SR), or currently taking glucose – lowering medications. Hypertension defined as BP ≥ 130 / ≥ 80 for those with diabetes or CKD, otherwise BP ≥ 140 / ≥ 90, or taking medication for hypertension. The table represents NHANES participants who are classified hypertensive (measured/ treated) but some of those are at target of blood pressure. Abbreviation: ACR, urine albumin / creatinine ratio; Af Am, African American; BMI, body mass index, BP, blood pressure; CKD, chronic kidney disease; eGFR, estimated glomerular filtration rate.

The frequency of hospitalizations and readmissions after hospitalization are indicative of disease severity.

With a decreasing renal function we observe a higher number of hospital admissions, after data analysis adjusted for age, race, sex, comorbidity.

CKD patients have a hospitalization rate of 0.40 per patient year overall—0.35 for Stages 1-2, 0.40 for Stage 3, and 0.55 for Stages 4-5 (0.39 where stage is not specified) [13].

The USRDS noted that the hospitalizations rate for CVD and infection increases with decreasing of Glomerular Filtration Rate (GFR) [10].

Table 2. Prevalences (%) of cardiovascular comorbidities, by CKD status, age, race and sex, 2012 (modified)

	Atherosclerotic heart disease (ASHD)		Acute myocardial infarction (AMI)		Congestive heart failure (CHF)	
	w/o CKD	Any CKD	w/o CKD	Any CKD	w/o CKD	Any CKD
Overall	17.4	42.9	2.4	10.6	6.7	30.1
66 – 69	11.6	35.2	1.7	9.7	3.3	22.2
70 – 74	15.4	39.5	2.1	9.7	4.5	24.3
75 – 84	20.6	44.8	2.7	10.6	7.6	29.4
85 +	23.1	46.1	3.3	11.8	14.0	39.5
White	17.9	43.9	2.5	11.0	6.7	30.1
Black /Af Am	14.2	36.4	1.9	8.9	8.1	32.3
Other	17.7	40.1	1.6	8.1	5.4	26.4
Male	23.2	50.2	3.1	12.6	6.9	30.2
Female	13.3	36.3	1.9	8.9	6.6	30.1
	Cerebrovascular accident/ transient ischemic attack (CVA – TIA)		Peripheral artery disease (PAD)		Atrial fibrillation (AIFB)	
	w/o CKD	Any CKD	w/o CKD	Any CKD	w/o CKD	Any CKD
Overall	7.5	19.1	9.1	26.4	9.6	24.2
66 – 69	4.3	14.7	4.6	19.5	4.3	14.1
70 – 74	5.9	16.2	6.4	22.4	6.6	18.2
75 – 84	9.1	20.0	10.5	26.8	11.9	25.0
85 +	12.1	21.9	17.9	32.0	18.0	32.3
White	7.5	18.9	9.2	26.6	10.3	26.0
Black /Af Am	8.5	21.4	10.1	26.2	4.8	14.6
Other	6.4	17.8	7.1	22.9	5.3	16.1
Male	7.5	19.0	9.2	27.3	10.8	26.5
Female	7.6	19.2	9.1	25.6	8.7	22.1
	Cardiac arrest and ventricular arrhythmias (SCA / VA)					
	w/o CKD	Any CKD				
Overall	1.3	4.5				
66 – 69	0.9	4.0				
70 – 74	1.2	4.5				
75 – 84	1.6	4.8				
85 +	1.6	4.3				
White	1.4	4.6				
Black /Af Am	1.1	4.5				
Other	0.8	2.9				
Male	1.9	6.2				
Female	0.9	3.0				

Data source: Medicare 5 percent sample. Patients age 66 and older, alive, without end – stage renal disease and residing in the U.S. on 12/31/2012 with fee – for service coverage for the entire calendar year. The denominators for all cardiovascular comorbidities are Medicare enrollees age 66 +.

Overall, hospitalizations increased in the presence of comorbidities, such as DM and CVD.

Table 3. Prevalences (%) of cardiovascular procedures, by CKD status, age, race and sex, 2012 (modified)

	Revascularization-percutaneous coronary interventions (PCI)		Revascularization-coronary artery bypass graft (CABG)		Implatable cardioverter defibrillators & cardiac resynchronization therapy with defibrillator (ICD/CRT-D)	
	w/o CKD	Any CKD	w/o CKD	Any CKD	w/o CKD	Any CKD
Overall	4.2	5.3	1.1	1.8	0.8	1.2
66 – 69	6.2	7.8	1.7	2.9	1.4	2.0
70 – 74	5.1	6.7	1.4	2.8	1.1	1.8
75 – 84	3.9	5.5	1.1	1.9	0.9	1.5
85 +	2.1	3.3	0.3	0.6	0.3	0.5
White	4.3	5.4	1.2	1.9	0.8	1.3
Black/ Af Am	3.5	4.7	0.8	1.3	0.5	0.9
Other	3.8	4.8	0.9	1.3	0.8	1.2
Male	4.7	5.9	1.4	2.2	1.3	1.9
Female	3.6	4.6	0.8	1.2	0.4	0.6

Data source: Medicare 5 percent sample. Patients age 66 and older, alive, without end – stage renal disease, and residing in the U.S. on 12/31/2012 with fee – for service coverage for the entire calendar year. The denominators for PCI and CABG are Medicare enrollees age 66 + with ASHD. The denominators for ICD/CRT-D are Medicare enrollees age 66 +with CHF.

Hospitalizations for CVD were 23% and 19% for infections, according to data reported in January 2012 from the Medicare database.

In 2012, 24% of CKD patients were readmitted to the hospital within thirty days after hospital discharge, while those without CKD had a 17% re-hospitalization rate [10]. As patients get closer to the pre-dialysis stages the frequency of readmissions increases gradually, peaking in the month preceding the start of dialysis.

CVD prevalence in CKD patients is double as compared to non-CKD patients (69.8% vs 34.8%) [10] (Table 2).

The coronary artery disease is the most common form of CVD exceeding the 40% in 2012, in CKD patients older than 66.

This is in relation with the increase of interventional procedures carried out in recent years (Table 3).

CKD occurrence worsens the prognosis in the short and long term of any CVD.

Over 40% of patients older than 66 have Congestive Heart Failure (CHF), which is the most frequent chronic form of heart disease related to CKD. Slightly more frequent systolic dysfunction is found as compared to diastolic dysfunction [10].

The heart-kidney relation is very complex and pathophysiologically well described in many recent studies. Certainly the common risk factors and the management of the fluid volume play an important role [14].

The occurrence of congestive heart failure (CHF) in CKD patients increases the risk of death from all causes more than twofold (odds ratio 2.6). At the same time the CKD increases the risk of death of 50% in the CHF group.

The USRDS Annual Data Report 2014 emphasizes the importance of Acute Renal Failure (AKI) [10].

In fact over the last decade there has been an increase in hospitalizations for AKIwhich is correlated with the increasing age of the population. It should be noted that in the first year after the AKI event, less than 20% of patients were -followed by a nephrologist.

The latest guidelines KDIGO 2013 on CKD stress the importance of albuminuria for the kidney disease diagnosis and prognosis [15]. Albuminuria correlates with kidney function loss. At lower levels of GFR there is a greater number of patients with high levels of albuminuria. This also correlates with the increased risk of disease progression to kidney death and renal replacement therapy.

6.5% of people with normal kidney-function have some evidence of albuminuria. The percentage increases for GFR between 60 and 90 ml/min, between 45 and 59 ml/min and between 30 and 44 ml/min with values of 9.4%, 22.2% and 46.7%, respectively.

More than 50% of population with micro or macro-albuminuria shows GFR levels lower than 30 ml/min.

From the Medicare database the mortality of CKD patients can be adressed.

In an unadjusted analysis, the cohort of patients aged 66 years or more shows a mortality decrease of about 42% from 1995 to 2012, moving from 245 deaths per 1000 patients/year to 143 deaths per 1000 patients/year.

Non-CKD-patients, however, show a mortality reduction in the same period by 16%, from 55 to 46 deaths per 1000 patients/year.

Adjusting the analysis for age, race, sex, state of health, the mortality rate in 2012 is reduced considerably for CKD patients, reaching 76 deaths per 1000 patients/year.

The factor most affecting the mortality difference between patients with and without CKD is the age difference of the study population.

In 2012 the average age of CKD-patients was 79.1 years, while the group without CKD had an average age of 76 years, the average of the entire group was 76.3 years.

As expected, all causes of mortality increase dramatically with increasing age. In the analysis adjusted for sex, race, and comorbidities, the mortality rate increases by 4.5 times, from 36/1000 patients/year to 162/1000 patients/year for patients aged between 66 and 69 and patients 85 and older, respectively.

Mortality is higher in males and in the white race.

DM and CVD co-occurrence doubles the mortality rate of CKD patients with CKD [10].

CONCLUSION

CKD despite being a serious disease that worsens the prognosis of any other concomitant illness, still it does not have a system of epidemiological observation institutionalized in each country.

In order to implement the appropriate strategies for the prevention and treatment of this disease, it would be essential to learn more about the risk factors, the geographical distribution, the true incidence and prevalence of the disease as well as its complications.

Optimizing CKD management would result in significant savings by the healthcare systems and a better quality of life for all patients.

REFERENCES

[1] NCD global monitoring framework indicator definitions and specifications. Geneva: *World Health Organization*; 2014.

[2] Mathers CD, Loncar D projections of global mortality and burden of disease 2002–2030. PLoS Med. 2006;3(11): e442. doi:10.1371/journal. pmed.0030442.

[3] Global status report on noncommunicable diseases 2014 WHO.

[4] Projections of mortality and causes of death, 2015 and 2030 (http://www.who.int/healthinfo/global_burden_disease/projections/en/, http://www.who.int/gho/ncd/mortality_morbidity/en/, accessed 4 November 2014).

[5] Ref. Lysaght MJ. Maintenance dialysis population dynamics: current trends and long-term implications. *J. Am. Soc. Nephrol.* 2002; 13 (Suppl 1): S37–S40.

[6] Coresh J, Astor BC, Greene T et al. Prevalence of chronic kidney disease and decreased kidney function in the adult US population: Third National Health and Nutrition Examination Survey. *Am. J. Kidney Dis.* 2003; 41: 1–12.

[7] Coresh J, Selvin E, Stevens LA et al. Prevalence of chronic kidney disease in the United States. *JAMA* 2007; 298: 2038–2047.

[8] Astor BC, Matsushita K, Gansevoort RT, van der Velde M, Woodward M, Levey AS, de Jong E, Coresh and CKD Prognosis Consortium. Lower estimated glomerular filtration rate and higher albuminuria are associated with mortality and end-stage renal disease. A collaborative meta-analysis of kidney disease population cohorts. *Kidney Intl.* 2011;79: 1331-1340.

[9] Centers for Disease Control and Prevention. National Diabetes Statistics Report: Estimates of Diabetes and Its Burden in the United States, 2014. Atlanta, GA: *U.S. Department of Health and Human Services*, 2014.

[10] Saran R, Li Y, Robinson B, et al. US Renal Data System 2014 annual data report: epidemiology of kidney disease in the United States. *Am. J. Kidney Dis.* 2015;66(1)(suppl 1): S1-S306.

[11] Tseng CL, Kern EF, Miller DR, Tiwari A, Maney M, Rajan M, Pogach L. Survival benefit of nephrologic care in patients with diabetes mellitus and chronic kidney disease. *Arch. Intern. Med.* 2008 Jan 14;168(1): 55-62.

[12] Jones C, Roderick P, Harris S, Rogerson M. Decline in kidney function before and after nephrology referral and the effect on survival in moderate to advanced chronic kidney disease. *Nephrol. Dial. Transplant.* 2006 Aug; 21(8): 2133-43.

[13] Go AS, Chertow GM, Fan D, McCulloch CE, Hsu C. Chronic kidney disease and the risks of death, cardiovascular events, and hospitalization. *N. Engl. J. Med.* 2004; 351(13): 1296-1305.

[14] Di Lullo L, House A, Gorini A, Santoboni A, Russo D, Ronco C. Chronic kidney disease and cardiovascular complications. *Heart Fail Rev.* 2015 May;20(3): 259-72.

[15] Kidney Disease: Improving Global Outcomes (KDIGO) CKD Work Group. KDIGO 2012 clinical practice guideline for the evaluation and management of chronic kidney disease. *Kidney Int. Suppl.* 2013;3(1):1–150.

In: Comorbidities in Chronic Kidney Disease
Editor: Luca Di Lullo

ISBN: 978-1-63485-070-4

Chapter 2

HYPERTENSION AND CHRONIC KIDNEY DISEASE

Antonio De Pascalis*
Nephrology and Dialysis Unit, V. Fazzi Hospital, Lecce, Italy

ABSTRACT

The progression of chronic kidney disease (CKD) is largely independent of the underlying kidney disorder once renal function has fallen below a critical level. Hypertension is an independent risk factor for disease progression in both adult and pediatric patients with kidney disorders. Optimal blood pressure control (<130/80mm Hg) represents a main goal of conservative therapy in patients with chronic kidney disease (CKD) but it is rarely achieved in clinical practice. Angiotensin-converting enzyme inhibitors and angiotensin receptor blockers are more effective than other drugs in slowing progression of proteinuric CKD. Dietary salt restriction (≤100 mEq/d of NaCl) may be useful to correct the extracellular volume expansion. If this intervention fails, hypertension can be treated by thiazide diuretics in patients with mild CKD, whereas loop diuretics at adequate doses are indicated in patients with more advanced CKD.

Keywords: CKD, hypertension, diuretics, RAS inhibitors

INTRODUCTION

The elevation of blood pressure (BP) is a major risk factor in chronic kidney disease (CKD). The main factors involved in the pathogenesis of hypertension in CKD are listed in Table 1. The prevalence of hypertension increases linearly from65% to 95% as the glomerular filtration rate (GFR) declines from 85 to 15 mL/min/1.73 m² [1]. Correction of hypertension has been identified as an important intervention because uncontrolled hypertension is a recognized determinant of worsening renal function [2, 3] and it also likely represents a major risk factor for the extraordinarily high mortality observed in these patients [6-8]. Both effects

* Corresponding author: Antonio DePascalis, MD, Nephrology and Dialysis Unit, V. Fazzi Hospital, PiazzettaMuratore, 73100 - Lecce (LE), Italy.

have been provenin the long term [9]. Accordingly, current guidelines now strongly suggest optimal BP control, i.e., to less than 130/80 mm Hg, in CKD [10]. Unfortunately, the achievement of optimal BP values remains dramatically low in clinical practice despite the prevalent use of inhibitors of the renin-angiotensin system (RAS) [11].

TREATMENT

Renin-Angiotensin System (RAS) Inhibitors. RAS is an important therapeutic target and drugs that block this system have been extensively developed, such as ACE inhibitors (ACE-i) and Angiotension II receptor blockers (ARB). This blocking has been postulated as the first choice for treatment of hypertension in CKD patients [13]. Several ARB inhibitor trials for CKD patients were conducted and showed a slower decline in renal function with the use of this class of antihypertensive medication related mainly to proteinuria reduction than to intensive blood pressure control [14-18]. The antiproteinuric effect which is postulated to be the main cause oftheir renoprotective action, is more prominent when patients are kept on a low sodium diet or are treated with diuretics because relative volume depletion results in enhanced angiotensin II dependence of the glomerular microcirculation. The combination of ECV depletion and RAS inhibition in proteinuric CKD is strongly recommended because interventions that lower both BP and proteinuria lead to better renal outcome [19].

In diabetic nephropathy, RAS inhibitors are highly effective in reducing protein excretion and progression from microalbuminuria to overt proteinuria as well as in slowing the rate of decline in GFR [20, 21]. This benefit also holds true in patients who are not hypertensive. The renoprotective effectiveness of ARBs has been clearly shown in type 2 diabetic nephropathy [22, 23]. A critical issue is the role of ACE.i plus ARB combination therapy. Additive antiproteinuric effect and concomitant increased efficacy in terms of slowing CKD progression has been reported in proteinuric nondiabetic CKD patients affectedby glomerular nephropathies such as IgA nephropathy [13]. Indeed, this approach may be considered in the majority of CKD patients because the desired reduction of proteinuria to less than 500 mg/d is infrequently achieved by administration of ACE-I alone [24]. The safety of combinationtherapy depends on the preliminary exclusion of patients suffering adverse effects ofstrong RAS inhibition (hyperkalemia, marked increase in serum creatinine concentration) and on the extensive use of diuretics that may have accounted for the absence of hyperkalemic episodes. Plasma creatinine and potassium concentrations should be measured in the first weeks of therapy.

Table 1. Selected factors implicated with Hypertension in CKD

Factor	Dominant mechanism
Impaired Na excretion	Expansion of ECF volume
Activation of RAS	Direct vasoconstriction Sympathetic activation
Sympathetic activation	Direct vasoconstriction Stimulation of renin release
Imbalance in PG or kinins	Vasoconstriction
Endothelin	Direct vasoconstriction Renal injury
Reduced nitric oxide	Loss of vasodilator effect

Salt restriction. In CKD impairment of renal function causes fluid retention. Sodium retention is of primary importance in the pathogenesis of hypertension, even if the degree of extracellular volume (ECV) expansion is insufficient to induce edema, as usually occurs in the absence of heart failure. Sodium retention, which can be evaluated by urinary fractional excretion of sodium, increases exponentially as GFR declines and may preclude an adequate control of BP, especially during pharmacological treatment with RAS inhibitors [25]. In patients with CKD, moderate reduction of salt intake allows a much greater BP decrease in comparison with hypertensive patients with normal GFR undergoing major restriction of salt intake [26–28]. The different response to salt reduction is probably caused by the basal ECV. Therefore, the sensitivity of BP to sodium restriction is greatly increased in patients with advanced CKD.

Despite the evidence on the beneficial effects of salt restriction in CKD, compliance with the dietary prescription is generally poor in the setting of clinical practice. The determination of urinary excretion of sodium (target: ≤100 mEq/d, equal to ≤6 g NaCl/d), is very important to monitor the patient's adherence to dietary prescriptions, specifically reducing added salt in the diet, cooking with spices rather than salt, choosing fresh food, eating low-salt bread.

Diuretic Treatment. In the presence of poor adherence to salt restriction (urinary sodium excretion >100 mEq/d), natriuretic agents become the cornerstone of treatment of hypertension secondary to CKD [29]. In patients with mild renal impairment (GFR >40 mL/min), thiazide diuretics are indicated. It is well known, in fact, that these agents restore the antiproteinuric effect of ACE-I in patients not compliant to a low-salt diet and are useful in preventing the development of cardiovascular events in older persons with systolic hypertension and mild renal insufficiency. Of note, thiazide diuretics diminish BP levels also by mechanisms other than reduction of volemia [30]. Loop diuretics are indicated in CKD patients with a GFR of 40 mL/min or lower. They should be titrated upwards until BP is normalized (<130/80 mm Hg) or the patient reaches the "dry weight" that, in the presence of persistent hypertension, is defined as the weight at which further fluid losses will lead either to symptoms (orthostatic hypotension, cramps) or to decreased tissue perfusion as evidenced by an otherwise unexplained elevation of azotemia and plasma creatinine concentration. Recently, clinical studies showed that torasemide, 40 mg/d, or furosemide, 80 mg /day, in patients with a mean GFR of 45 mL/min induces a similar antihypertensive effect, which is strictly correlated to natriuretic response and contraction of ECV [31]. Of note, after correction of sodium retention (induction phase), which is shown by the achievement of normal BP or dry weight during up-titration of loop diuretic, the physician must down-titrate the dose of loop diuretic so that the value of dry body weight can be steadily maintained (maintenance phase). Obviously, the maintenance dose of loop diuretic is lower than that of the induction phase. It is important to remember that the efficacious dose of furosemide is characterized by a large inter-individual variability secondary to the very different bioavailability. Therefore, it is useful to begin with a low dose and gradually increase the dose to obtain the progressive reduction of body weight in the range of daily and cumulative values reported previously, up to the achievement of normal BP or dry weight. Conversely, in the maintenance phase, it is necessary to adequately down titrate the dose of loop diuretic to detect the lowest dose capable of maintaining steady body weight and target BP.

Disappointingly, nephrologists are reluctant to "adequately" use loop diuretics in their hypertensive CKD patients, probably because of the fear of side effects but if patients are carefully followed, adverse effects will be less frequent and dangerous than expected.

Independent of the specific agent used, a major adverse effect can be avoided if renal function and serum electrolyte levels are periodically checked in the first weeks of treatment.

Aldosterone antagonists. In CKD, the major emphasis has been on using aldosterone antagonists to reduce urine albumin levels and as an adjunct to other antihypertensive agents in treating resistant hypertension. Aldosterone antagonists are of proven benefit in non-CKD patients with heart failure, including heart failure after myocardial infarction. Because of the risk of hyperkalemia and reduction in GFR, they should be used at lower doses (i.e., 25-50 mg/d) and with caution in CKD patients.

Other antihypertensive drugs. RAS inhibitors and diuretics are the cornerstones of therapy in hypertensive CKD patients. Additional agents should be chosen based on cardiovascular disease-specific indications to achieve therapeutic and preventive targets and to avoid side-effects and interactions [32]. A proposed algorithm of hypertension treatment is reported in Figure 1.

Beta blockers. Beta-blockers are beneficial in patients with a prior history of angina, myocardial infarction, congestive heart failure (due to diastolic dysfunction and for certain agents also for systolic dysfunction), resting tachycardia, migraine headaches, and glaucoma. Conversely, beta-blockers should in general not be used in patients with bradycardia, second- or third-degree heart block, asthma, chronic obstructive pulmonary disease, severe peripheral vascular disease, or depression, as ß-adrenergic tone is beneficial in these circumstances. Beta receptors also stimulate cellular uptake of glucose and potassium. Beta-blockers in CKD patients can cause hyperkalemia due to altered transcellular distribution of potassium. Selective beta-blockers may cause lesser elevation in serum potassium than non-selective beta-blockers. All beta-blockers can cause an increase in serum levels of plasma glucose and triglyceride levels and in insulin resistance and a decrease in HDL cholesterol levels.

Calcium channel blockers. The nondihydropyridine calcium-channel blockers have beneficial effects on CKD and cardiovascular disease. Diltiazem and verapamil are effective in decreasing proteinuria in diabetic kidney disease [32]. Nondihydropyridine calcium-channel blockers can diminish cardiac contractility and slow cardiac conduction. Therefore, these agents should not be used in patients with severe left ventricular dysfunction, sick sinus syndrome, or second- or third-degree heart block. In addition, constipation can be seen in up to 25% of patients prescribed verapamil. There are a large number of dihydropyridine agents. Some have cardiac depressant activity, such as short-acting nifedipine; long-acting agents that do not have cardiac depressant effects include amlodipine and lacidipine. In general, longer acting agents without cardiac depressant effects are preferred. The dihydropyridines are associated with a number of other side-effects due to direct vasodilatation and can cause peripheral edema, dizziness, headache, and flushing.

Alpha-adrenergic agents (methyldopa, doxazosine, clonidine). In general, these agents should not be used as a first-line therapy for hypertension due to the relatively high incidence of side-effects. Side-effects of the centrally acting agents include dry mouth, sedation, and sexual dysfunction. Side-effects of the selective α-1 blockers include headache, weakness, dizziness, and, on rare occasions, syncope. Dizziness and syncope can be minimized by starting with a low dose of a long-acting agent such as doxazosin and administering the initial dose at bedtime.

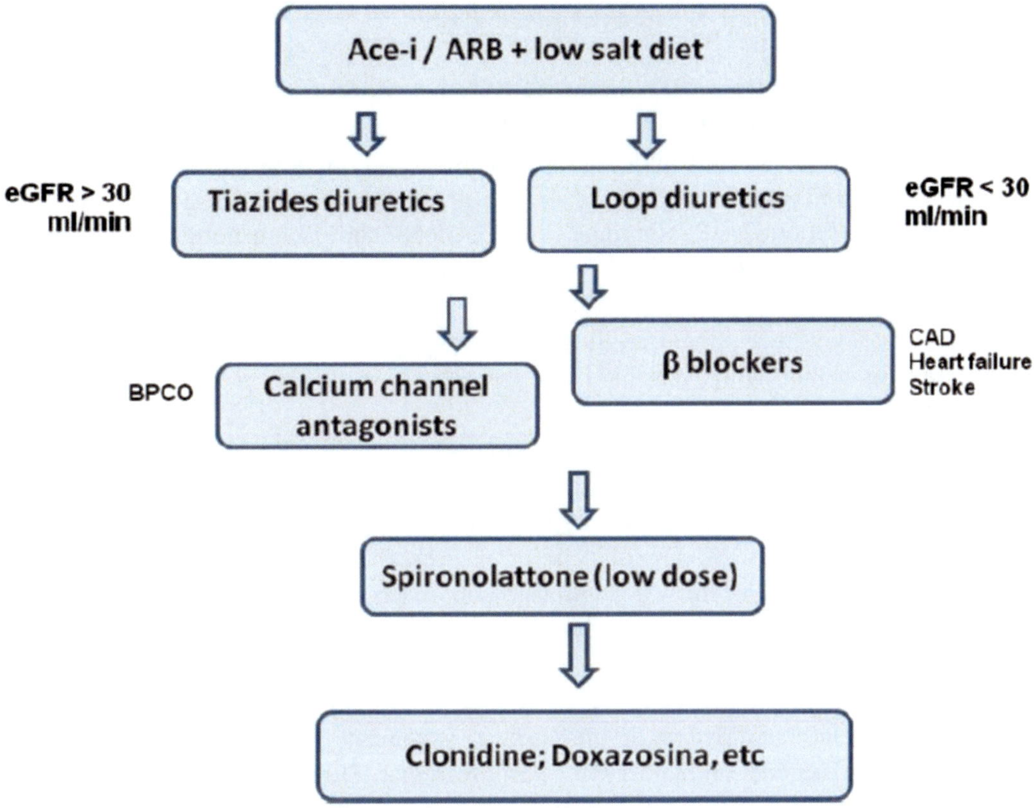

Figure 1. Algorithm of hypertension treatment in CKD proteinuric patients.

Peripheral vasodilators. Minoxidil is a powerful vasodilator that can cause lower extremity edema, tachycardia, hirsutism, and, in rare cases, pleural or pericardial effusions, at therapeutic doses. This agent is almost always used in combination with a beta-blocker and loop diuretic in order to minimize reflex tachycardia and lower extremity edema. Minoxidil should be reserved for those patients who cannot obtain blood pressure control with the preferred agent and at least three of the other recommended agents.

Conclusion

Management of hypertension represents the main intervention in CKD patients for both renal and cardiovascular protection. Nevertheless, the achievement of BP goals remains low in clinical practice despite the availability of several drug classes. Moreover the management of hypertension in CKD patients appears extremely different when comparing recent observational studies, witnessing the real world of clinical practice, with the main randomized control trials carried out in the last several years. Greater effort should be made, therefore, to increase the use of antihypertensive agents other than RAS inhibitors. Overall, these findings identify the correction of volume expansionby salt restriction and adequate use of diuretics and the increased number of prescribed antihypertensive drugs are major areas of improvement in the conservative care of CKD from moderate to advanced stages.

REFERENCES

[1] Buckalew, VM; Jr Berg, RL; Wang, SR; et al. Prevalence of hypertension in 1,795 subjects with chronic renal disease: the modification of diet in renal disease study baseline cohort. Modification of Diet in Renal Disease Study Group. *Am J Kidney Dis*, 1996, 28,811–821.

[2] De Nicola, L; Minutolo, R; Chiodini, P; et al. Global approach to cardiovascular risk in chronic kidney disease: reality and opportunities for intervention. *Kidney Int*, 2006, 69, 538–545.

[3] Bakris, GL; Weir, MR; Shanifar, S; et al. Effects of blood pressure level on progression of diabetic nephropathy: results from the RENAAL study. *Arch Int Med*, 2003, 163,1555–1565.

[4] Jafar, TH; Stark, PC; Schmid, CH; et al. Progression of chronic kidney disease: the role of blood pressure control, proteinuria, and angiotensin-converting enzyme inhibition: a patient-levelmeta-analysis. *Ann Inter Med*, 2003, 139, 244–252.

[5] Bakris, GL; Williams, M; Dworkin, L; et al. Preserving renal function in adults with hypertension and diabetes: a consensus approach. National Kidney Foundation Hypertension and Diabetes Executive Committee Working Group. *Am J Kidney Dis*, 2000, 36, 646–661.

[6] Sarnak, MJ; Levey, AS; Schoolwerth, AC; et al. Kidney disease as a risk factor for development of cardiovascular disease: a statement from the American Heart Association Councils on Kidney in Cardiovascular Disease, High Blood Pressure Research, Clinical Cardiology, and Epidemiology and Prevention. *Circulation*, 2003, 108, 2154–2169.

[7] Keith, DS; Nichols, GA; Gullion, CM; et al. Longitudinal follow-up and outcomes among a population with chronic kidney disease in a large managed care organization. *Arch Inter Med*, 2004, 164, 659–663.

[8] Go, AS; Chertow, GM; Fan, D; et al. Chronic kidney disease and the risks of death, cardiovascular events, and hospitalization. *N Engl J Med*, 2004, 351, 1296–1305.

[9] Sarnak MJ; Greene, T; Wang, X; et al. The effect of a lower target blood pressure on the progression of kidney disease: long-term follow-up of the modification of diet in renal disease study. *Ann Int Med*, 2005, 142, 342–351.

[10] K/DOQI clinical practice guidelines on hypertension and antihypertensive agents in chronic kidney disease. *Am J Kidney Dis*, 2004, 43(5 Suppl 1), S1–S290.

[11] Marin, R; Fernandez-Vega, F; Gorostidi, M; et al. Blood pressure control in patients with chronic renal in sufficiency in Spain: a cross-sectional study. *J Hypertens*, 2006, 24, 395–402.

[12] Management of Hypertension in chronic kidney disease. Zamboli, P; De Nicola, L; Minutolo, R; et al. *Current Hypertension Reports*, 2006, 8, 497–501.

[13] Ruggenenti, P; Schieppati, A; Remuzzi, G. Progression, remission, regression of chronic renal diseases. *Lancet*. 2001, 357, 1601–1608.

[14] Klahr, S; et al. The effects of dietary protein restriction and blood pressure control on the progression of chronic kidney disease. *N Engl J Med*, 1994, 330, 877-884.

[15] Ruggenenti, P; et al. Bllod pressure control for renoprotection in patients with non diabetic chronic renal disease (REIN 2): multicentre, randomised controlled trial. *Lancet*, 2005, Mar 12-18, 365, 939-46.

[16] Wright, JT; Jr, Bakris G; et al. Effect of blood pressure lowering and anti hypertensive drug class on progression of hypertensive kidney disease: results from the AASK trial *JAMA*. 2002 Nov 20, 288(19), 2421-31.

[17] Sarnak, MJ; Greene, T; et al. The effect of a lower target blood pressure on the progression of kidney disease: long-term follow-up of the modification of diet in renal disease study. *Ann Intern Med.*, 2005 Mar 1, 142(5), 342-51.

[18] Appel, LJ; Wright, JT; Jr, Greene, T; et al. Intensive blood-pressure control in hypertensive chronic kidney disease. *N Engl J Med.*, 2010 Sep 2, 363(10), 918-29.

[19] Klosa, N; Bakris, G. Lessons learned from recent hypertension trials about kidney disease. *Clin J Am Soc Nephrol*, 2006, 1, 229–235.

[20] Lewis, EJ; Hunsicker, LG; Bain, RP; Rhode, RD. The effect of angiotensin-converting-enzyme inhibition on diabetic nephropathy. The Collaborative Study Group. *N Engl J Med*, 1993, 329, 1456–1462.

[21] Barnett, AH; Bain, SC; Bouter, P; et al. Angiotensin-receptor blockade versus converting enzyme inhibition in type 2 diabetes and nephropathy. *N Engl J Med*, 2004, 351, 1952–1961.

[22] Brenner, BM; Cooper, ME; De Zeeuw, D; et al. Effects of losartan on renal and cardiovascular outcomes in patients with type 2 diabetes and nephropathy. *N Engl J Med*, 2001, 345, 861–869.

[23] Lewis, EJ; Hunsicker, LG; Clarke, WR; et al. Renoprotective effect of the angiotensin-receptor antagonist irbesartan in patients with nephropathy due to type 2 diabetes. *N Engl J Med*, 2001, 345, 851–860.

[24] Di Iorio, BR; Minutolo, R; De Nicola, L; et al. Supplemented very low protein diet ameliorates responsiveness to erythropoietin in chronicrenal failure. *Kidney*, Int 2003, 64, 1822–1828.

[25] Vasawada, N; Agarwal, R. Role of excess volume in the pathophysiology of hypertension in chronic kidney disease. *Kidney Int*, 2003, 64, 1772–1779.

[26] He, FJ; MacGregor, GA. Effect of modest salt reduction on blood pressure: a meta-analysis of randomized trials. Implications for public health. *J Hum Hypertens*, 2002, 16, 761–770.

[27] Cianciaruso, B; Bellizzi, V; Minutolo, R; et al. Renal adaptation to dietary sodium restriction in moderate renal failure resulting from chronic glomerular disease. *J Am Soc Neprol*, 1996, 7, 306–313.

[28] Koomans, HA;Roos, JC; Dorhout Mees, EJ; Delawi, IM. Sodium balance in renalfailure: A comparison of patients with normal subjects under extremes of sodium intake. *Hypertension*, 1985, 7, 714–721.

[29] Dorhout, Mees EJ. Volaemia and blood pressure in renalfailure: Have oldtruths been forgotten? *Nephrol Dial Transplant*, 1995, 10, 1297–1298.

[30] Brater, DC. Diuretic therapy. *N Engl J Med*, 1998, 339, 387–395.

[31] Vasavada, N; Saha, C;Agarwal, R. A double-blind randomized crossover trail of two loop diuretics in chronic kidney disease. *Kidney Int*, 2003, 64, 632–640.

[32] National Kidney Foundation. K/DOQI clinical practice guidelines for chronic kidney disease: evaluation, classification, and stratification. *Am J Kidney Dis*., 2002, 39, 2 Suppl 1, S1–S266.

In: Comorbidities in Chronic Kidney Disease
Editor: Luca Di Lullo
ISBN: 978-1-63485-070-4

Chapter 3

Atherosclerosis, Dyslipidemia and Chronic Kidney Disease

Vincenzo Panichi**, Alessia Scatena and Massimiliano Migliori
Nephrology and Dialysis, Versilia Hospital, Italy

Abstract

Cardiovascular disease (CVD) is the most common cause of morbidity and mortality in Chronic Kidney Disease (CKD) patients. CVD mortality is 3- to 6- fold above age- and risk-adjusted mortality in the general population, and on average is 10-fold higher in dialysis-treated patients.

Multiple nontraditional risk factors for coronary artery disease (CAD) are present in CKD patients, including insulin resistance, increased oxidative stress, inflammation, anemia, endothelial dysfunction and reduced nitric oxide availability.

The relationship between cholesterol levels and increased CAD risk seen in the general population has been difficult to establish in CKD patients, most notably in patients undergoing haemodialysis treatment. Lipid abnormalities in CKD patients are characterized more by qualitative rather than quantitative abnormalities of cholesterol-containing lipoproteins.

Keywords: dyslipidemia, atherosclerosis, chronic kidney disease

Introduction

Cardiovascular disease (CVD) is the most common cause of morbidity and mortality in Chronic Kidney Disease (CKD) patients [1-3]. CVD mortality is 3- to 6- fold above age- and risk-adjusted mortality in the general population, and on average is 10-fold higher in dialysis-treated patients.

* Corresponding author: Vincenzo Panichi, Nephrology and Dialysis Dept., Versilia Hospital, Ausl 12 di Viareggio - Via Aurelia 335, Lido di Camaiore (LU), Phone +39 0584 605 8652 – E-mail- v.panichi@usl12.toscana.it.

Several risk factors have been involved in the pathogenesis of the high CVD mortality and morbidity of the uremic syndrome and traditional Framingham risk factors are not able to fully explain these data; multiple putative nontraditional risk factors for coronary artery disease (CAD) are present in CKD patients, including insulin resistance, increased oxidative stress, inflammation, anemia, endothelial dysfunction and reduced nitric oxide availability [4, 5].

However, dyslipidemia has also been linked to an increased risk of CAD in CKD patients in both predialysis and haemodialysis patients [6-8], although some studies have demonstrated that cardiac-related causes of death in patients with CKD are not all directly related to the atherosclerotic process [9].

The relationship between cholesterol levels and increased CAD risk seen in the general population has been difficult to establish in CKD patients, most notably in patients undergoing haemodialysis treatment [10]. Moreover, lipid abnormalities in CKD patients are characterized more by qualitative rather than quantitative abnormalities of cholesterol-containing lipoproteins.

These changes depend on the stage of the disease but are present throughout all natural history, from its earliest stages to the ESRD replacement therapy.

Normal Structure and Function of Lipoproteins

As the name implies, the lipoproteins are macromolecular complexes composed of lipids and proteins (known as apolipoproteins or apoproteins; Apo) and have the function of transporting water-insoluble lipids (triglycerides (TG), cholesterol, cholesterol esters (CE) and phospholipids (PL); no the fatty acids (FFA)) in the bloodstream, from the sites of absorption (gut) and/or synthesis (liver) to the sites of utilization (peripheral tissues) or processing.

The major types of the plasma lipoproteins, in order of increasing density, are: Chylomicron (CM), Very low-density lipoprotein (VLDL), Intermediate-density lipoprotein (IDL; not a "true" class of lipoproteins), Low-density lipoprotein (LDL) and High-density lipoprotein (HDL).

CM lipoproteins are produced in enterocytes and provide the *lipid exogenous pathway* (Figure1a). Their core consists of lipids that are absorbed from the intestine (TG, CE and PL) while in the surface are present mainly apoproteins B-48, and also C-II, C-III, A-IV, E (Table 1). Main function of these lipoproteins is transport of dietary TG to muscle tissue (for energy production) and adipose tissue (for energy storage) and the cholesterol to the liver [11, 12].

Nascent CM reach the circulation through the intestinal lymphatics and thoracic duct and enrich Apo E and Apo C removing them to other lipoproteins, including HDL. Once in circulation, the Lipoprotein Lypase (LPL) cleaves TG so that the FFA are released and can enter in adipose and muscular tissues [13, 14]. During this catabolic process, CM diminish in size and become chylomicron remnants, normally removed by hepatic LDL receptor-related protein (LRP) or LDL receptor (LDL-R) after further hydrolysis of the TG and PL by hepatic lipase (HL). Instead cholesterol will be released to the liver where is added to hepatic cholesterol pool or secreted into the bile and then re-absorbed in the intestine [11].

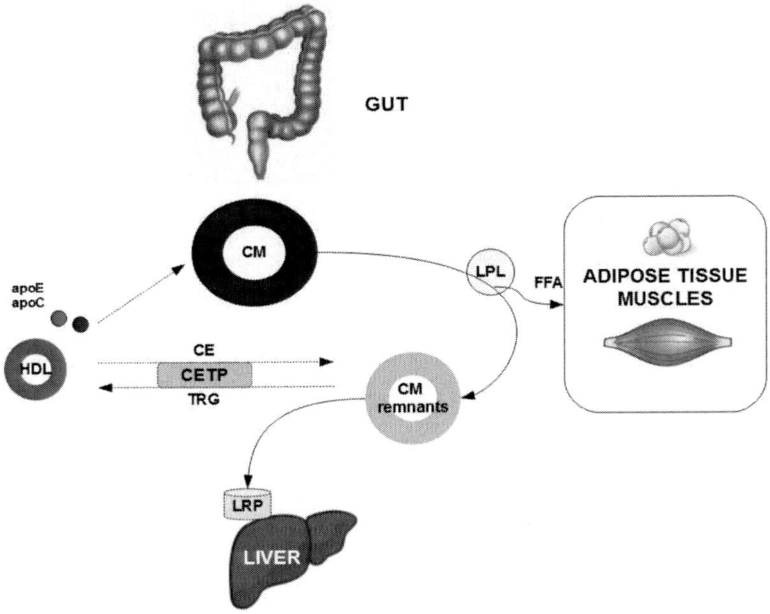

Figure 1a. Lipid exogenous pathway.

VLDL lipoproteins represent the *lipidic endogenous pathway* (Figure 1b), are synthesized and secreted by liver and are useful to transport endogenous lipids to peripheral tissues. In the core of these particles are TG, CE and PL de novo synthesis and/or captured by circulating lipoproteins. The outer layer is composed mainly by apoproteins B100, but also C-II, C-III, E (Table 1) [11].

The TG within the VDLD are hydrolyzed by LPL and FFA are taken up by adipocytes or myocytes. VLDL particles are so reduced to VLDL remnants or IDL. On adipocytes and skeletal muscle are present VLDL receptor which have the task of removing these particles [14]. IDL can be taken up by the liver or can be further hydrolyzed to LDL particles that will be taken up by LDL-R and LRP.

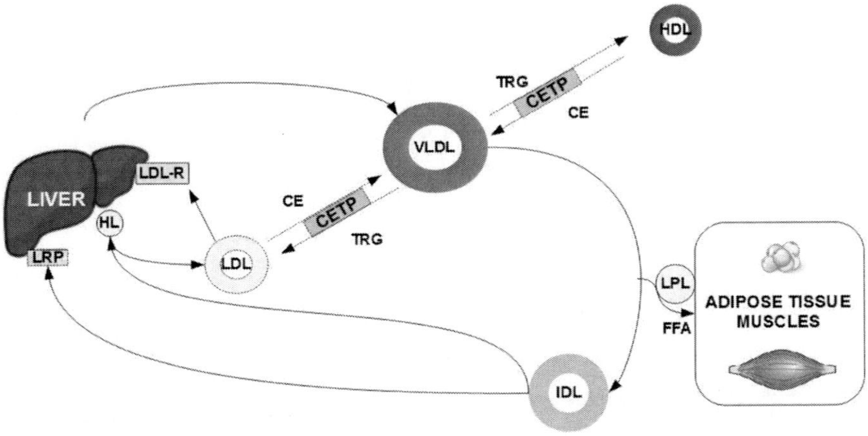

Figure 1b. Lipid endogenous pathway.

IDL are intermediary of VLDL metabolism; usually present in small concentrations in plasma but elevated in kidney failure. The apoprotein present on these particles are B-100 and E.

LDL transports cholesterol primarily to hepatocytes but also to peripheral tissues. Apo B-100 is the apoprotein presents on the surface of these particle, and is responsible for the recognition and uptake of LDL by the LDL-R, which clears approximately 60 to 80% of LDL in normal individuals. The remaining LDL is removed by other specific receptors, such as LRP, or by scavenger receptors [16]. When LDL becomes lipid depleted, small dense LDL (sdLDL) is generated, which has lower affinity for the LDL-R but is more susceptible to oxidative modification and more atherogenic.

HDL escreted by liver are involved in reverse cholesterol transport, removing cholesterol surplus from tissue and vascular vessels [17]. HDL bind cholesterol released into the plasma from the cell turnover and bring him back to the liver where the breakdown occurs or to steroidogenic tissue.

HDL particles are protectives, reducing atherogenic plaques formation, reducing inflammatory process and limiting oxidative stress. Apo A-I, A-II, A-IV are the apoproteins of these particles (Table 1).

HDL precursor particles are secreted as disc-shaped structures by the liver and intestine and can absorb free cholesterol from cell membranes, a process that is mediated by ATP binding cassette transporter 1, apoA-I, and apoA-IV. By acquisition of additional apolipoproteins, cholesteryl esters, and triglycerides, HDL3 particles are transformed into larger HDL2 particles [18]. Reverse cholesterol transport can take three different routes. First, large HDL particles with multiple copies of apoE can be taken up by the liver *via* the LDL receptor [17]. Second, the accumulated cholesteryl esters from HDL can be selectively taken up by the liver mediated by scavenger receptor B1 [19]. This receptor is expressed primarily in liver and nonplacental steroidogenic tissues. Third, cholesteryl esters are transferred by the cholesteryl ester transfer protein from HDL to triglyceride-rich lipoproteins [17]. Plasma HDL cholesterol levels are influenced by the complexity of these reverse cholesterol transport processes.

The process of exogenous and endogenous pathways of lipid metabolism is a complicated phenomenon in both normal and abnormal conditions. A schematic presentation of both pathways is shown in Figure 1a-b.

Table 1. Apoprotein functions

ApoA-I is the major apolipoprotein of HDL and an activator of LCAT, which catalyzes the esterification and hence the reverse transport of cholesterol from periphery to liver.
ApoA-II is an activator of the hepatic lipase, which also hydrolyzes TG from lipoproteins.
ApoA-IV is an activator of LCAT and lipoprotein lipase.
ApoB is a ligand for cellular receptors for lipoprotein uptake; Apo B48 for CM and Apo B-100 for VLDL.
ApoC-II is an activator of lipoprotein lipase that hydrolyzes triglycerides.
ApoC-III is an inhibitor of the lipases.
ApoE is a ligand for hepatic receptors that mediate the uptake of VLDL and IDL.

LIPID ABNORMALITIES IN CKD PATIENTS

The spectrum of dyslipidemia in renal patients is distinct from that of the general population. It involves all lipoprotein classes and shows considerable variations depending on the stage of disease (see Table 2). These changes may actively participate in the pathogenesis of serious complications such as atherosclerotic vascular disease.

The nature of dyslipidemia can be significantly influenced by several intrinsic (nephrotic range proteinuria, concomitant diseases such as diabetes mellitus, hereditary disorders of lipid metabolism) or exogenous (epoietin administration, drugs such as steroids, calcineurin inhibitors, etc.) factors.

Notably, total and LDL-cholesterol levels are usually within normal limits or slightly reduced in predialysis or hemodialysis patients, and increased in patients with marked proteinuria or in peritoneal dialysis (PD).

The most common *quantitative* lipid abnormalities in these patients are:

1. Hypertriglyceridemia
2. Accumultion of Apo B lipoproteins (VLDL apolipoprotein B 100 of hepatic synthesis and CM apolipoprotein B48 intestinal-derived) and accumulation of VLDL and CM remnants, with high athcrogenic power
3. Reduction of HDL cholesterol, with a consequent increase in the LDL /HDL ratio.

In addition to these quantitative changes, CKD patients are also characterized by *qualitative* lipid dysregulation:

1. Increased levels of Lp (a): LDL plus Apo-A.
2 Increased in sd-LDL.

Quantitative Changes

Hypertriglyceridemia and Apo B Lipoproteins Accumulation

Plasma triglycerides start to increase in early stages of CKD (Table 2) and show the highest concentrations in nephrotic syndrome and in dialysis patients, especially those in peritoneal dialysis (PD).

Increased levels of TG, CM and VLDL in CKD is due to the impairment of various steps involved in the metabolism or clearance of these lipoproteins [20]. Furthermore an increased production of TG-rich lipoproteins is possibly as consequence of impaired carbohydrate tolerance and enhanced hepatic VLDL synthesis [21].

The reduced fractional catabolic rate is likely due to the decreased activity of two endothelium-associated lipases, namely, LPL and HL, which have the primary physiologic function of cleaving triglycerides into FFA for energy production or storage.

In CKD patients LPL deficiency is linked to:

Table 2. Lipid abnormalities in renal patient

	LDL-C	sdLDL	TRG	HDL-C	Lp(a)
CKD 1-4	↔ or ↓	↑	↑	↓	↑[a]
Nephrotic syndrome	↑	↑	↔ or ↑	↓or ↔ or ↑	↑
Hemodialysis	↔ or ↓	↑	↑	↓	↑
Peritoneal dialysis	↑	↑	↑	↓	↑

CKD = Chronic Kidney Disease; LDL-C = low-density lipoprotein-cholesterol; sdLDL = small, dense LDL subfractions; TRG = triglycerides; HDL-C = high-density lipoprotein-cholesterol; Lp(a) = lipoprotein(a).

↑Increase;↔No change;↓Decrease.

[a] Mainly in individual with high-molecular-weight apolipoprotein (a) phenotypes.

- presence of excess of Apo CI, the removal of which, for example by dialysis, can increase the activity of LPL.
- increase in the plasma apoC-III/apoC-II ratio. ApoC-II is an activator of LPL, whereas apoC-III is an inhibitor of LPL. The increased apoC-III/apoC-II ratio is usually due to a disproportionate increase in plasma apoC-III [22].
- decrease in LPL synthesis as a result of secondary hyperparathyroidism or suppressed insulin level [23]
- heparin treatment, in hemodialysis (HD) patients [24].

The accumulation of TG-rich lipoproteins, as a result of the decreased activity of the LPL, causes a consequent decrease in the delivery of lipids to adipocytes and myocytes, predisposing CKD patients to cachexia and the inability to perform normal physical activity.

Incomplete catabolism results in the accumulation of CM remnants and IDL that contribute to the heterogeneity of the plasma pool of triglyceride-rich lipoproteins, with different sites of origin, sizes, compositions [25], and degrees of atherogenicity [26]. These remnants are rich in apoE, a ligand that is critical for the removal of the particles from the circulation by binding to LRP [27]. The arterial wall therefore is exposed to high plasma levels of remnant lipoproteins for prolonged durations, which may predispose to atherogenesis.

The decreased activity of HL is partially due to secondary hyperparathyroidism and dysregulation of cytosolic Ca^{2+} present in CKD patients [28, 29]. It has been demonstrated that HL activity after injection of heparin is reduced in CKD [30]. This defect was apparently due to the rise in calcium content of the liver mediated by the state of secondary hyperparathyroidism of CKD [30]. An increase in calcium content of the liver may reflect an elevation in cytosolic calcium of hepatocytes. Indeed, CKD is associated with sustained elevation in Ca2+ of many cells [31], including hepatocytes [32], and the high Ca2+ is a major factor underlying cell dysfunction in CKD [31]. A decrease in the activity of hepatic lipase in CKD could be due to a decrease in the production of the enzyme, an inhibition of the enzyme activity, an impairment in its release from the liver, or to any combination of such potential derangements.

Recent data have demonstrated that the elevation in Ca^{2+} downregulates the mRNA of many proteins such as the receptors of parathyroid hormone (PTH)-PTHrP, angiotensin II, or vasopressin in hepatocytes [33] and of PTH-PTHrP in kidney [33-35] and heart [36]. It is theoretically possible that the elevation in Ca2+ of hepatocytes in CKD exerts a similar effect on the mRNA of hepatic lipase. Such a potential action could cause a decrease in the production of the enzyme.

HDL Cholesterol Reduction

In CKD patients generally plasma HDL cholesterol concentrations is reduced compared with non-uremic individuals. Furthermore, the distribution of HDL sub fractions is different.

In CKD patients reverse cholesterol transfer is reduced because: hepatic ApoA-I synthesis is decreased and its catabolism is also increased; binding between ApoA-I and ABCA is reduced; lecithin cholesterol acyltransferase (LCAT) activity is reduced.

This decreased ability of the HDL particles to carry cholesterol leads to an impairment in the reverse cholesterol transport from peripheral cells to the liver, thereby burdening the vasculature with cholesterol and promoting atherosclerosis [37-39].

Another important component of HDL is paraoxonase, an enzyme that inhibits the oxidation of LDL. Plasma paraoxonase activity is reduced in patients with CKD [40], thereby predisposing the LDL and possibly also HDL particles to oxidation.

Furthermore, infection-associated or uremia-associated inflammation might convert HDL from an antioxidant into a prooxidant particle [41, 42]. All of these may contribute to atherogenesis in CKD. Furthermore in CKD patients, triglyceride-rich HDL is increased due to reduced HL expression and is poorly cleared. TG-rich HDL is subjected to greater modification and becomes more dysfunctional.

Qualitative Changes

Increased Levels of Lp (a)

Increased levels of Lp(a) are independent risk factor for atherosclerosis and CVD in general population; however, a direct causal relationship has not been established [43, 44]. Few studies have covered the association between Lp(a) and kidney dysfunction but elevated serum Lp(a) levels have been consistently reported in CKD patients on dialysis and in those with nephrotic syndrome [10, 45, 46].

Lp(a) is a modified low-density lipoprotein particle covalently linked to the highly polymorphic apolipoprotein(a) [apo (a)], a glycoprotein of genetically-variable protein length that varies widely among individuals [47-50]. Apo (a) shows a high degree of genetic polymorphism, resulting from a variable number of kringle-IV type 2 (K-IV type 2) repeats. At least thirty-four different apo(a) isoforms have been identified which can be grouped into low (LMW) and high molecular weight (HMW) isoforms according to the number of K-IV repeats in the apo(a) molecule [51]. The number of kringle repeats is genetically determined and the levels of Lp (a) are determined by the size of the apo(a) isoform inherited. In healthy individuals increased levels of Lp(a) are inversely associated with low molecular weight isoforms as a result of increased synthesis.

Adult Lp(a) levels are attained in early childhood and remain constant in healthy individuals throughout life, and are usually not affected by diet, age, and other environmental factors [52].

Levels of Lp(a) are increased in patients with nephrotic syndrome and those with CKD, independent of the isoform inherited, because the concentration of the high molecular weight isoforms of Lp(a) is also increased [53, 54]. High levels of Lp(a) are attributed to increased synthesis in nephrotic syndrome patients [55], while in dialysis patients impaired clearance due to decreased catabolism is believed to be the predominant mechanism [56]. Although high molecular weight isoforms of Lp (a) are increased in CKD patients, CVD risk is primarily associated with high levels of the lower molecular weight isoform in these patients [46].

However, CKD is an important non-genetic, secondary cause of increase in plasma Lp(a) levels [57], which start rising in early stages and become more pronounced in later stages (48, 56). There are no suitable interventions or therapies available to decrease plasma Lp(a) levels; however, we have shown a variable decrease in plasma Lp(a) after starting maintenance hemodialysis (58). The reasons for variable increase in Lp(a) levels in kidney disease and decline in response to hemodialysis are not clear. Dieplinger et al. [59] have reported apo(a) phenotype-dependent alterations in Lp(a) levels in patients with renal disease, showing that patients with HMW apo(a) isoforms have elevated Lp(a) levels as compared to apo(a) phenotype-matched controls. Kronenberg et al. [60], have also shown higher Lp(a) levels in CKD which negatively correlated with glomerular filtration rate (GFR) only in patients with HMW apo(a) isoforms. Parsons et al., [61] have also reported higher median Lp(a) levels in patients with CKD having HMW apo(a) isoforms; however, in their study, a significant proportion of CKD patients with HMW isoforms had Lp(a) levels lower than 10 mg/dl. However, the reason for this discrepancy has not been elucidated.

Increased in Small, Dense LDL Particles

CKD patients exhibit important disturbances in the density distribution of LDL sub fractions that is characterized by a predominance of sdLDL [62, 63].

sdLDL particles results more atherogenic than the large thanks to have altered apo B conformation, lowered affinity for the LDL receptor and a greater affinity for macrophages.

Oxidized LDL (ox-LDL) in particular can be taken up by scavenger receptors on macrophages and vascular smooth muscle cells. When these macrophages become overloaded with cholesteryl esters, they transform into foam cells, which is a major step in the development of atherosclerotic plaque [16, 64-66].

LDL leak across the endothelium and accumulate in the subendothelial space, in part through binding to proteoglycans. Over time, exposure to oxygen radicals results in oxidation of polyunsaturated fatty acids within LDL and modification of the apolipoprotein.

Macrophages have on their surface scavenger receptors that cause them to take up oxidized lipoproteins, becoming “foam cells” that have many cytoplasmic lipid droplets. Although in humans foam cells mainly develop from macrophages, smooth muscle cells may also migrate into the subendothelial space and transition into foam cells.

Foam cells aggregate within the developing arterial plaque. Within the plaque core foam cells eventually undergo necrotic death, releasing harmful cellular contents that can promote plaque rupture and development of blood clots.

THE EFFECT OF DIALYSIS

The patho physiological mechanisms that underlie the alterations in lipoprotein metabolism in HD patients are generally similar with those described in CKD I-IV patients. However, the dialysis procedure may result in additional defects in lipid homeostasis (such as increased catabolic rate of apolipoprotein AI) [67] that reinforce the clinical expression of these mechanisms. Despite the neutral effect of dialysis on serum lipid profile, certain dialysis-related parameters may significantly affect lipoprotein metabolism and modify the features of dyslipidemia in HD patients. Thus, it has been shown that the use of high-flux polysulfone or cellulose triacetate membranes instead of low-flux membranes is accompanied by a significant reduction in serum triglyceride levels as well as by an increase in apolipoprotein AI and HDL-cholesterol levels [68]. This improvement could, at least in part, be attributed to an increase in the apolipoprotein C-II/C-III ratio which increases the activity of lipoprotein lipase and facilitates the intravascular lipolysis of triglyceride rich-lipoproteins [79]. In addition, the type of dialysate may also significantly affect the serum levels of lipoproteins in HD patients. Indeed, it has been shown that the use of bicarbonate dialysate may result in higher HDL-cholesterol concentrations than the use of acetate dialysate [70]. Another factor that can potentially affect lipoprotein metabolism in HD patients is the repeated use of heparin as an anticoagulant. Heparin releases lipoprotein lipase from the endothelial surface and thus its chronic use may result in lipoprotein lipase depletion and defective catabolism of triglyceride-rich lipoproteins. However, the studies that tested the role of heparin in the pathogenesis of HD-induced dyslipidemia revealed contradictory results [71-73]. In addition, controversy exists as to whether low-molecular weight heparins have a more favorable effect on the lipid profile of HD patients compared to standard unfractionated heparin [74, 75]. Finally, recent studies indicate that the use of the phosphate-binder sevelamer hydrochloride significantly reduces the concentrations of total cholesterol and apolipoprotein B in HD patients [76]. Obviously, the cholesterol-lowering properties of this compound are irrelevant to phosphate reduction and can be mainly attributed to its bile acid sequestrating properties.

In contrast to HD patients whose serum lipoprotein concentrations resemble those of predialysis renal failure subjects, continuous ambulatory peritoneal dialysis (CAPD) patients usually exhibit a more atherogenic lipid profile that is characterized by higher total and LDL-cholesterol values, increased apolipoprotein B concentrations, and more pronounced hypertriglyceridemia [77, 78]. In addition, CAPD patients have increased concentrations of sdLDL, higher Lp(a) values and reduced HDL-cholesterol concentrations compared to healthy age- and sex-matched individuals [79] (Table 2). The pathophysiological mechanisms that exacerbate dyslipidemia in CAPD individuals are not well characterized. However, a number of factors have been proposed to play contributory roles in this exacerbation. It is well known that CAPD patients lose substantial amount of proteins into the peritoneal dialysate, resembling the protein losses observed in nephrotic syndrome. This protein loss may, in turn, stimulate the hepatic production of albumin and cholesterol-enriched lipoproteins thus leading to elevated concentrations of LDL-cholesterol and Lp (a) [80-83]. In addition, the absorption of glucose from the dialysis fluid and the resultant increase in insulin levels may enhance the hepatic synthesis and secretion of VLDL and possibly that of other lipoproteins such as Lp (a) [85]. Although no direct correlation has been observed between peritoneal glucose absorption and serum lipid levels in peritoneal dialysis patients, recent studies indicate that the reduction in glucose load with the use of less absorbed icodextrin-containing dialysis solution instead of glucose for the overnight dwell sufficiently reduces the serum levels of total and LDL-cholesterol as well as the concentrations of triglycerides and small, dense LDL particles [86, 87].

It should be noted that even though substantial amounts of apolipoproteins and intact lipoproteins (especially HDL) are lost via the peritoneal cavity in CAPD patients, the pathophysiological significance of these losses as well as their impact on lipoprotein metabolism remain indeterminate [88, 89]. In a recent study Tsimihodimos V et al. [90], investigated the efficiency of the phosphate-binder sevelamer hydrochloride in the treatment of hyperphosphatemia and its influence on serum lipid parameters in patients on CAPD. The data from this prospective, randomized, cross-over study indicate that, over a period of 8 weeks, the drug effectively lowered serum phosphorus and also had a significant beneficial effect on both total and LDL-cholesterol serum levels [91].

Dyslipidemia and CV Outcome in CKD

In the dialysis populations, the preponderance of the literature, including cross-sectional [39, 92, 94] and longitudinal [38, 47, 95-104] studies, does not support a strong association between dyslipidemia and CVD. The precise contributions of lipids to atherogenicity should probably be evaluated longitudinally using multiple measurements over time, because the plasma lipid patterns change substantially as kidney disease progresses, as illustrated by the decline of plasma LDL levels from the nephrotic stage to the HD stage (Table 2). Furthermore, the atherogenic potential of dyslipidemia in CKD may depend more on the apolipoprotein than on lipid abnormalities and may not always be recognized by measurement of plasma lipids alone, as suggested by Attman and Alaupovic [105]. Moreover, in many dialysis patients, CVD is caused or accentuated by other risk factors, such as volume overload, medial calcification, and arrhythmogenicity, and may not necessarily be related to atherosclerosis.

Total Cholesterol

In large administrative databases, the relationship between plasma total cholesterol and mortality in HD patients has been found to be U-shaped [106, 107]. The group with total cholesterol between 200 and 250 mg/dl had the lowest risk for death, whereas those with levels #350 mg/dl had a relative risk of 1.3-fold and those with levels #100 mg/dl had a relative risk of 4.2-fold. The association between low total cholesterol and increased mortality, however, was reduced after statistical adjustment for plasma albumin levels. Subgroup analysis provides further insights into the potential effects of plasma total cholesterol on clinical outcomes. A recent study of 1167 HD patients found that among those with low plasma albumin level (3.5 to 3.9 g/dl), low plasma total cholesterol levels were also associated with increased all-cause mortality. Among those with plasma albumin #4.5 g/dl, however, high plasma total cholesterol levels were associated with increased mortality [108], as observed in the general population. This dichotomous relationship was confirmed in the Choices for Healthy Outcomes in Caring for ESRD (**CHOICE**) study [109], which showed a non-significant negative association of cardiovascular mortality with plasma total as well as non–HDL cholesterol levels in the presence of inflammation and/or malnutrition; in contrast, there was a positive association between total and non–HDL cholesterol and mortality in the absence of inflammation or malnutrition. These observations are compatible with the hypothesis that the inverse association of total cholesterol levels with mortality in dialysis patients is mediated by the cholesterol-lowering effect of malnutrition and/or systemic inflammation and not due to a protective effect of high cholesterol concentrations.

IDL Cholesterol

In observational studies, high plasma IDL cholesterol levels have been shown to be a risk factor independent of LDL cholesterol for coronary artery disease in the general population [110] and may also be a predictor for aortic atherosclerosis in HD patients [111]. Furthermore IDL cholesterol is often elevated in uremia. Unfortunately, the current clinical assays do not differentiate between LDL cholesterol and IDL cholesterol. Therefore, current clinical assays may not accurately assess the atherosclerotic burden of plasma cholesterol in uremia.

Lp(a) Concentrations and Apo(a) Polymorphism

The association of Lp(a) with atherosclerotic complications has been investigated in numerous studies in dialysis patients. The results were inconsistent in prospective as well as in retrospective studies [96, 100, 112]. This inconsistency might have been due, at least in part, to the nonstandardized assay method for Lp (a) in the past. When apo(a) phenotyping was performed in conjunction with plasma Lp (a) concentrations, however, an association between the apo (a) K-IV repeat polymorphism and CV complications was consistently observed [96, 92, 100, 112-119]. A cross-sectional study in 607 HD patients showed an association between low molecular weight apo (a) phenotype with history of coronary events [39]. Two large prospective studies also found a clear association of the apo (a) polymorphism with coronary events and total mortality, respectively [96, 100, 112]. Kronenberg et al. [96] followed 440 HD patients for 5 yr and found a strong association between the low molecular weight apo (a) phenotype and severe coronary events. In contrast, plasma Lp (a) in those with clinical events showed only a trend toward elevated levels and did not reach statistical significance. Similarly, the CHOICE Study recently reported small apo (a) isoforms to be associated with total mortality in an inception cohort of #800 incident dialysis patients who were followed for a median of 33.7 mo [100, 112].

In that study, Lp (a) concentrations were associated with CV events [110] but not with total mortality [112].

Apolipoproteins

In the general population, plasma apoA-IV was reported to be lower in patients with CVD compared with control subjects, and this association was independent of HDL cholesterol and triglyceride concentrations [120, 121]. Similarly, participants in the Mild to Moderate Kidney Disease Study with CVD complications also had lower apoA-IV levels than those without [122]. More data in various stages of CKD are required to confirm these findings.

Lipid Management in CKD

Effect of Statins in Primary Prevention of CVD in ESRD Patients

Three large prospective randomized clinical trials have been conducted to determine the efficacy of different statins in reducing the risk of CVD in hemodialysis patients. The first among these trials was the **4D** (Die Deutsche Diabetes Dialyse) study [123]. This study enrolled 1, 255 hemodialysis patients with type 2 diabetes randomized to receive atorvastatin (20 mg/day) or placebo for 4 years. The study revealed no reduction in the risk of either death from cardiac causes or non-fatal MI. On the contrary, the study showed a significant increase in the risk of fatal stroke in the statin-treated patients.

The second trial was **AURORA** (A Study to Evaluate the Use of Rosuvastatin in Subjects on Regular Hemodialysis: An Assessment of Survival and Cardiovascular Events) which was a double-blind, randomized, placebocontrolled trial designed to compare the impact of rosuvastatin (10 mg/day) against placebo on cardiovascular morbidity and mortality in hemodialysis patients [124]. The study enrolled 2,776 hemodialysis patients aged 50–80 years with a mean baseline LDL cholesterol concentration of about 100 mg/dl. The mean duration of treatment was 2.4 years and the mean length of follow-up was 3.2 years. During the study period, close to 1,300 patients died and over 800 patients discontinued the treatment as a result of either adverse drug reactions or kidney transplantation.

Despite an impressive 43% reduction in serum LDL cholesterol, rosuvastatin therapy failed to reduce the incidence of major cardiovascular events including fatal and non-fatal myocardial infarction or overall mortality. In fact the drug significantly increased the rate of fatal hemorrhagic stroke in diabetic patients ($p = 0.03$), confirming the finding of the 4D study. The third large randomized stat in trial in patients with kidney disease was **SHARP** (the Study of Heart And Renal Protection) [125] which differed from the 4D and AURORA trials in that it included 3, 023 dialysis patients and a large cohort of 6, 247 CKD patients not requiring dialysis with an average estimated glomerular filtration rate of 27 ml/min/1.73 m 2. The enrolled patients were randomized to receive simvastatin 20 mg/day with or without ezetimibe 10 mg/day or placebo. The median duration of follow-up in this trial was 4.9 years. The trial intended to determine the efficacy of LDL cholesterol reduction on major atherosclerotic event including death due to coronary disease, myocardial infarction, nonhemorrhagic stroke, or need for revascularization procedures and the rate of decline in renal function in the CKD patients. The study showed 17% reduction in major atherosclerotic events, 25% reduction in non-hemorrhagic stroke, 21% reduction in coronary revascularization and a trend toward reduction in non-fatal myocardial infarction in the simvastatin- and ezetimibe-treated group.

However, as with the 4D and AURORA studies, cholesterol- lowering therapy failed to reduce either mortality rates or cardiovascular events in the dialysis patients enrolled in the SHARP trial. Thus the favorable effects reported in this study were due to the inclusion of a large cohort of patients with less advanced CKD in whom the pathophysiology of CVD more closely resembles that of the general population than the hemodialysis patients.

However, a meta-analysis of 25 studies involving 8289 dialysis patients found no benefit of statin therapy on major cardiovascular events, cardiovascular mortality, all-cause mortality or myocardial infarction, despite efficacious lipid lowering [126]. Nevertheless, a post-hoc analysis of the 4D study did demonstrate a benefit of statin therapy in the subgroup that had LDL cholesterol > 145 mg/dl (3.76 mmol/l) [127]. Although the use of statins in dialysis patients does not clearly cause harm, at present there is no indication for use in dialysis patients, with the exception of a possible benefit in those with significant elevation in LDL-cholesterol.

Given the robust data demonstrating statin efficacy in CVD risk reduction in virtually all other populations studied, the lack of efficacy in ESRD subjects in perplexing. However, it may be due to different mechanisms of disease progression in ESRD populations compared to other populations. In ESRD subjects there is increased inflammation and oxidative stress as well as increased non-lipid-associated pro-atherogenic factors, which may be the major cause of atherosclerosis development or progression in CKD subjects [for review see [128]]. The primary cause of atherosclerosis and CVD in this population is oxidative stress, inflammation [129-131], HDL deficiency and dysfunction [132-134], accumulation of IDL and chylomicrons remnants, and presence of small dense LDL [13]. These abnormalities cannot be corrected by inhibiting cholesterol synthesis. In addition disturbances of calcium and phosphate metabolism, hypertension, arrhythmogenic electrolyte disorders, hypervolemia, uremic toxins, anemia, comorbid conditions such as diabetes, etc. contribute to cardiovascular disease in this population which are likewise unrelated to cholesterol metabolism and are not amenable to statin administration. The differences in the disturbances in cholesterol metabolism between earlier stages of CKD particularly when accompanied by nephrotic proteinuria and advanced CKD contribute to the divergent response to statin therapy. Therefore, the relative impact of dyslipidemia on CVD development and progression in ESRD subjects may be less than in other CKD and non-CKD subjects, and thus the potential benefit of lipid lowering therapy is reduced. In ESRD subjects with significant hyperlipidemia (such as genetic hyperlipidemias) there may still be a role for statins, or other lipid lowering therapies. Furthermore, while no benefit has been found for statins in dialysis subjects, there is no evidence of increased harm, and thus consideration of lipid lowering medications in particular individuals with ESRD is warranted.

Non-Statins Lipid Lowering Agents

In patients that cannot tolerate or who have contra-indications to statin therapy, there may be some benefit from use other non-statin lipid lowering agents; until today there has been relatively little research into the use of these compound in CKD [135].

Nicotinic Acid

Nicotinic Acid, also known as vitamin B3 or Niacin, is an organic compound; pharmaceutical supplementary is primarily used to treat hypercholesterolemia and pellagra (niacin deficiency). Insufficient niacin in the diet can cause nausea, skin and mouth lesions, anemia, headaches, and tiredness. The lack of niacin may also be observed in pandemic deficiency disease, which is caused by a lack of five crucial vitamins (niacin, vitamin C, thiamin, vitamin D, and vitamin A) and is usually found in areas of widespread poverty and malnutrition. Niacin has not been found to be useful in decreasing the risk of cardiovascular disease in those already on a statin [136] but appears to be effective in those not taking a statin [137].

As Nicotinic Acid is not cleared via the kidney it is theoretically safe in CKD; however, its use is limited due to side effects (predominantly flushing) and a lack of data. Several short term studies have evaluated niacin in CKD patients and it is efficacious in lipid lowering. There is an emerging interest in use of niacin or its analog niacinimide in CKD and ESRD patients for their effects to decrease phosphate levels. A meta-analysis of randomized controlled trials of niacin and niacinamide in dialysis patients found that niacin reduced serum phosphorus but did not change serum calcium levels; furthermore niacin increased HDL levels but had no significant effect on LDL-cholesterol, triglycerides or total cholesterol levels; no CVD outcomes data were provided [138]. Animal studies have suggested a beneficial effect of niacin on renal outcomes [139], and clinical literature is suggestive that this may occur in humans. A database study of niacin in veterans reported that niacin may slow progression of chronic kidney disease (reported at the 2014 Kidney Week meeting (140), but this data is not yet published and further study is needed. Kang et al. treated patients with CKD stages 2-4 with niacin 500mg/d x 6 months; niacin led to increased HDL-cholesterol and decreased triglyceride levels, and improved GFR compared to baseline levels [141].

However, Nicotinic Acid in cholesterol lowering doses (500–2000 mg per day) causes facial flushes by stimulating biosynthesis of prostaglandin D2 (PGD2), especially in the skin. PGD2 dilates the blood vessels via activation of prostaglandin D2 receptors (DP1), increasing blood flow and thus leading to flushes.

Laropiprant was a drug used in combination with Nicotinic Acid to reduce blood cholesterol (LDL and VLDL) that is no longer sold, due to increases in side-effects with no cardiovascular benefit. Laropiprant itself has no cholesterol lowering effect, but it reduces facial flushes induced by Nicotinic Acid. Laropiprant has been developed as an inhibitor of prostaglandin-medicated niacin-induced flushing. In a sub-study examining the use of niacin with laropiprant in dyslipidemic subjects with impaired renal function, the use of niacin resulted in a mean decrease in serum phosphorus of 11% with similar effects between those with eGFR above or below 60 ml/min/1.73 m2 [142]; the parent study reported significant reduction in lipid parameters including a decrease in LDL-cholesterol of 18%, decrease in triglycerides of 25% and an increase in HDL of 20% [142]. Thus, there may be an indication for use of niacin in CKD subjects beyond lipid lowering considerations. However, cardiovascular outcome studies evaluating the combination of statin plus niacin have not found any additional benefit compared to statin alone [144, 145]; thus, at this time further research is needed in CKD subjects to determine if niacin may be more beneficial than statins, or if the addition of niacin to statin may confer non-CVD benefit, for example, from phosphorus lowering.

Fibrates

Fibrates are generally effective in lowering elevated plasma triglycerides and cholesterol. The most pronounced effects of fibrates are a decrease in plasma triglyceride-rich lipoproteins. Moreover, fibrate treatment results in a reduction of the LDL fraction of atherogenic small, dense particles with an equivalent increase in the intermediate subfraction [146-148].

As fibric acid derivatives are used primarily to raise HDL-cholesterol and lower triglycerides; thus, they target two major components of CKD associated dyslipidemia. However, fibrates are known to decrease renal blood flow and glomerular filtration and they are cleared renally [149]; therefore, there is significant concern re their use in CKD. Furthermore, the fibric acid derivatives raise serum creatinine levels and may thus trigger medical investigations into renal disease progression. Thus, there is concern regarding their use in CKD. However, there is a potential for fibric acid derivatives to improve both CVD and CKD outcomes. The acute changes in serum creatinine do not necessarily indicate adverse renal effects. A meta-analysis [150] examined the use of fibrates in CKD subjects and reported beneficial effects to reduce total cholesterol and triglyceride levels and raise HDL-cholesterol levels with no effect on LDL-cholesterol levels. In addition, 3 trials reporting on > 14,000 patients reported that fibrates reduced risk of albuminuria progression in diabetic subjects, with 2 trials (>2,000 patients) reporting albuminuria regression [151-153]. This was associated with a reduction in major cardiovascular events, CVD death, stroke and all-cause mortality in subjects with moderate renal dysfunction, but not in those with eGFR > 60 ml/min/1.73m2. Thus, despite the elevations in serum creatinine seen with fibrates, there is the potential for both cardiac and renal benefit, and further studies specifically designed to evaluate these outcomes in CKD subjects are urgently needed. At this point, providers are encouraged to consider fibrate therapy for appropriate subjects, especially if statins are not tolerated or are contra-indicated.

Ezetimibe

Ezetimibe is presently the only member of the class of cholesterol absorption inhibitors. As monotherapy it can lower LDL approximately 15%; however, the majority of research has examined ezetimibe in combination with a statin (primarily simvastatin) where the addition of ezetimibe can induce a further 25% lowering of LDL cholesterol. Ezetimibe is metabolized through intestinal and hepatic metabolism, and does not require any dose adjustment in CKD or ESRD, making it potentially attractive therapy in CKD. Recently, the results of the Improved Reduction of Outcomes: Vytorin Efficacy International Trial (IMPROVE IT) study were presented [154] demonstrating that the combination of statin + ezetimibe led to further LDL lowering and improved CVD outcomes compared to statin alone in high risk patients [155]. The Study of Heart and Renal Protection (SHARP) compared CVD and renal effects in CKD patients treated with statin plus ezetimibe versus placebo. There was a reduction in CVD events [156]; however, there was no effect on renal disease progression [157]. Note, neither of these studies included an ezetimibe only arm; thus, the effects of ezetimibe monotherapy on outcomes are unknown, although it can be expected to reduce CVD events in proportion to its degree of LDL-cholesterol lowering. A small study evaluating ezetimibe monotherapy in CKD patients found it safe and effective [158]. Thus, the use of ezetimibe with or without statin is likely to benefit pre-end stage CKD patients in terms of CVD outcomes (given that the impact of ezetimibe is on lowering LDL-cholesterol we can anticipate lack of CVD benefit in ESRD subjects based on the statin studies and SHARP).

Fish Oil

Fish oil is oil derived from the tissues of oily fish. Fish oils contain the omega-3 fatty acids eicosapentaenoic acid and docosahexaenoic acid, precursors of eicosanoids that are known to lower triglyceride levels, making them a potential therapy in CKD. The role of fish oil/omega-3 supplements in the general population for prevention of CVD events remains unclear, with some studies suggesting benefit but others finding no CVD protection. A recent meta-analysis found no evidence for CVD protection [159]. In CKD patients there is little data and it is conflicting. A small randomized study evaluated omega-3 fish oil supplements, coenzyme Q10, or both in subjects with CKD stage 3 for 8 weeks. The group that received the omega-3 supplements had decreased heart rate and blood pressure and triglycerides, but there was no effect on renal function (eGFR, or albuminuria) [160]. Conversely, a study evaluating dietary omega-3 intake found that higher consumption was associated with reduced likelihood of CKD. Fish oil supplementation has not been found to have any clear benefit on hemodialysis arteriovenous graft function (161) or on cardiovascular events or mortality in hemodialysis patients [162]. Thus, there is no clear benefit to the use of fish oil supplements in CKD, but further research is needed.

Bile Acid Resins

Bile acid resins or gels are sometimes called sequestrants; these compounds bind to bile acids in the intestine and prevent them from being reabsorbed into the blood. The liver then produces more bile to replace the bile that has been lost. Because the body needs cholesterol to make bile, the liver uses up the cholesterol in the blood, which reduces the amount of LDL cholesterol circulating in the blood.

The bile acid resins tend to be used less commonly than other classes of lipid lowering agents overall, and their use in CKD is limited by a lack of data. Bile acid resins as a class can lower LDL-cholesterol by 10-20% so they are less effective than statins; furthermore, they can raise triglyceride levels and their use is contra-indicated with elevated triglyceride levels, for example > 400-500 mg/dl (>4.5 – 5.6 mmol/L). Thus, overall bile acid resins are rarely used in CKD patients. However, their metabolism is intestinal and thus there are no required modifications for their use in mild-moderate CKD. Although there are no theoretical concerns regarding their use in ESRD there is no data to address safety or efficacy. Today cholestyramine and colestipol are hardly used anymore for lowering cholesterol because their intake frequently causes gastrointestinal side effects (e.g., nausea, gastrointestinal discomfort) [163]. However, the novel bile acid resin colesevelam appears to have fewer side effects [163].

PCSK9 Inhibitors

Proprotein convertase subtilisin/kexin type 9 (PCSK9) is generated by liver cells and emitted to the cells surface. By binding to hepatic LDL-R and promoting their lysosomal degradation, PCSK9 reduces LDL uptake, leading to an increase in LDL cholesterol concentrations. Gain-of-function mutations in PCSK9 associated with high LDL cholesterol and premature cardiovascular disease have been causally implicated in the pathophysiology of autosomal-dominant familial hypercholesterolemia. In contrast, the more commonly expressed loss-of-function mutations in PCSK9 are associated with reduced LDL cholesterol and cardiovascular disease risk [164, 165].

Two recent meta-analyses evaluated the clinical potential of antibody PCSK9 inhibition in >10,000 patients who participated in over 20 phase II and III trials [166, 167]. These meta-analyses included data from most of the available studies with alirocumab and evolocumab. Another PCSK9 inhibitor, Bococizumab is close to finish a first phase III study [168].

All trials confirmed the beneficial effect of PCSK9 inhibition on LDL-C levels. The use of PCSK9 monoclonal antibodies was associated with mean LDL-C reductions of approximately 50% [166, 167]. These results persisted during follow-up, and were similar across different doses, patient populations, and in patients with or without background statin therapy [166, 169].

In addition to their LDL-C lowering effect, PCSK9 inhibitors consistently increased high-density lipoprotein cholesterol by approximately 6% (95% CI, 6–7%) and lowered lipoprotein(a) by approximately 26% (95% CI, 23–30%) both in placebo- and ezetimibe-controlled trials [166]. The effects on lipid levels were similar in trials on evolocumab, alirocumab, and bococizumab [166-170]; good compatibility and little adverse effects has been foud. Furthermore, these preliminary analyses suggest a statistically significant reduction in all-cause mortality and a non-significant reduction in CVD mortality.

PCSK9 inhibitors have just received approval for the treatment of FH and clinical atherosclerotic disease, and patients not at target under maximally tolerated statin therapy or intolerant to statins.

Others Therapies

There are a number of new and pending therapies for the treatment of dyslipidemia, including mipomersen (an anti-sense oligonucleotide against apoB-100) [171, 172], lomitapide (a microsomal triglyceride transfer protein inhibitor) [173], and evacetrapib and anacetrapib (cholesterol ester transfer protein [CETP] inhibitors) [174, 175]. However, to date none of these agents have been studied in CKD; thus, there is no data available to assess their potential use in this population.

Mipomersen and lomitapide are both FDA approved for use in homozygous familial hypercholesterolemia (FH). The clinical impact of the lipid-modifying effects of anacetrapib is being evaluated in the cardiovascular disease outcomes trial, Randomized EValuation of the Effects of Anacetrapib though Lipid-modification (REVEAL).

In HD can also be used extracorporeal therapies to reduce lipid levels.

Use of a vitamin E–coated membrane (VEM) dialyzer results in a significant reduction in ox-LDL or malondialdehyde-rich LDL compared to the ordinary cellulose membrane dialyzer and an attenuation of the increase in aortic calcification index after 24 months [176]. In another recent study the use of VEM and simvastatin resulted in similar anti-inflammatory and anti-oxidative effects which, however, appeared more directly and immediately with the VEM treatment compared to the simvastatin treatment. Simvastatin, on the other hand, caused a more intense anti-inflammatory response, which was in part correlated with its preceding lipid-lowering effects [177].

Lipid apheresis is very effective in lowering plasma LDL cholesterol and, depending on the technique, can also lower plasma Lp(a), triglycerides, and fibrinogen [178].

Although previous and recent studies have suggested that LDL apheresis exerts beneficial effects on the peripheral circulation in dialysis patients suffering from peripheral artery disease, probably through a reduction of not only serum lipids but also of inflammatory or coagulatory factors and oxidative stress, the precise molecular mechanisms underlying the long-term effects of LDL apheresis on the improvement of the peripheral circulation remains unclear and warrants further investigation [179].

REFERENCES

[1] McCullough, PA. Cardiovascular disease in chronic kidney disease from a cardiologist's perspective. *Curr Opin Nephrol Hyperten*, 2004, 13, 591-600.

[2] Ronco, C; Haapio, M; House, AA; Anavekar, N; Bellomo, R. Cardiorenal Syndrome. *J Am Coll Cardiol*, 2008, 52, 1527-1539.

[3] McCullough, PA; Verrill, TA. Cardiorenal interaction: appropriate treatment of cardiovascular risk factors to improve outcomes in chronic kidney disease. *Postgrad Med*, 2010, 122, 25-34.

[4] Harper, CR; Jacobson, TA. Managing dyslipidemia in chronic kidney disease. *J Am Coll Cardiol*, 2008, 51, 2375-2384.

[5] Lacquaniti, A; Bolignano, D; Donato, V; Bono, C; Razio, MR; Buemi, M. Alterations of Lipid Metabolism in Chronic Nephrothies: Mechanisms, Diagnosis and Treatment. *Kidney Blood Press Res*, 2010, 33, 100-110.

[6] Foley, RN; Murray, AM; Li, S; Herzog, CA; McBean, AM; Eggers, PW; Collins, AJ. Chronic kidney disease and the risk for cardiovascular disease, renal replacement, and death in the United States Medicare population, 1998 to 1999. *J Am Soc Nephrol*, 2005, 16, 489-495.

[7] Muntner, P; He, J; Astor, BC; Folsom, AR; Coresh, J. Traditional and nontraditional risk factors predict coronary heart disease in chronic kidney disease: results from the atherosclerosis risk in communities study. *J Am Soc Nephrol*, 2005, 16, 529-538.

[8] Shoji, T; Masakane, I; Watanabe, Y; Iseki, K; Tsubakihara, Y. Elevated non-high-density lipoprotein cholesterol (non-HDL-C) predicts atherosclerotic cardiovascular events in hemodialysis patients. *Clin J Am Soc Nephrol*, 2011, 6, 1112-1120.

[9] Reiner, Z; Catapano, AL; De Backer, G; Graham, I; Taskinen, MR; Wiklund, O; Agewall, S; Alegria, E; Chapman, MJ; Durrington, P; Erdine, S; Halcox, J; Hobbs, R; Kjekshus, J; Filardi, PP; Riccardi, G; Storey, RF; Wood, D; Bax, J; Vahanian, A; Auricchio, A; Baumgartner, H; Ceconi, C; Dean, V; Deaton, C; Fagard, R; Filippatos, G; Funck-Brentano, C; Hasdai, D; Hobbs, R; Hoes, A; Kearney, P; Knuuti, J; Kolh, P; McDonagh, T; Moulin, C; Poldermans, D; Popescu, BA; Reiner, Z; Sechtem, U; Sirnes, PA; Tendera, M; Torbicki, A; Vardas, P; Widimsky, P; Windecker, S; Funck-Brentano, C; Poldermans, D; Berkenboom, G; De Graaf, J; Descamps, O; Gotcheva, N; Griffith, K; Guida, GF; Gulec, S; Henkin, Y; Huber, K; Kesaniemi, YA; Lekakis, J; Manolis, AJ; Marques- Vidal, P; Masana, L; McMurray, J; Mendes, M; Pagava, Z; Pedersen, T; Prescott, E; Rato, Q; Rosano, G; Sans, S; Stalenhoef, A; Tokgozoglu, L; Viigimaa, M; Wittekoek, ME; Zamorano, JL. ESC/EAS Guidelines for the management of dyslipidaemias: the Task Force for the management of dyslipidaemias of the European Society of Cardiology (ESC) and the European Atherosclerosis Society (EAS). *Eur Heart J*, 2011, 32, 1769-1818.

[10] Kaysen, GA. Lipid and Lipoprotein Metabolism in Chronic Kidney Disease. *J Ren Nutr*, 2009, 19, 73-77.
[11] Kruit, JK; Groen, AK; van Berkel, TJ; Kuipers, F. Emerging roles of the intestine in control of cholesterol metabolism. *World J Gastroenterol*, 2006, 12, 6429-6439.
[12] Redgrave, TG. Chylomicron metabolism. *Biochem Soc Trans*, 2004, 32, 79-82.
[13] Vaziri, ND; Norris, K. Lipid Disorders and Their Relevance to Outcomes in Chronic Kidney Disease. *Blood Purif*, 2011, 31, 189-196.
[14] Vaziri, ND. Dyslipidemia of chronic renal failure: the nature, mechanisms, and potential consequences. *Am J Physiol Renal Physiol*, 2006, 290, F262-F272.
[15] Vaziri, ND; Liang, KH. Down-regulation of VLDL receptor expression in chronic experimental renal failure. *Kidney Int*, 1997, 51, 913-919.
[16] Brown, MS; Goldstein, JL. Lipoprotein metabolism in the macrophage: Implications for cholesterol deposition in atherosclerosis. *Annu Rev Biochem*, 52, 223–261, 1983.
[17] Bruce, C; Chouinard, RA; Jr. Tall, AR. Plasma lipid transfer proteins; high-density lipoproteins, and reverse cholesterol transport. *Annu Rev Nutr* 18, 297–330, 1998.
[18] Dieplinger, H; Zechner, R; Kostner, GM. The *in vitro* formation of HDL2 during the action of LCAT: The role of triglyceride-rich lipoproteins. *J Lipid Res*, 26, 273–282, 1985.
[19] Acton, S; Rigotti, A; Landschulz, KT; Xu, S; Hobbs, HH; Krieger, M. Identification of scavenger receptor SR-BI as a high density lipoprotein receptor. *Science*, 271, 518–520, 1996.
[20] Batista, MC; Welty, FK; Diffenderfer, MR; Sarnak, MJ; Schaefer, EJ; Lamon-Fava, S; Asztalos, BF; Dolnikowski, GG; Brousseau, ME; Marsh, JB. Apolipoprotein A-I, B-100, and B-48 metabolism in subjects with chronic kidney disease, obesity, and the metabolic syndrome. *Metabolism*, 53, 1255–1261, 2004.
[21] Appel, G. Lipid abnormalities in renal disease. *Kidney Int*, 39, 169–183, 1991.
[22] Senti, M; Romero, R; Pedro-Botet, J; Pelegri, A; Nogues, X; Rubies-Prat, J. Lipoprotein abnormalities in hyperlipidemic and normolipidemic men on hemodialysis with chronic renal failure. *Kidney Int*, 41, 1394–1399, 1992.
[23] Cryer, A. Tissue lipoprotein lipase activity and its action in lipoprotein metabolism. *Int J Biochem*, 13, 525–541, 1981.
[24] Arnadottir, M. Pathogenesis of dyslipoproteinemia in renal insufficiency: The role of lipoprotein lipase and hepatic lipase. *Scand J Clin Lab Invest*, 57, 1–11, 1997.
[25] Brown, MS; Goldstein, JL. A receptor-mediated pathway for cholesterol homeostasis. *Science*, 232, 34–47, 1986.
[26] McNamara, JR; Shah, PK; Nakajima, K; Cupples, LA; Wilson, PW; Ordovas, JM; Schaefer, EJ. Remnant-like particle (RLP) cholesterol is an independent cardiovascular disease risk factor in women: results from the Framingham Heart Study. *Atherosclerosis*, 154, 229–236, 2001.
[27] Leary, ET; Wang, T; Baker, DJ; Cilla, DD; Zhong, J; Warnick, GR; Nakajima, K; Havel, RJ. Evaluation of an immunoseparation method for quantitative measurement of remnantlike particle-cholesterol in serum and plasma. *Clin Chem*, 44, 2490–2498, 1998.
[28] Klin, M; Smogorzewski, M; Ni, ZM; Zhang, GX; Massry, SG. Abnormalities in hepatic lipase in chronic renal failure - Role of excess parathyroid hormone. *J Clin Investig*, 1996, 97, 2167-2173.

[29] Liang, K; Vaziri, ND. Down-regulation of hepatic lipase expression in experimental nephrotic syndrome. *Kidney Int*, 1997, 51, 1933-1937.

[30] Akmal, MS; Perkins, SE; Kasim, HY; Oh, M. Smogorzewski, and S.G. Massry. 1993. Verapamil prevents chronic renal failure-induced abnormalities in lipid metabolism. *Am. J. Kidney Dis*. 22,158–163.

[31] Massry, SG; Smogorzewski, M; 1994. Mechanisms through which parathyroid hormone mediates its deleterious effects on organ function in uremia. Sem. *Nephrol*, 14, 219–231.

[32] Klin, MM; Smogorzewski, SG. Massry. 1995. Chronic renal failure increases cytosolic [Ca]i of hepatocytes. *Am. J. Physiol*, 269, G103–G109.

[33] Massry, SG; Klin, M; Ni, Z; Tian, J; Kedes, L; Smogorzewski, M. 1995. Impaired agonist-induced calcium signaling in hepatocytes from chronic renal failure. *Kidney Int*, 48, 1324–1331.

[34] Tian, J; Smogorzewski, M; Kedes, L; Massry, SG. 1995. PTH- PTHrP receptor is down-regulated in chronic renal failure. *Am. J. Nephrol*, 14, 41–46.

[35] Urena, P; Kubrusly, M; Mannstadt, M; Hruley, M; Tan, MMTT; Silve, C; LaCour, B; Abou-Samara, AB; Segre, GV; Drueke, T. 1994. The renal PTH/PTHrP receptor is down-regulated in rats with chronic renal failure. *Kidney Int*, 45, 605–611.

[36] Smogorzewski, M; Tian, J; Massry, SG. 1995. Downregulation of PTH-PTHrP receptor in heart in CRF: Role of [Ca]i. *Kidney Int*, 47, 1182–1186.

[37] Cheung, AK; Wu, LL; Kablitz, C; Leypoldt, JK. Atherogenic lipids and lipoproteins in hemodialysis patients. *Am J Kidney Dis*, 22, 271 –276, 1993.

[38] Cressman, MD; Heyka, RJ; Paganini, EP; O'Neil, J; Skibinski, CI; Hoff, HF. Lipoprotein(a) is an independent risk factor for cardiovascular disease in hemodialysis patients. *Circulation*, 86, 475 –482, 1992.

[39] Koch, M; Kutkuhn, B; Trenkwalder, E; Bach, D; Grabensee, B; Dieplinger, H; Kronenberg, F. Apolipoprotein B, fibrinogen, HDL cholesterol, and apolipoprotein(a) phenotypes predict coronary artery disease in hemodialysis patients. *J Am Soc Nephrol*, 8, 1889 –1898, 1997.

[40] Dantoine, TF; Debord, J; Charmes, JP; Merle, L; Marquet, P; Lachatre, G; Leroux-Robert, C. Decrease of serum paraoxonase activity in chronic renal failure. *J Am Soc Nephrol*, 9, 2082 –2088, 1998.

[41] Navab, M; Hama, SY; Reddy, ST; Ng, CJ; Van Lenten, BJ; Laks, H; Fogelman, AM. Oxidized lipids as mediators of coronary heart disease. *Curr Opin Lipidol*, 13, 363 – 372, 2002.

[42] Solakivi, T; Jaakkola, O; Salomaki, A; Peltonen, N; Metso, S; Lehtimaki, T; Jokela, H; Nikkari, ST. HDL enhances oxidation of LDL *in vitro* in both men and women. *Lipids Health Dis*, 4, 25, 2005.

[43] Danesh, J; Collins, R; Peto, R. Lipoprotein(a) and coronary heart disease. Meta-analysis of prospective studies. *Circulation*, 2000, 102, 1082-1085.

[44] Erqou, S; Kaptoge, S; Perry, PL; Di Angelantonio, E; Thompson, A; White, IR; Marcovina, SM; Collins, R; Thompson, SG; Danesh, J. Lipoprotein(a) concentration and the risk of coronary heart disease, stroke, and non-vascular mortality. *JAMA*, 2009, 302, 412-423.

[45] Kaysen, GA. New Insights into Lipid Metabolism in Chronic Kidney Disease: What Are the Practical Implications *Blood Purif*, 2009, 27, 86-91.

[46] Longenecker, JC; Klag, MJ; Marcovina, SM; Liu, YM; Jaar, BG; Powe, NR; Fink, NE; Levey, AS; Coresh, J. High lipoprotein(a) levels and small apolipoprotein(a) size prospectively predict cardiovascular events in dialysis patients. *J Am Soc Nephrol*, 2005, 16, 1794-1802.

[47] Clarke, R; Peden, JF; Hopewell, JC; Kyriakou, T; Goel, A; et al. Genetic variants associated with Lp(a) lipoprotein level and coronary disease. *N Engl J Med*, 2009, 361, 2518–28.

[48] Kamstrup, PR; Tybjaerg-Hansen, A; Nordestgaard, BG. Genetic Evidence That Lipoprotein(a) Associates With Atherosclerotic Stenosis Rather Than Venous Thrombosis. *Arterioscler Thromb Vasc Biol*, 2012, 32, 1732–41.

[49] Kronenberg, F; Utermann, G; Dieplinger, H. Lipoprotein(a) in renal disease. *Am J Kidney Dis*, 1996, 27, 1–25.

[50] Lin, J; Reilly, MP; Terembula, K; Wilson, FP. Plasma Lipoprotein(a) Levels Are Associated with Mild Renal Impairment in Type 2 Diabetics Independent of Albuminuria. *PLoS ONE*, 2014, 9, e114397.

[51] Sandholzer, C; Hallman, DM; Saha, N; Sigurdsson, G; Lackner, C; Császár, A; et al. Effects of the apolipoprotein(a) size polymorphism on the lipoprotein(a) concentration in 7 ethnic groups. *Hum Genet*, 1991, 86, 607–14.

[52] Rifai, N; Heiss, G; Doetsch, K. Lipoprotein(a) at birth; in blacks and whites. *Atherosclerosis*, 1992, 92, 123–9.

[53] Kronenberg, F; Kuen, E; Ritz, E; Junker, R; Konig, P; Kraatz, G; Lhotta, K; Mann, JF; Muller, GA; Neyer, U; Riegel, W; Reigler, P; Schwenger, V; von Eckardstein, A. Lipoprotein(a) serum concentrations and apolipoprotein(a) phenotypes in mild and moderate renal failure. *J Am Soc Nephrol*, 2000, 11, 105-115.

[54] Kuboyama, M; Ageta, M; Ishihara, T; Fujiura, Y; Kashio, N; Ikushima, I. Serum lipoprotein(a) concentration and Apo(a) isoform under the condition of renal dysfunction. *J Atheroscler Thromb*, 2003, 10, 283-289.

[55] de Sain-van der Velden, MG; Reijngoud, DJ; Kaysen, GA; Gadellaa, MM; Voorbij, H; Stellaard, F; Koomans, HA; Rabelink, TJ. Evidence for increased synthesis of lipoprotein(a) in the nephrotic syndrome. *J Am Soc Nephrol*, 1998, 9, 1474-1481.

[56] Frischmann, ME; Kronenberg, F; Trenkwalder, E; Schaefer, JR; Schweer, H; Dieplinger, B; Koenig, P; Ikewaki, K; Dieplinger, H. *In vivo* turnover study demonstrates diminished clearance of lipoprotein(a) in hemodialysis patients. *Kidney Int*, 2007, 71, 1036-1043.

[57] Elisaf, MS; Millionis, HJ; Siamopoulos, KC. Increased serum lipoprotein (a) levels in patients with early renal failure. *Ann Intern Med*, 1999, 130, 1028–9.

[58] Kalra, OP; Khaira, A; Gambhir, JK; Agarwal, S; Bhargava, SK. Lipoprotein (a) in chronic renal failure: effect of maintenance hemodialysis. *Hemodial Int*, 2003, 7, 326–31.

[59] Dieplinger, H; Lackner, C; Kronenberg, F; Sandholzer, C; Lhotta, K; Hoppichler, F; et al. Elevated plasma concentrations of lipoprotein(a) in patients with end-stage renal disease are not related to the size polymorphism of apolipoprotein(a) *J Clin Invest*, 1993, 91, 397–401.

[60] Kronenberg, F; Kuen, E; Ritz, E; Junker, R; König, P; Kraatz, G; et al. Lipoprotein(a) serum concentrations and apolipoprotein(a) phenotypes in mild and moderate renal failure. *J Am Soc Nephrol*, 2000, 11, 105–15.

[61] Parsons, DS; Reaveley, DA; Pavitt, DV; Misra, M; Brown, EA. Lipoprotein(a) levels in those with high molecular weight apo(a) isoforms may remain low in a significant proportion of patients with end-stage renal disease. *Nephrol Dial Transplant*, 2003, 18, 1848–53.

[62] Rajman, I; Harper, L; McPake, D; Kendall, MJ; Wheeler, DC. Low-density lipoprotein sub-fraction profiles in chronic renal failure. *Nephrol Dial Transplant*, 1998, 13, 2281–2287.

[63] Deighan, CJ; Caslake, MJ; McConnell, M; Boulton-Jones, JM; Packard, CJ. Atherogenic lipoprotein phenotype in end-stage renal failure: origin and extent of small dense low- density lipoprotein formation. *Am J Kidney Dis*, 2000, 35, 852–862.

[64] St Pierre, AC; Cantin, B; Dagenais, GR; Mauriege, P; Bernard, PM; Despres, JP; Lamarche, B. Low-density lipoprotein subfractions and the long-term risk of ischemic heart disease in men: 13-year follow-up data from the Quebec Cardiovascular Study. *Arterioscler Thromb Vasc Biol*, 2005, 25, 553–559.

[65] Austin, MA; King, MC; Vranizan, KM; Krauss, RM. Atherogenic lipoprotein phenotype. A proposed genetic marker for coronary heart disease risk. *Circulation*, 82, 495–506, 1990.

[66] Okubo, K; Ikewaki, K; Sakai, S; Tada, N; Kawaguchi, Y; Mochizuki, S. Abnormal HDL apolipoprotein A-I and A-II kinetics in hemodialysis patients: a stable isotope study. *J Am Soc Nephrol*, 2004, 15, 1008–1015.

[67] Blankestijn, PJ; Vos, PF; Rabelink, TJ; van Rijn, HJ; Jansen, H; Koomans, HA. High-flux dialysis membranes improve lipid profile in chronic hemodialysis patients. *J Am Soc Nephrol*, 1995, 5, 1703–1708.

[68] Docci, D; Capponcini, C; Mengozzi, S; Baldrati, L; Neri, L; Feletti, C. Effects of different dialysis membranes on lipid and lipoprotein serum profiles in hemodialysis patients. *Nephron*, 1995, 69, 323–326.

[69] Wanner, C; Bahner, U; Mattern, R; Lang, D; Passlick-Deetjen, J. Effect of dialysis flux and membrane material on dyslipidaemia and inflammation in haemodialysis patients. *Nephrol Dial Transplant*, 2004, 19, 2570– 2575.

[70] Jung, K; Scheifler, A; Schulze, BD; Scholz, M. Lower serum high-density lipoprotein-cholesterol concentration in patients undergoing maintenance hemodialysis with acetate than with bicarbonate. *Am J Kidney Dis*, 1995, 25, 584–588.

[71] Mordasini, R; Frey, F; Flury, W; Klose, G; Greten, H. Selective deficiency of hepatic triglyceride lipase in uremic patients. *N Engl J Med*, 1977, 297, 1362–1366.

[72] Shoji, T; Nishizawa, Y; Nishitani, H; Yamakawa, M; Morii, H. Impaired metabolism of high density lipoprotein in uremic patients. *Kidney Int*, 1992, 41, 1653–1661.

[73] Huttunen, JK; Pasternack, A; Vanttinen, T; Ehnholm, C; Nikkila, EA. Lipoprotein metabolism in patients with chronic uremia. Effect of hemodialysis on serum lipoproteins and postheparin plasma triglyceride lipases. *Acta Med Scand*, 1978, 204, 211–218.

[74] Katopodis, KP; Elisaf, M; Balafa, O; Nikolopoulos, P; Bairaktari, E; Katsaraki, A; Siamopoulos, KC. Influence of the type of membrane and heparin on serum lipid parameters during a dialysis session: a pilot study. *Am J Nephrol*, 2004, 24, 469–473.

[75] Schrader, J; Stibbe, W; Armstrong, VW; Kandt, M; Muche, R; Kostering, H; Seidel, D; Scheler, F. Comparison of low molecular weight heparin to standard heparin in hemodialysis/hemofiltration. *Kidney Int*, 1988, 33, 890–896.

[76] Chertow, GM; Burke, SK; Raggi, P. Sevelamer attenuates the progression of coronary and aortic calcification in hemodialysis patients. *Kidney Int*, 2002, 62, 245–252.

[77] Attman, PO; Samuelsson, OG; Moberly, J; Johansson, AC; Ljungman, S; Weiss, LG; Knight-Gibson, C; Alaupovic, P. Apolipoprotein B containinglipoproteins in renal failure: the relation to mode of dialysis. *Kidney Int*, 1999, 55, 1536–1542.

[78] Kronenberg, F; Lingenhel, A; Neyer, U; Lhotta, K; Konig, P; Auinger, M; Wiesholzer, M; Andersson, H; Dieplinger, H. Prevalence of dyslipidemic risk factors in hemodialysis and CAPD patients. *Kidney Int Suppl*, 2003, 84, S113–S116.

[79] Deighan, CJ; Caslake, MJ; McConnell, M; Boulton-Jones, JM; Packard, CJ. Atherogenic lipoprotein phenotype in end-stage renal failure: origin and extent of small dense lowdensity lipoprotein formation. *Am J Kidney Dis*, 2000, 35, 852–862.

[80] Wheeler, DC. Abnormalities of lipoprotein metabolism in CAPD patients. *Kidney Int Suppl*, 1996, 56, S41–S46.

[81] Heimburger, O; Stenvinkel, P; Berglund, L; Tranoeus, A; Lindholm, B. Increased plasma lipoprotein(a) in continuous ambulatory peritoneal dialysis is related to peritoneal transport of proteins and glucose. *Nephron*, 1996, 72, 135–144.

[82] Wanner, C; Bartens, W; Walz, G; Nauck, M; Schollmeyer, P. Protein loss and genetic polymorphism of apolipoprotein(a) modulate serum lipoprotein(a) in CAPD patients. *Nephrol Dial Transplant*, 1995, 10, 75–81.

[83] Kagan, A; Bar-Khayim, Y; Schafer, Z; Fainaru, M. Heterogeneity in peritoneal transport during continuous ambulatory peritoneal dialysis and its impact on ultrafiltration; loss of macromolecules and plasma level of proteins, lipids and lipoproteins. *Nephron*, 1993, 63, 32–42.

[84] Siamopoulos, KC; Elisaf, M. Is CAPD atherogenic? *Perit Dial Int*, 1997, 17, 227–231.

[85] Johansson, AC; Samuelsson, O; Attman, PO; Haraldsson, B; Moberly, J; Knight-Gibson, C; Alaupovic, P. Dyslipidemia in peritoneal dialysis– relation to dialytic variables. *Perit Dial Int*, 2000, 20, 306–314.

[86] Bredie, SJ; Bosch, FH; Demacker, PN; Stalenhoef, AF; van Leusen, R. Effects of peritoneal dialysis with an overnight icodextrin dwell on parameters of glucose and lipid metabolism. *Perit Dial Int*, 2001, 21, 275–281.

[87] Babazono, T; Nakamoto, H; Kasai, K; Kuriyama, S; Sugimoto, T; Nakayama, M; Hamada, C; Furuya, R; Hasegawa, H; Kasahara, M; Moriishi, M; Tomo, T; Miyazaki, M; Sato, M; Yorioka, N; Kawaguchi, Y. Effects of icodextrin on glycemic and lipid profiles in diabetic patients undergoing peritoneal dialysis. *Am J Nephrol*, 2007, 27, 409–415.

[88] Kagan, A; Bar-Khayim, Y; Schafer, Z; Fainaru, M. Kinetics of peritoneal protein loss during CAPD. II. Lipoprotein leakage and its impact on plasma lipid levels. *Kidney Int*, 1990, 37, 980–990.

[89] Kandoussi, A; Cachera, C; Reade, R; Pagniez, D; Fruchart, JC; Tacquet, A. Apo AIV in plasma and dialysate fluid of CAPD patients: comparison with other apolipoproteins. *Nephrol Dial Transplant*, 1992, 7, 1026–1029.

[90] Tsimihodimos, V; Dounousi, E; Siamopoulos, KC. Dyslipidemia in chronic kidney disease: an approach to pathogenesis and treatment. *Am J Nephrol*, 2008, 28(6), 958-73.

[91] Katopodis, KP; Andrikos, EK; Gouva, CD; Bairaktari, ET; Nikolopoulos, PM; Takouli, LK; Tzallas, CS; Elisaf, MS; Pappas, MV; Siamopoulos, KC. Sevelamer hydrochloride

versus aluminum hydroxide: effect on serum phosphorus and lipids in CAPD patients. *Perit Dial Int*, 2006, 26, 320–327.

[92] Stack, AG; Bloembergen, WE. Prevalence and clinical correlates of coronary artery disease among new dialysis patients in the United States: A cross-sectional study. *J Am Soc Nephrol*, 12, 1516–1523, 2001.

[93] Cheung, AK; Sarnak, MJ; Yan, G; Dwyer, JT; Heyka, RJ; Rocco, MV; Teehan, BP; Levey, AS. Atherosclerotic cardiovascular disease risks in chronic hemodialysis patients. *Kidney Int*. 58, 353–362, 2000.

[94] Guz, G; Nurhan Ozdemir, F; Sezer, S; Isiklar, I; Arat, Z; Turan, M; Haberal, M. Effect of apolipoprotein E polymorphism on serum lipid, lipoproteins, and atherosclerosis in hemodialysis patients. *Am J Kidney Dis*, 36, 826–836, 2000.

[95] Degoulet, P; Legrain, M; Reach, I; Aime, F; Devries, C; Rojas, P; Jacobs, C. Mortality risk factors in patients treated by chronic hemodialysis. Report of the Diaphane collaborative study. *Nephron*, 31, 103–110, 1982.

[96] Kronenberg, F; Neyer, U; Lhotta, K; Trenkwalder, E; Auinger, M; Pribasnig, A; Meisl, T; Konig, P; Dieplinger, H. The low molecular weight apo(a) phenotype is an independent predictor for coronary artery disease in hemodialysis patients: A prospective follow-up. *J Am Soc Nephrol*, 10, 1027–1036, 1999.

[97] Zimmermann, J; Herrlinger, S; Pruy, A; Metzger, T; Wanner, C. Inflammation enhances cardiovascular risk and mortality in hemodialysis patients. *Kidney Int*, 55, 648–658, 1999.

[98] Iseki, K; Fukiyama, K. Predictors of stroke in patients receiving chronic hemodialysis. *Kidney Int*, 50, 1672–1675, 1996.

[99] Liu, Y; Coresh, J; Eustace, JA; Longenecker, JC; Jaar, B; Fink, NE; Tracy, RP; Powe, NR; Klag, MJ. Association between cholesterol level and mortality in dialysis patients: Role of inflammation and malnutrition. *JAMA*, 291, 451–459, 2004.

[100] Koda, Y; Nishi, S; Suzuki, M; Hirasawa, Y. Lipoprotein (a) is a predictor for cardiovascular mortality of hemodialysis patients. *Kidney Int Suppl*, 71, S251–S253, 1999.

[101] Ohashi, H; Oda, H; Ohno, M; Watanabe, S; Sakata, S. Lipoprotein(a) as a risk factor for coronary artery disease in hemodialysis patients. *Kidney Int Suppl*, 71, S242–S244, 1999.

[102] Shoji, T; Emoto, M; Shinohara, K; Kakiya, R; Tsujimoto, Y; Kishimoto, H; Ishimura, E; Tabata, T; Nishizawa, Y. Diabetes mellitus, aortic stiffness, and cardiovascular mortality in end-stage renal disease. *J Am Soc Nephrol*, 12, 2117–2124, 2001.

[103] Hocher, B; Ziebig, R; Altermann, C; Krause, R; Asmus, G; Richter, CM; Slowinski, T; Sinha, P; Neumayer, HH. Different impact of biomarkers as mortality predictors among diabetic and nondiabetic patients undergoing hemodialysis. *J Am Soc Nephrol*, 14, 2329–2337, 2003.

[104] Schwaiger, JP; Lamina, C; Neyer, U; Konig, P; Kathrein, H; Sturm, W; Lhotta, K; Grochenig, E; Dieplinger, H; Kronenberg, F. Carotid plaques and their predictive value for cardiovascular disease and all-cause mortality in hemodialysis patients considering renal transplantation: A decade follow-up. *Am J Kidney Dis*, 47, 888–897, 2006.

[105] Attman, PO; Alaupovic, P. Lipid and apolipoprotein profiles of uremic dyslipoproteinemia: Relation to renal function and dialysis. *Nephron*, 57, 401–410, 1991.

[106] Lowrie, EG; Lew, NL. Commonly measured laboratory variables in hemodialysis patients: Relationships among them and to death risk. *Semin Nephrol*, 12, 276–283, 1992.

[107] Lowrie, EG; Lew, NL. Death risk in hemodialysis patients: The predictive value of commonly measured variables and an evaluation of death rate differences between facilities. *Am J Kidney Dis*, 15, 458–482, 1990.

[108] Iseki, K; Yamazato, M; Tozawa, M; Takishita, S. Hypocholesterolemia is a significant predictor of death in a cohort of chronic hemodialysis patients. *Kidney Int*, 61, 1887–1893, 2002.

[109] Longenecker, JC; Coresh, J; Powe, NR; Levey, AS; Fink, NE; Martin, A; Klag, MJ. Traditional cardiovascular disease risk factors in dialysis patients compared with the general population: The CHOICE Study. *J Am Soc Nephrol*, 13, 1918–1927, 2002.

[110] Tatami, R; Mabuchi, H; Ueda, K; Ueda, R; Haba, T; Kametani, T; Ito, S; Koizumi, J; Ohta, M; Miyamoto, S; Nakayama, A; Kanaya, H; Oiwake, H; Genda, A; Takeda, R. Intermediatedensity lipoprotein and cholesterol-rich very low density lipoprotein in angiographically determined coronary artery disease. *Circulation*, 64, 1174–1184, 1981.

[111] Shoji, T; Nishizawa, Y; Kawagishi, T; Kawasaki, K; Taniwaki, H; Tabata, T; Inoue, T; Morii, H. Intermediate-density lipoprotein as an independent risk factor for aortic atherosclerosis in hemodialysis patients. *J Am Soc Nephrol*, 9, 1277–1284, 1998.

[112] Longenecker, JC; Klag, MJ; Marcovina, SM; Powe, NR; Fink, NE; Giaculli, F; Coresh, J. Small apolipoprotein(a) size predicts mortality in end-stage renal disease: The CHOICE study. *Circulation*, 106, 2812–2818, 2002.

[113] Auguet, T; Senti, M; Rubies-Prat, J; Pelegri, A; Pedro-Botet, J; Nogues, X; Romero, R. Serum lipoprotein(a) concentration in patients with chronic renal failure receiving haemodialysis: Influence of apolipoprotein (a) genetic polymorphism. *Nephrol Dial Transplant*, 8, 1099–1103, 1993.

[114] Kronenberg, F; Kathrein, H; Konig, P; Neyer, U; Sturm, W; Lhotta, K; Grochenig, E; Utermann, G; Dieplinger, H. Apolipoprotein(a) phenotypes predict the risk for carotid atherosclerosis in patients with end-stage renal disease. *Arterioscler Thromb*, 14, 1405–1411, 1994.

[115] Wanner, C; Bartens, W; Walz, G; Nauck, M; Schollmeyer, P. Protein loss and genetic polymorphism of apolipoprotein(a) modulate serum lipoprotein(a) in CAPD patients. *Nephrol Dial Transplant*, 10, 75–81, 1995.

[116] Emanuele, E; Lusignani, LS; Peros, E; Montagna, G; D'Angelo, A; Montagna, L; Geroldi, D. Lipoprotein(a)-associated atherothrombotic risk in hemodialysis patients. *Am J Nephrol*, 24, 221–229, 2004.

[117] Iliescu, EA; Marcovina, SM; Morton, AR; Lam, M; Koschinsky, ML. Apolipoprotein(a) phenotype and lipoprotein(a) level predict peritoneal dialysis patient mortality. *Perit Dial Int*, 22, 492–499, 2002.

[118] Webb, AT; Reaveley, DA; O'Donnell, M; O'Connor, B; Seed, M; Brown, EA. Lipids and lipoprotein(a) as risk factors for vascular disease in patients on renal replacement therapy. *Nephrol Dial Transplant*, 10, 354–357, 1995.

[119] Gazzaruso, C; Bonetti, G; Garzaniti, A; Pini, G; Ragazzoni, A; Bianchi, C; Jucci, A; Buscaglia, P; Geroldi, D. Increased plasma concentrations of lipoprotein(a) for every

phenotype of apolipoprotein(a) in patients with chronic renal failure treated by hemodialysis. *Nutr Metab Cardiovasc Dis*, 6, 203–210, 1996.
[120] Kronenberg, F; Stuhlinger, M; Trenkwalder, E; Geethanjali, FS; Pachinger, O; von Eckardstein, A; Dieplinger, H. Low apolipoprotein A-IV plasma concentrations in men with coronary artery disease. *J Am Coll Cardiol*, 36, 751–757, 2000.
[121] Warner, MM; Guo, J; Zhao, Y. The relationship between plasma apolipoprotein A-IV levels and coronary heart disease. *Chin Med J (Engl)*, 114, 275–279, 2001.
[122] Kronenberg, F; Kuen, E; Ritz, E; Konig, P; Kraatz, G; Lhotta, K; Mann, JF; Muller, GA; Neyer, U; Riegel, W; Riegler, P; Schwenger, V; von Eckardstein, A. Apolipoprotein A-IV serum concentrations are elevated in patients with mild and moderate renal failure. *J Am Soc Nephrol*, 13, 461–469, 2002.
[123] Wanner, C; Krane, V; Marz, W; et al. Atorvastatin in patients with type 2 diabetes mellitus undergoing hemodialysis. *N Engl J Med.*, 2005, 353, 238–248].
[124] Fellstrom, BC; Jardine, AG; Schmieder, RE; et al. Rosuvastatin and cardiovascular events in patients undergoing hemodialysis. *N Engl J Med.*, 2009, 360, 1395–1407.
[125] Baigent, C; Landray, MJ; Reith, C; et al. The effects of lowering LDL cholesterol with simvastatin plus ezetimibe in patients with chronic kidney disease (Study of Heart and Renal Protection): a randomized placebo-controlled trial. *Lancet.*, 2011, 377, 2181–2192.
[126] Palmer, SC; Navaneethan, SD; Craig, JC; Johnson, DW; Perkovic, V; Nigwekar, SU; Hegbrant, J; Strippoli, GF. 2013. HMG CoA reductase inhibitors (statins) for dialysis patients. Cochrane Database Syst Rev.
[127] Marz, W; Genser, B; Drechsler, C; Krane, V; Grammer, TB; Ritz, E; Stojakovic, T; Scharnagl, H; Winkler, K; Holme, I; Holdaas, H; Wanner, C; German, D; Dialysis Study, I. 2011. Atorvastatin and low-density lipoprotein cholesterol in type 2 diabetes mellitus patients on hemodialysis. *Clin J Am Soc Nephrol*, 6, 1316-1325.
[128] Vaziri, ND; Norris, KC. 2013. Reasons for the lack of salutary effects of cholesterol-lowering interventions in end-stage renal disease populations. *Blood purification*, 35, 31-36.
[129] Himmelfarb, J; Stenvinkel, P; Ikizler, TA; Hakim, R. The elephant in uremia: Oxidant stress as a unifying concept of cardiovascular disease in uremia. *Kidney Int.*, 2002, 62, 1524–1538.
[130] Stenvinkel, P; Alvestrand, A. Inflammation in end-stage renal disease: Sources; consequences; and therapy. *Semin Dial.*, 2002, 15, 329–337.
[131] Vaziri, ND. Oxidative stress in chronic renal failure: The nature; mechanism and consequences. *Semin Nephrol.*, 2004, 24, 469–473.
[132] Vaziri, ND; Navab, M; Fogelman, AM. HDL metabolism and activity in chronic kidney disease. *Nature, Reviews Nephrology.*, 2010, 6(5), 287–296.
[133] Kalantar-Zadeh, K; Kopple, JD; Kamranpour, N; Fogelman, AM; Navab, M. HDL-inflammatory index correlates with poor outcome in hemodialysis patients. *Kidney Int.*, 2007, 72, 1149–1156.
[134] Vaziri, ND; Moradi, H; Pahl, MV; Fogelman, AM; Navab, M. *In vitro* stimulation of HDL antiinflammatory activity and inhibition of LDL pro-inflammatory activity in the plasma of patients with end-stage renal disease by an apoA-1 mimetic peptide. *Kidney Int.*, 2009, 76, 437–444.

[135] Tannock, L. Dyslipidemia in Chronic Kidney Disease. In: De Groot LJ; Beck-Peccoz P; Chrousos G; Dungan K; Grossman A; Hershman JM; Koch C; McLachlan R; New M; Rebar R; Singer F; Vinik A; Weickert MO; editors, 2015.

[136] Keene, D; Price, C; Shun-Shin, MJ; Francis, DP. Effect on cardiovascular risk of high density lipoprotein targeted drug treatments niacin; fibrates; and CETP inhibitors: meta-analysis of randomised controlled trials including 117, 411 patients. *BMJ (Clinical research ed.)*, 2014, 349, g4379. doi:10.1136/bmj.g4379.

[137] Bruckert, Eric; Labreuche, Julien; Amarenco, Pierre. Meta-analysis of the effect of nicotinic acid alone or in combination on cardiovascular events and atherosclerosis. *Atherosclerosis*, 2010, 210 (2), 353–361. doi:10.1016.

[138] He, YM; Feng, L; Huo, DM; Yang, ZH; Liao, YH. 2014. Benefits and harm of niacin and its analog for renal dialysis patients: a systematic review and meta-analysis. *Int Urol Nephrol*, 46, 433-442.

[139] Cho, KH; Kim, HJ; Kamanna, VS; Vaziri, ND. 2010. Niacin improves renal lipid metabolism and slows progression in chronic kidney disease. *Biochim Biophys Acta*, 1800, 6-15.

[140] Charnow, JA. 2014. Niacin may slow chronic kidney disease progression. In Renal & Urology News.

[141] Kang, HL; Kim, DY; Lee, SM; Kim, KH; Han, SH; Nam, HK; Kim, KH; Kim, SE; Son, YK; An, WS. 2013. Effect of low-dose niacin on dyslipidemia; serum phophorus levels and adverse effects in patients with chornic kidney disease. *Kidney Res Clin Pract*, 32, 21-26.

[142] Maccubbin, D; Tipping, D; Kuznetsova, O; Hanlon, WA; Bostom, AG. 2010. Hypophosphatemic effect of niacin in patients without renal failure: a randomized trial. *Clin J Am Soc Nephrol*, 5, 582-589.

[143] Maccubbin, D; Bays, HE; Olsson, AG; Elinoff, V; Elis, A; Mitchel, Y; Sirah, W; Betteridge, A; Reyes, R; Yu, Q; Kuznetsova, O; Sisk, CM; Pasternak, RC; Paolini¸ JF. 2008. Lipid-modifying efficacy and tolerability of extended-release niacin/laropiprant in patients with primary hypercholesterolaemia or mixed dyslipidaemia. *International journal of clinical practice*, 62, 1959-1970.

[144] Boden, WE; Probstfield, JL; Anderson, T; Chaitman, BR; Desvignes-Nickens, P; Koprowicz, K; McBride, R; Teo, K; Weintraub, W. 2011. Niacin in patients with low HDL cholesterol levels receiving intensive statin therapy. *N Engl J Med*, 365, 2255-2267.

[145] Group, HTC; Landray, MJ; Haynes, R; Hopewell, JC; Parish, S; Aung, T; Tomson, J; Wallendszus, K; Craig, M; Jiang, L; Collins, R; Armitage, J. 2014. Effects of extended-release niacin with laropiprant in high-risk patients. *N Engl J Med*, 371, 203-212.

[146] Caslake, M; Packard, C; Gaw, E; Murray, E; Griffin, B; Vallance, B; Shepherd, J. Fenofibrate and LDL metabolic heterogeneity in hypercholesterolemia. *Arterioscler Thromb.*, 1993, 13, 702–711.

[147] Bruckert, E; Dejager, S; Chapman, M. Ciprofibrate therapy normalises the atherogenic low-density lipoprotein subspecies profile in combined hyperlipidemia (published erratum appears in Atherosclerosis. 1993 102:129). *Atherosclerosis.*, 1993, 100, 91–102.

[148] de Graaf, J; Hendriks, J; Demacker, P; Stalenhoef, A. Identification of multiple dense LDL subfractions with enhanced susceptibility to *in vitro* oxidation among

hypertriglyceridemic subjects: normalization after clofibrate treatment. *Arterioscler Thromb.*, 1993, 13, 712–719.

[149] Sica, DA. 2009. Fibrate therapy and renal function. *Curr Atheroscler Rep*, 11, 338-342.

[150] Jun, M; Zhu, B; Tonelli, M; Jardine, MJ; Patel, A; Neal, B; Liyanage, T; Keech, A; Cass, A; Perkovic, V. 2012. Effects of fibrates in kidney disease: a systematic review and meta-analysis. *J Am Coll Cardiol*, 60, 2061-2071.

[151] Davis, TM; Ting, R; Best, JD; Donoghoe, MW; Drury¸ PL; Sullivan, DR; Jenkins, AJ; O'Connell, RL; Whiting, MJ; Glasziou, PP; Simes, RJ; Kesaniemi, YA; Gebski, VJ; Scott, RS; Keech, AC; Fenofibrate, I; Event Lowering in Diabetes Study, i. 2011. Effects of fenofibrate on renal function in patients with type 2 diabetes mellitus: the Fenofibrate Intervention and Event Lowering in Diabetes (FIELD) Study. *Diabetologia*, 54, 280-290.

[152] Tonelli, M; Collins, D; Robins, S; Bloomfield, H; Curhan, GC. 2004. Gemfibrozil for secondary prevention of cardiovascular events in mild to moderate chronic renal insufficiency. *Kidney Int*, 66, 1123-1130.

[153] Ting, RD; Keech, AC; Drury, PL; Donoghoe¸ MW; Hedley¸ J; Jenkins, AJ; Davis, TM; Lehto, S; Celermajer, D; Simes, RJ; Rajamani, K; Stanton, K. 2012. Benefits and safety of long-term fenofibrate therapy in people with type 2 diabetes and renal impairment: the FIELD Study. *Diabetes Care*, 35, 218-225.

[154] Špinar, J; Špinarová, L; Vítovec, J. IMProved Reduction of Outcomes: Vytorin Efficacy International Trial (studie IMPROVE-IT). *Vnitr Lek.*, 2014 Dec, 60(12), 1095-101.

[155] Haynes; R; Lewis¸ D; Emberson, J; Reith, C; Agodoa, L; Cass, A; Craig, JC; de Zeeuw, D; Feldt-Rasmussen, B; Fellstrom, B; Levin, A; Wheeler, DC; Walker, R; Herrington, WG; Baigent, C; Landray, MJ; Group, SC; Group, SC. 2014. Effects of lowering LDL cholesterol on progression of kidney disease. *J Am Soc Nephrol*, 25, 1825-1833.

[156] Baigent, C; Landray, MJ; Reith¸ C; Emberson, J; Wheeler, DC; Tomson, C; Wanner, C; Krane, V; Cass, A; Craig, J; Neal, B; Jiang, L; Hooi, LS; Levin, A; Agodoa, L; Gaziano, M; Kasiske, B; Walker¸ R; Massy, ZA; Feldt-Rasmussen, B; Krairittichai, U; Ophascharoensuk, V; Fellstrom, B; Holdaas, H; Tesar, V; Wiecek, A; Grobbee, D; de Zeeuw, D; Gronhagen-Riska, C; Dasgupta, T; Lewis, D; Herrington, W; Mafham, M; Majoni, W; Wallendszus, K; Grimm, R; Pedersen, T; Tobert, J; Armitage, J; Baxter, A; Bray, C; Chen, Y; Chen, Z; Hill, M; Knott, C; Parish, S; Simpson, D; Sleight, P; Young, A; Collins, R. 2011. The effects of lowering LDL cholesterol with simvastatin plus ezetimibe in patients with chronic kidney disease (Study of Heart and Renal Protection): a randomised placebo-controlled trial. *Lancet*, 377, 2181-2192.

[157] Morita, T; Morimoto, S; Nakano, C; Kubo, R; Okuno, Y; Seo, M; Someya, K; Nakahigashi, M; Ueda, H; Toyoda, N; Kusabe, M; Takahashi, FJoN; Iwasaka, T; Shiojima, I. 2014. Renal and vascular protective effects of ezetimibe in chronic kidney disease. *Internal medicine*, 53, 307-314.

[158] Rizos, EC; Ntzani, EE; Bika, E; Kostapanos, MS; Elisaf, MS. 2012. Association between omega-3 fatty acid supplementation and risk of major cardiovascular disease events: a systematic review and meta-analysis. *JAMA*, 308, 1024-1033.

[159] Mori, TA; Burke, V; Puddey, I; Irish, A; Cowpland, CA; Beilin, L; Dogra, G; Watts, GF. 2009. The effects of [omega]3 fatty acids and coenzyme Q10 on blood pressure

and heart rate in chronic kidney disease: a randomized controlled trial. *J Hypertens*, 27, 1863-1872.

[160] Gopinath, B; Harris, DC; Flood, VM; Burlutsky, G; Mitchell, P. 2011. Consumption of long-chain n-3 PUFA; alpha-linolenic acid and fish is associated with the prevalence of chronic kidney disease. *The British journal of nutrition*, 105, 1361-1368.

[161] Lok, CE; Moist, L; Hemmelgarn, BR; Tonelli¸ M; Vazquez, MA; Dorval; M; Oliver, M; Donnelly, S; Allon, M; Stanley, K. 2012. Effect of fish oil supplementation on graft patency and cardiovascular events among patients with new synthetic arteriovenous hemodialysis grafts: a randomized controlled trial. *Jama*, 307, 1809-1816.

[162] Svensson, M; Schmidt, EB; Jorgensen, KA; Christensen, JH. 2006. N-3 fatty acids as secondary prevention against cardiovascular events in patients who undergo chronic hemodialysis: a randomized; placebo-controlled intervention trial. *Clin J Am Soc Nephrol*, 1, 780-786.

[163] Out, C; Groen, AK; Brufau, G. Bile acid sequestrants: more than simple resins. *Curr Opin Lipidol*, 23 (2012), 43–55.

[164] Stoekenbroek, RM; Kastelein, JJ; Huijgen, R. PCSK9 inhibition: the way forward in the treatment of dyslipidemia. *BMC Med.*, 2015 Oct 12, 13, 258.

[165] Gencer, B; Lambert, G; Mach, F. PCSK9 inhibitors. *Swiss Med Wkly.*, 2015, 145, w14094.

[166] Navarese, EP; Kolodziejczak, M; Schulze, V; Gurbel, PA; Tantry, U; Lin, Y; et al.. Effects of proprotein convertase subtilisin/kexin type 9 antibodies in adults with hypercholesterolemia: a systematic review and meta-analysis. *Ann Intern Med.*, 2015, 163, 40-51.

[167] Zhang, XL; Zhu, QQ; Zhu, L; Chen, JZ; Chen, QH; Li, GN; et al. Safety and efficacy of anti-PCSK9 antibodies: a meta-analysis of 25 randomized; controlled trials. *BMC Med.*, 2015, 13, 123.

[168] Ballantyne, CM; Neutel, J; Cropp, A; Duggan, W; Wang, EQ; Plowchalk, D; Sweeney, K; Kaila, N; Vincent, J; Bays, H. Results of bococizumab; a monoclonal antibody against proprotein convertase subtilisin/kexin type 9; from a randomized; placebo-controlled; dose-ranging study in statin-treated subjects with hypercholesterolemia. *Am J Cardiol.*, 2015 May 1, 115(9), 1212-21.

[169] Sabatine, MS; Giugliano, RP; Wiviott, SD; Raal, FJ; Blom, DJ; Robinson, J; et al. Open-Label Study of Long-Term Evaluation against LDL Cholesterol (OSLER) Investigators. Efficacy and safety of evolocumab in reducing lipids and cardiovascular events. *N Engl J Med.*, 2015, 372, 1500-9.

[170] Ballantyne, CM; Neutel, J; Cropp, A; Duggan, W; Wang, EQ; Plowchalk, D; et al.. Results of bococizumab; a monoclonal antibody against proprotein convertase subtilisin/kexin type 9; from a randomized; placebo-controlled; dose-ranging study in statin-treated subjects with hypercholesterolemia. *Am J Cardiol.*, 2015, 115, 1212-21.

[171] Visser, ME; Wagener, G; Baker, BF; Geary, RS; Donovan, JM; Beuers, UH; Nederveen, AJ; Verheij, J; Trip, MD; Basart, DC; Kastelein, JJ; Stroes, ES. Mipomersen; an apolipoprotein B synthesis inhibitor; lowers low-density lipoprotein cholesterol in high-risk statin-intolerant patients: a randomized; double-blind; placebo-controlled trial. *Eur Heart J.*, 2012 May, 33(9), 1142-9.

[172] Panta, R; Dahal, K; Kunwar, S. Efficacy and safety of mipomersen in treatment of dyslipidemia: a meta-analysis of randomized controlled trials. *J Clin Lipidol.*, 2015 Mar-Apr, 9(2), 217-25.

[173] Roeters van Lennep, J; Averna, M; Alonso, R. Treating homozygous familial hypercholesterolemia in a real-world setting: Experiences with lomitapide. *J Clin Lipidol.*, 2015 Jul-Aug, 9(4), 607-17.

[174] Nicholls, SJ; Brewer, HB; Kastelein, JJ; Krueger, KA; Wang, MD; Shao, M; Hu, B; McErlean, E; Nissen, SE. Effects of the CETP inhibitor evacetrapib administered as monotherapy or in combination with statins on HDL and LDL cholesterol: a randomized controlled trial. *JAMA.*, 2011 Nov 16, 306(19), 2099-109.

[175] Brinton, EA; Kher, U; Shah, S; Cannon, CP; Davidson, M; Gotto, AM; Ashraf, TB; McCrary Sisk, C; Dansky, H; Mitchel, Y; Barter, P DEFINE Investigators. Effects of anacetrapib on plasma lipids in specific patient subgroups in the DEFINE (Determining the Efficacy and Tolerability of CETP INhibition with AnacEtrapib) trial. *J Clin Lipidol.*, 2015 Jan-Feb, 9(1), 65-71.

[176] Mune, M; Yukawa, S; Kishino, M; Otani, H; Kimura, K; Nishikawa, O; Takahashi, T; Kodama, N; Saika, Y; Yamada, Y. Effect of vitamin E on lipid metabolism and atherosclerosis in ESRD patients. *Kidney Int Suppl*, 71, S126 –S129, 1999.

[177] Kirmizis, D; Papagianni, A; Dogrammatzi, F; Belechri, AM; Alexopoulos, E; Efstratiadis, G; Memmos, D. The effects of vitamin E-coated membrane dialyzer compared to simvastatin in patients on chronic hemodialysis. *Ren Fail.*, 2012, 34(9), 1135-9.

[178] Bosch, T; Gahr, S; Belschner, U; Schaefer, C; Lennertz, A; Rammo, J. Direct adsorption of low-density lipoprotein by DALI-LDL-apheresis: Results of a prospective long-term multicenter follow-up covering 12;291 sessions. *Ther Apher Dial*, 10, 210 – 218, 2006.

[179] Tamura, K; Tsurumi-Ikeya, Y; Wakui, H; Maeda, A; Ohsawa, M; Azushima, K; Kanaoka, T; Uneda, K; Haku, S; Azuma, K; Mitsuhashi, H; Tamura, N; Toya, Y; Tokita, Y; Kokuho, T; Umemura, S. Therapeutic potential of low-density lipoprotein apheresis in the management of peripheral artery disease in patients with chronic kidney disease. *Ther Apher Dial.*, 2013 Apr, 17(2), 185-92.

In: Comorbidities in Chronic Kidney Disease
Editor: Luca Di Lullo

ISBN: 978-1-63485-070-4

Chapter 4

CHRONIC KIDNEY DISEASE – MINERAL BONE DISEASE (CKD-MBD): PRESENT AND FUTURE PERSPECTIVES

Antonio Bellasi[1, 2,*], Mario Cozzolino[1] and Andrea Galassi[3]
[1]Department of Health Sciences, Renal Division, San Paolo Hospital, University of Milan, Italy
[2]U.O.C. di Nefrologia, Dialisi, Ospedale Sant'Anna, Azienda Ospedaliera Sant'Anna, Como, Italy
[3]Renal and Dialysis Unit, Department of Medicine, Desio Hospital, Desio, Italy

ABSTRACT

Chronic Kidney Disease-Mineral Bone Metabolism (CKD-MBD) is a prevalent comorbid condition linked with unfavorable outcome. This syndrome encompasses laboratory, bone tissue derangements as well as cardiovascular and soft tissue calcification. Epidemiological studies suggest that as the glomerular filtration rate declines (GFR), several laboratory abnormalities become progressively more prevalent. Although it isn't clear at the current time what is the *primum movens*, it has been repeatedly documented that serum levels of vitamin D, parathyroid hormone (PTH), calcium, phosphate and fibroblast growth factor 23 (FGF23) are commonly disrupted since the earlier stages of CKD. Of importance, *in vitro* evidence suggest that calcium, phosphate, vitamin D promote vascular calcification supporting the notion of a plausible link between serum biomarkers and soft tissue as well as vascular calcification occurrence. In turn, vascular calcification reduces large artery compliance and is associated with the occurrence of major cardiovascular events and the risk of death.

Herein is reviewed current evidence on CKD-MBD physiopathology as well as treatments and therapeutic strategies for CKD-MBD.

---

* Corresponding author: Antonio Bellasi, MD, PhD, UOC di Nefrologia e Dialisi, Ospedale Sant'Anna, Azienda Ospedaliera Sant'Anna- Como, Via Ravona 20, 22020 San Fermo della battaglia (CO), Italy Tel: 031.585.9966 E-mail: antoniobellasi@gmail.com.

Keywords: calcium and phosphate balance, parathyroid hormone, vitamin D, CKD-MBD Treatment

INTRODUCTION

Chronic Kidney Disease- Mineral Bone Metabolism (CKD-MBD) is a prevalent comorbid condition [1] that portends poor quality and reduced life expectancy [2-4]. This syndrome encompasses laboratory, bone tissue derangements as well as cardiovascular and soft tissue calcification (Figure 1) [5]. Epidemiological studies suggest that as the glomerular filtration rate declines (GFR), several laboratory abnormalities become progressively more prevalent (Figure 2) [6, 7]. Notably, numerous reports suggest a considerable risk burden associated with these abnormalities in chronic kidney disease patients as well as normal renal function individuals [2, 5, 8].

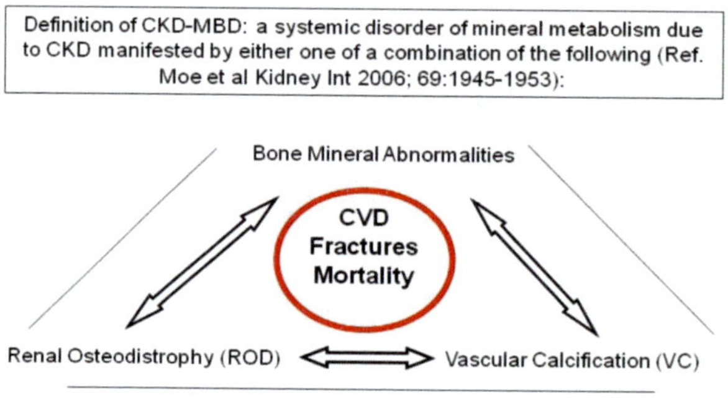

Figure 1. According to the definition of Chronic Kidney Disease Mineral Bone Disorder (CKD-MBD); this syndrome encompasses abnormal serum levels of different biomarkers; renal osetodistrophy (ROD) and vascular calcification (VC). In turn these abnormalities are linked with the risk of fractures; cardiovascular (CV) event and poor prognosis.

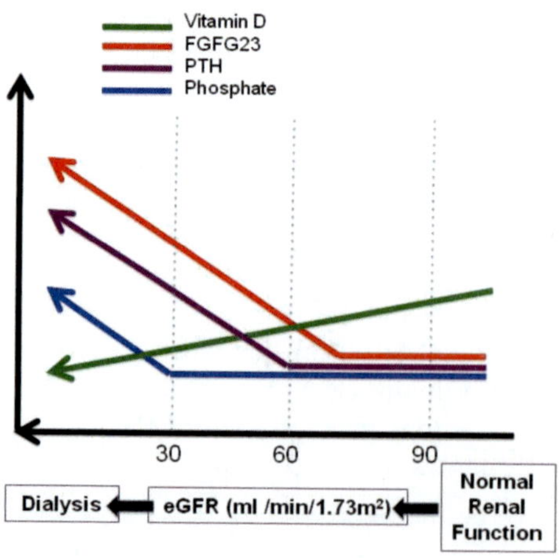

Figure 2. The prevalence of altered serum biomarkers of CKD-MBD increases as the glomerular filtration rate (GFR) declines.

Although it isn't clear at the current time what is the *primum movens*, it has been repeatedly documented that serum levels of vitamin D, parathyroid hormone (PTH), calcium, phosphate and fibroblast growth factor 23 (FGF23) are commonly disrupted since the earlier stages of CKD (Figure 2) [6, 7]. Of importance, in vitro evidence suggest that calcium, phosphate, vitamin D promote vascular calcification supporting the notion of a plausible link between serum biomarkers and soft tissue as well as vascular calcification occurrence [5]. In turn, vascular calcification reduces large artery compliance and is associated with the occurrence of major cardiovascular events and the risk of death [9].

Therapeutic strategies rely on dialysis optimization, phosphate and calcium balance neutralization, vitamin D supplementation as well as drugs targeting the parathyroid glands (i.e., calcimimentics)

Calcium, Phosphate, PTH and Vitamin D Homeostasis in Normal Renal Function Condition

Calcium and phosphate homeostasis is maintained through a complicated interplay of different hormones such as vitamin D, PTH and FGF23 that regulates calcium and phosphate absorption, excretion as well as accumulation in the bones [10].

Phosphorous (P^-) is one of the most prevalent cation in the body [11-13]. In normal condition, phosphate is stored in bone and teeth (≈85% of the total body pool), interstitial or intracellular space (≈14% of the total body pool) and only a minor part is dissolved in serum (≈1% of the total body pool). This cation is essential for life and is involved in several key biological systems such as adenosine triphosphate (ATP) or deoxyribonucleic acid (DNA) metabolism. It is a cell membranes constituent and a substrate for various kinases involved in numerous metabolic pathways [14]. In western countries it is estimated that about 800-1800 mg per day is ingested with various food and additives. This amount is largely absorbed (60-80%) in the gastrointestinal tract and partially excreted in feces (≈4-500 mg/day). Of note, vitamin D and other factors such as vegetarian or animal food sources may variably affect gastrointestinal absorption [15]. The amount absorbed is partially exchanged with bones and excreted in urine (≈750-850 mg/day) to maintain a neutral balance [16-18]. It is estimated that ≈80-95% of the filtered load is reabsorbed in the proximal tubule via the type II sodium and phosphate co-transporter (NaPi-2a) [16]. Although mechanisms need to be elucidated, several factors such as parathyroid hormone (PTH) and/or fibroblast growth factor (FGF23) reduce phosphate reabsorption and increase phosphaturia to maintain a neutral phosphate balance [10].

Data on calcium (Ca^{2+}) intake and balance suggest that in normal kidney function individuals a calcium intake of 750-1750 mg/day (usual intake in the western countries) is required to achieve a neutral balance (National Institute of Health: http://ods.od.nih.gov/ factsheets/Calcium-HealthProfessional/). As per phosphorous, a substantial variability (from 10-60% of the daily intake) in calcium absorption in the gastrointestinal tract has been documented. Indeed, factors such as vitamin D or different food sources (vegetable vs animal nutrients) may variably affect calcium absorption and availability. Consistently, a considerable variability in 24-hours calcium excretion in urine (100-300 mg/day) and feces

(900-1800 mg/day) is required to balance the amount absorbed as well as subject's need[19, 20].

As mentioned, vitamin D regulates and increases calcium and phosphate intestinal absorption [21]. Two forms of vitamin D namely cholecalciferol (vitamin D3) and ergocalciferol (vitamin D2) are ingested from different dietary sources (meat, fish liver, eggs, fish oils) (Figure 3) [21]. Cholecalciferol is also produced in the skin from 7-dehydrocholesterol (pre-vitamin D3), through the nonenzymatic effect of sunlight ultraviolet B rays (UVB, wavelengths 295-305 nm). Cholecalciferol, ergocalciferol are enzymatically hydroxylated at carbon 25 in the liver and at carbon 1 in kidney tubules (Figure 3) [13, 21]. Of note, both parathyroid hormone (PTH) and hypophosphatemia regulate vitamin D activation enhancing the renal 1a-hydroxylase but not the liver 25-hydroxylase activity. The final product, 1, 25-dihydroxycholecalciferol (1, 25(OH) 2D), is the active metabolite of vitamin D and is also called calcitriol. 1, 25(OH) 2D promotes active and passive intestinal absorption of calcium and phosphate, and bone mineralization. Conversely, 1,25 (OH)2D suppresses PTH synthesis and parathyroid cell proliferation through a genomic activity modulated by a specific cytosolic receptor for vitamin D (VDR) [13, 21]. The monohydroxylated metabolite, 25-hydroxycholecalciferol (25(OH) D also called calcidiol), is 500 times less active than 1,25 (OH)2D, but its serum concentration is the best indicator of vitamin D body stores (Figure 3). In spite of its low affinity for VDR, 25(OH)D maintains some biological effects, because its serum concentrations are 1000 times higher than those of 1,25(OH)2D, thus compensating for the low affinity for VDR [13, 21]. The physiopathological relevance of 25(OH)D has been recently revaluated in population studies showing that low serum concentrations of 25(OH)D were associated with higher serum PTH, lower bone mineral density (BMD) and osteopenia, increased risk of bone fractures and adverse outcome also in healthy individuals [13, 21].

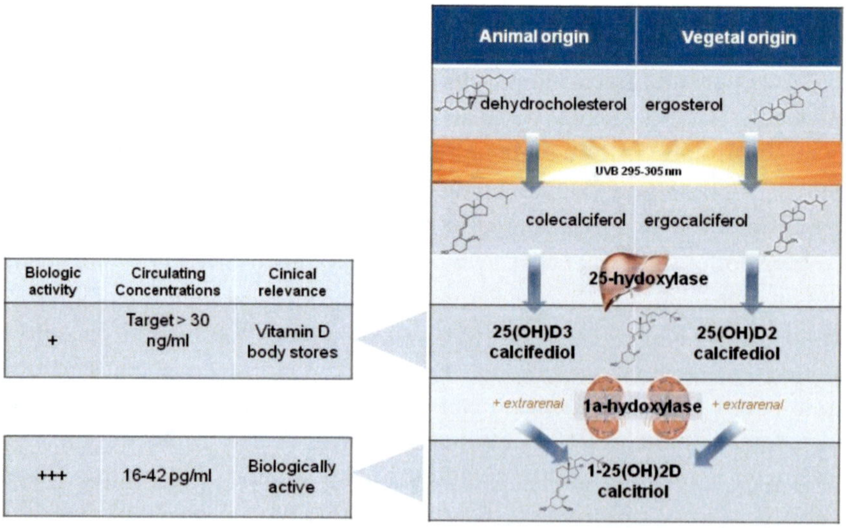

Figure 3. Vitamin D metabolism. Active Vitamin D (1-25(OH)2D) derives from the non-enzymatic activation of its two precursors (7-dehydrocholesterol and ergosterol) and from their further hepatic hydroxylation. Circulating levels of 25(OH)D are an accepted indicator of Vitamin D body stores; with a biologic activity 500 times lower than 1-25(OH)2D.

Parathyroid hormone (PTH) is a key regulator of calcium metabolism. PTH promotes bone resorption, controls calcium and phosphorus blood levels, and regulates calcitriol production [22]. Under physiologic conditions, fluctuations in serum levels of calcium are sensed by the calcium-sensing receptor (CaSR) located on the chief cells of the parathyroid gland [23]. An increase in serum calcium levels stimulates CaSR activation that in turn inhibits PTH gene expression, synthesis, and secretion. On the other hand, a decrease in serum calcium levels result in reduced CaSR activity, which promotes PTH synthesis and secretion [23]. Hence, disruption of calcium homeostasis, triggers PTH secretion modulation that regulates calcium removal from the bone as well as calcium excretion by the kidney to modulate the amount of calcium dissolved in the serum. Of interest, vitamin D deficiency and phosphate overload may promote PTH synthesis and release by the parathyroid glands although more studies are needed to better elucidate the molecular mechanisms responsible for these effects.

Bone Mineral Abnormalities in Chronic Kidney Disease: The Phosphorocentric Paradigm

A large and expanding body of evidence suggests the existence of different mechanisms aimed at controlling phosphorous homeostasis. Indeed, PTH, fibroblast growth factor 23 (FGF23) and other phosphatonins such as fibroblast growth factor 7 (FGF7) as well as 1, 25 (OH) 2D are among the most studied factors that regulate intestinal and renal phosphate handling [10, 14, 16].

In chronic kidney disease (CKD), the overall amount of phosphate filtered every day falls together with the GFR decline (Figure 4). Hence, phosphorous reabsorption in the proximal tubules of residual nephrons decreases to maintain a neutral balance and avoid hyper-phosphatemia. Though the mechanisms are only partly elucidated, FGF23 and its co-receptor agonist Klotho regulate proximal tubular phosphate reabsorption by inhibiting the NaPi2a co-transporter [10, 14]. Activation of the FGF23/Klotho axis also induces renal tubular calcium absorption as well as inhibition of the 1-25-OH2-hydroxylase and activation of the 24-OH-hydroxylase, the key enzymes responsible for vitamin D activation and deactivation, respectively. The final result of the FGF23/Klotho axis activation is an increase of phosphate excretion per nephron as well as reduced intestinal phosphate absorption at the cost of reduced vitamin D activation [10, 14].

Later in the course of CKD, vitamin D deficiency and perhaps the need to further enhance phosphorous excretion, stimulates the release of other phosphaturic hormones such as PTH [6]. Consistently, epidemiological data suggest that overt hyperphosphatemia (i.e., serum phosphorus greater than 4.5 mg/dl) ensues only late in the course of CKD, usually when the GFR drops below ≈30 ml/min and serum levels of FGF23, vitamin D and PTH are already altered (Figure 2).

The persistence of a high phosphate intake as well as vitamin D deficiency eventually promote parathyroid gland hyperplasia [22] (Figure 4). Although FGF23 and calcitriol inhibit PTH secretion, hyperplastic parathyroid glands become resistant to FGF23 and/or vitamin D treatment and loose the normal feedback controls on PTH secretion leading to parathyroid glad adenoma and secondary hyperparatiroidism [22].

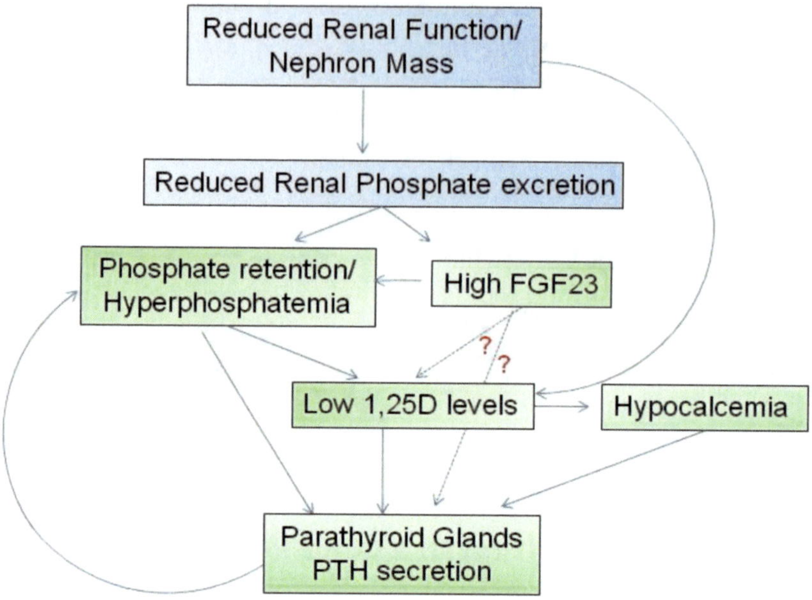

Figure 4. The phosphorocentric paradigm. As the renal function and mass decline; the overall amount of phosphate filtered every day falls. Hence; phosphorous reabsorption in the proximal tubules of residual nephrons decreases to maintain a neutral balance and avoid hyper-phosphatemia Activation of the FGF23/Klotho axis also induces renal tubular calcium absorption as well as inhibition of the 1-25-OH2-hydroxylase and activation of the 24-OH-hydroxylase; the key enzymes responsible for vitamin D activation and deactivation; respectively. The final result of the FGF23/Klotho axis activation is an increase of phosphate excretion per nephron as well as reduced intestinal phosphate absorption at the cost of reduced vitamin D activation and parathyroid gland activation and PTH secretion.

In essence, basic science and clinical data corroborates the hypothesis that the human body has several adaptive mechanisms aimed at controlling and adjusting phosphorous absorption and excretion to maintain a neutral phosphate balance. However, in conditions such as renal mass and function reduction, these adaptive mechanisms may turn into maladaptive mechanisms and potentially mediated the astonishing cardiovascular deterioration and risk seen in CKD patients.

Clinical Consequences of CKD-MBD

CKD-MBD can result in serious clinical *sequelae*. Data from the Dialysis Outcomes and Practice Patterns Study (DOPPS) in patients on maintenance hemodialysis (i.e., for more than 180 days) document a substantial risk of cardiovascular and all-cause mortality in patients with increased calcium (>10 mg/dL), phosphorus (>7 mg/dL), and PTH levels (>600 pg/mL) [8, 24]. Although the mechanisms that link mineral bone metabolism with unfavorable outcome are still largely speculative, it is plausible that both skeletal and extra-skeletal complications of deranged bone metabolism contribute to the abysmal risk at which CKD patients are exposed.

Bone-associated consequences include diseases associated with renal osteodystrophy (ROD) and bone fractures, while non-skeletal consequences include above all cardiovascular calcification and soft-tissue calcification as well as left ventricular hypertrophy (LVH) [9, 25, 26]. Other clinical consequences that have been associated with CKD-MBD are endocrine disturbances, compromised immune system, neurobehavioral changes, and altered erythropoiesis [27-29], although the link with CKD-MBD is less clear.

Renal osteodystrophy (ROD) refers to a bone disorder that occurs in patients with CKD, characterized by abnormal bone turnover, mineralization and volume secondary to vitamin D and PTH impaired synthesis and/or secretion [25]. According to the prevalent abnormal feature, ROD is characterized by five types of bone lesions. Osteitis fibrosa and mixed osteodystrophy are high-turnover bone diseases. Osteomalacia, aluminum-induced bone disease, and adynamic bone disease are low-turnover bone diseases [25]. High-turnover bone diseases are characterized by rapid bone turnover induced by high serum PTH levels and abnormal mineralization. Conversely, low-turnover bone diseases are caused by over-suppression of PTH or by the presence of aluminum at the site of bone mineralization [25]. ROD is contributor and likely a modifiable risk factor for the increased risk of bone deformities and fracture described in the CKD population [30].

Cardiovascular calcification and left ventricular hyperthrophy likely represent the most worrisome non-skeletal consequence of the bone mineral abnormalities that ensues as the GFR declines. In the last ten years, several studies pointed out that presence and extent of vascular calcification are markers of cardiovascular disease severity and portend poor CV prognosis in the general as well as dialysis population [9]. In vitro evidence suggests that vascular smooth muscle cells differentiate into osteoblast-like cells when incubated in calcium and phosphorous enriched media supporting the role of mineral metabolism imbalances in the pathogenesis of vascular calcification [2]. Clinical observations suggest that 60-80% of dialysis patients develop extensive medial calcification. In turn, calcification of compliance artery predisposes to increased arterial stiffness, prolonged QT tract on EKG, abnormal myocardial perfusion as well as high morbidity and mortality due to major cardiovascular events [9]. A multiplicity of factors is associated with vascular calcification in dialysis patients (time on dialysis, uremic toxins, history of diabetes, inflammation) however, abnormalities in bone mineral metabolism and likely some of current treatments undoubtedly play a critical role [9, 31]. Whether fibroblast growth factor 23 (FGF23) promotes vascular and cardiac valve calcification is still unclear. Nevertheless, clinical and experimental studies have shown that FGF23 induces left ventricular hyperthrophy and portend poor prognosis in CKD subjects [26]. Notably, a recent *post hoc* analysis of a large trial also suggest that FGF23 reduction maybe associated with increased survival in prevalent hemodialysis patients [32].

TREATMENT STRATEGIES IN CKD-MBD

Several decades ago Nephrologists started correcting deranged mineral bio-markers of CKD-MBD (hypocalcemia, hyperphosphatemia, hyperparathyroidism and Vitamin D insufficiency), with the specific intention to improve symptomatic, clinically relevant end eventually life-threatening complications. In spite of the great effort made to improve the understanding of CKD-MBD, the range of normality (and thus the therapeutic targets) of calcium (Ca^{2+}), phosphate (P), Vitamin D and parathyroid hormone (PTH) in different stages of CKD has never been identified through a rigorous methodology. Indeed, rather than testing the impact of the achievement of different serum targets on hard end-points such as cardiovascular disease, hospitalization, quality of life and/or survival, the majority of randomized clinical trials (RCT) conducted in CKD-MBD has been designed to compare safety and efficiency of different compounds to achieve non-validated surrogate outcome, such as levels of Ca^{2+}, P, PTH, vitamin D and/or vascular calcification progression attenuation. Furthermore, evidence on the association between improved survival and specific therapies for CKD-MBD is still scanty, mainly based on observational studies.

These limitations and uncertainties have always to be taken into account when discussing CKD-MBD therapies as well as when treating patients in the real world settings. Apart from dialysis, available therapeutic strategies for CKD-MBD are currently based on nutritional therapy and phosphate binders to achieve calcium and phosphate neutral balance, vitamin D compounds and calcimimetic to correct vitamin D deficiency and secondary hyperparathyroidism.

Dialysis

In anuric patients, renal phosphate (P) and calcium (Ca^{2+}) excretion is null. Thus, in dialysis dependent subjects, P clearance is only guaranteed by dialysis treatment. However, phosphate dialysis clearance is limited by (a) the presence of an aqueous cover that increases the P molecular diameter with consequent clearance behavior typical of middle molecules, (b) the intracellular distribution of P leading to multi-compartmental kinetic, (c) the fact that about 5% circulating P is bound to sodium, Ca and magnesium salts [33]. A standard 4-hour bicarbonate dialysis session removes approximately 800-1000 mg of P [34]. The slow inter-compartmental movement of P induces a very rapid fall in serum levels during the first 2 hours of dialysis session, followed by a sudden increase (more than 30% of the final value) toward the end of the dialysis session and a significant post-dialytic rebound [35]. It has been suggested that 38 hours per week of standard dialysis would be necessary to achieve a neutral P balance without the use of P binders [33, 34].

Short daily dialysis improves weekly P clearance. Extended duration of dialysis session up to 6-8 hours significantly improves dialytic P removal approaching 8.000 mg of P cleared per week with nocturnal hemodialysis. Patients treated with nocturnal hemodialysis experience P binder withdrawal and, in some instances, P supplements are needed to avoid unwanted negative P balance. Finally, convective techniques have been shown more effective than standard dialysis in phosphate removal. Physical activity during dialysis improves muscle perfusion, thus increasing the rate of P removal from peripheral tissues. Intra-dialytic motor driven passive leg cycling and transcutaneous electrical muscle stimulation increased P removal up to a total of 3.5 g/week and 3.6 g/week respectively in patients undergoing standard thrice weekly hemodialysis [33, 34].

Particularly in peritoneal dialysis patients, residual renal function significantly contributes to systemic P clearance, especially at the beginning of dialysis where it accounts for up to 65% of total P clearance [34]. Phosphate clearance in peritoneal dialysis is substantially lower (2.700 ± 1.000 g/week) than hemodialysis and is influenced by peritoneal membrane transport characteristics as well as peritoneal dialysis schedule and technique [34]. The increase of dwell times and transfer to CAPD are effective strategies to improve phosphate handling in patients with inadequate phosphate control on automated PD. The inclusion of a day dwell is associated with a descriptively higher peritoneal P clearance among patients receiving automated peritoneal dialysis. In high membrane transporters P clearance may resemble the clearance of creatinine and small molecules, while in the remaining membrane transport categories P clearance resembles the clearance of middle molecules and small proteins. However, circulating P levels are correlated with peritoneal P clearance but not with creatinine clearance, underlining the importance of assessing peritoneal P clearance to optimize P balance in peritoneal dialysis patients [33, 34].

In conclusion, P clearance in dialysis represents an unmet and tough goal, due to the molecular characteristics of P molecule and its multi-compartmental distribution. Currently, extending time and frequency of dialysis sessions and preferring hemodiafiltration (HDF) compared to standard bicarbonate dialysis may improve P clearance in hemodialysis. Peritoneal dialysis prescription, driven by careful membrane transport evaluation, is similarly required to improve P clearance in peritoneal dialysis patients.

Nutritional Therapy

A balanced intake of calories, proteins, Ca^{2+} and P^- is of importance in the general population as well as in CKD patients.

The suggested daily intake of elemental Ca^{2+} by National Institute of Health (NIH) in normal renal function individuals is 1.0 g in men and women aged 19-70 years and shortly larger intake of 1.2 g/day in older individuals, suggesting not to exceed 2.5 g daily in 19-50 years old subjects and 2.0 g daily in those older than 50 years (National Institute of Health: http://ods.od. nih.gov/factsheets/Calcium-HealthProfessional/). In contrast, the Kidney Disease Outcomes Quality Initiative guidelines issued by the National Kidney Foundation (NKF-KDOQI) mandate to reduce the daily intake of elemental Ca^{2+} coming from food as well as from calcium-containing phosphate binders to less than 2.0 g in CKD stage 3-5 patients. While no specific recommendation in normal renal function subjects is available, the NKF-KDOQI suggest to restrict phosphorous intake to 0.8-1.0 g/day in CKD patients [36]. Calcium and phosphate recommendations in CKD should not be achieved at the cost of inadequate caloric intake. The K/DOQI guidelines suggest to prescribe a daily caloric intake of 35 kCal/Kg in individuals younger than 60 years old and of 30-35 kCal/Kg in those individuals older than 60 years [37].

Controlling nutritional P intake since the earlier CKD stages is a crucial approach to prevent CKD-MBD [33]. Protein-rich food groups, including dairy products, meat, cheese, egg yolk and fish are the main nutritional sources of P. Almost 60% of P present in animal nutrients is absorbed in the intestine. However, in patients receiving calcitriol the absorption rate may approach 80%. Unlikely animal nutrients, P present in plants as phytate is poorly absorbed due to the absence of phytase in humans (absorption rate < 40%) [15, 33]. Finally, food additives represent a hidden source of P. Of note, inorganic P is almost entirely (≅ 90%) absorbed, limiting the efficacy of P-binders [33]. For instance, 300 mg of inorganic

P introduced with processed foods may neutralized the maximum dose of 3 g/day of lanthanum carbonate, one of the most potent phosphate binder currently available.

Cooking methods are essential to limit phosphorous intake. Boiling results in a 51%, 48%, 38%, 70% and 19% reduction of the amount of phosphate contained in vegetables, legumes, meat, flour and cheese, respectively Of note, this is achieved without a significant loss of nitrogen and thus of net protein intake [33, 38].

The management of P intake significantly changes at dialysis inception. Indeed, the coexistence of P and proteins in nutrients suggest the use of low protein intake until dialysis is established [39]. However, to counteract the hyper-catabolic uremic state, a higher protein intake is suggested in hemodialysis (1.2 g/Kg/day) and peritoneal dialysis (1.2-1.3 g/Kg/day) [37] leading to a high risk of positive P balance [33]. Thus, it is advisable to choose proteins with a low P content (10-12 mg of P per g of proteins) and to avoid preservative enriched foods in dialysis patients [37]. Though indispensable, nutritional therapy alone is not enough to maintain a neutral P balance in End Stage Renal Disease (ESRD). For example, a 70 Kg dialysis patient, ingesting 1.2 g/Kg/day of proteins with a low P content (10-12 mg/g) and undergoing 4 hours of standard bicarbonate dialysis thrice weekly, is exposed to a net P load of about 100 mg/day [33]. Hence, to preserve a neutral P balance in dialysis a multifaceted intervention that encompasses nutritional therapy, P binders and high efficiency dialysis use is required.

Adherence and compliance to nutritional therapy is a tough as vital goal in clinical practice. A teamwork involving nephrologists, renal nurses and dietitians is often required to provide patients with adequate counselling and develop educational programs that have been proven to effectively lower circulating P levels in persistently hyperphosphatemic CKD patients [40].

PHOSPHATE BINDERS

Phosphate binders are considered a cornerstone treatment to control P load. As previously mentioned, the efficacy of P binders on hard end-points as survival, hospitalizations, cardiovascular events and quality of life has never been tested against placebo in dedicated randomized clinical trials (RCTs). Observational studies showed better survival in pre-dialysis and dialysis patients receiving P binders, independently from case-mix and binder characteristics [41]. Notably, P binders were associated with a reduced mortality risk also among dialysis patients with P levels within the normal laboratory range [41]. Consistently, the Kidney Disease: Improving Global Outcomes (KDIGO) guidelines on mineral metabolism management suggest to administer P binders to hyperphosphatemic patients to maintain P levels within the normal range in CKD stage 3-5 and toward the normal range in dialysis patients [42].

Although different classes of P binders are currently available, the best choice for each individual patient remains uncertain. When prescribing P binders, the following characteristics should be considered: (1) presence of aluminum or calcium salts, (2) additive effects, (3) P binding capacity and (4) pill burden, (5) tolerability.

Current guidelines recommend to avoid aluminum administration in CKD 3-5D patients [42] and to limit the intake of elemental calcium with P binders to 1 g/day [36], especially in the presence of hypercalcemia, persistently low PTH levels and/or vascular calcification [42]. Indeed, evidence suggests a safer profile of calcium-free vs calcium-containing phosphate binder [31]. A relevant trend toward a slower progression of vascular calcification has been repeatedly observed in pre-dialysis as well as dialysis patients receiving calcium-free vs calcium-based phosphate binders [43]. Finally, a recent meta-analysis documents a significant 22% (risk ratio 0.78, 95% Confidence Interval: 0.61-0.98) risk reduction of all-cause mortality associated with the use of calcium-free vs calcium-based phosphate binders [31].

Based on these considerations, several Authors suggest to limit the use of calcium-based P binders in patients at high cardiovascular risk, elderly, post-menopausal women as well as diabetic patients and subjects with evidence of low bone turnover renal osteodistrophy, vascular or valvular calcification and inflammation [44]. Hence, several non-aluminum and calcium-free phosphate binders have been developed and are currently available on the market (sevelamer carbonate, sevelamer HCl, lanthanum carbonate, magnesium carbonate, PA21 and ferric citrate). Various additive effects of different P binders have been reported. Sevelamer and lanthanum, but not calcium salts, induced a significant reduction of FGF23 levels among normo-phosphatemic pre-dialysis CKD patients [45, 46]. Notably, this effect seems associated with the type of binder and independent P control. Further investigations are required to establish the clinical relevance of FGF23 variations on hard end-points. Sevelamer carbonate was repeatedly associated with a better anti-inflammatory profile compared to calcium-based binders and to a mild cholesterol binding activity [47]. Magnesium is gaining momentum as calcium-free P binder and is available on the market in formulation with calcium acetate. Calcium acetate-magnesium carbonate resulted non inferior to sevelamer HCl in controlling serum P levels among hemodialysis patients [48]. Magnesium supplementation could be beneficial in terms of mineral metabolism, cardiovascular stability and insulin sensitivity[49]. Preliminary data observed a favorable trend toward vascular calcification and intima-media thickness reduction in hemodialys patients receiving magnesium salts[49]. Aside of phosphate lowering, iron compounds may ameliorate sideropenic anemia [50]. PA21 (sucroferric oxyhydroxide), a new iron-based P binder, showed protective effects against vascular calcification in experimental models [51]. Although intriguing, clinical data are still insufficient to recommend the use one P binder over another based on plausible but hypothetic positive additive effects.

Phosphate binding capacity (PBC) represents the mg of P bound by 1 g of a certain P binder [52]. The highest and the lowest PBC is observed with lanthanum (135 mg of P bound by 1 g of lanthanum) and sevelamer (63 mg bound by 2.4 g of sevelamer carbonate), respectively [52]. One gram of elemental calcium, delivered as calcium carbonate, binds almost 111 mg of P [52] while 3 pills of calcium acetate-magnesium carbonate bind 138 mg of P, delivering only 330 mg of elemental calcium [52]. No data is reported for iron-based compounds.

Pill burden is a considerable matter in CKD patients, being negatively associated with therapeutic compliance. Phosphate binders significantly affect the pill burden. International data document a mean pill number of prescribed P binders ranging from 3.9 to 7.4[53], with lower number of pills observed among patients receiving phosphate binders with the highest PBC.

Tolerability is another key feature of P binders that affects patients' adherence and compliance to therapy and consequently P binding efficacy. P binders are currently available as pills and even as soluble (sevelamer) and non-soluble (lanthanum) powder.

In essence, P binder prescriptions should fit as much as possible with patients' characteristics, P intake as well as subjective tolerance to the compound and social habits.

VITAMIN D

Vitamin D is an established treatment for secondary hyperparathyrodism (SHPT) in CKD [42]. Different forms of vitamin D (Figure 3) as well as vitamin D analogues exist accounting for the complexity of this treatment that should aim at restoring and maintaining adequate levels of 25(OH) D and prevent SHPT and its clinical *sequelae*. In these regards, observational data document a better all-cause survival in dialysis patients receiving vs not receiving vitamin D [54]. Furthermore, pleiotropic effects of selective vitamin D receptor activators (VDRA) may also provide with some renal and cardiovascular protection, although more efforts are needed in this domain to establish the net benefit associated with these molecules.

A consensus on the desirable levels of 25(OH) D to be achieved and maintained to prevent or treat SHPT and improve survival in CKD patients is still lacking. Three nutritional molecules are currently available for 25(OH)D replenishment: the two pro-drugs cholecalciferol and ergocalciferol (requiring hepatic 25-alpha-hydroxylase to be converted in $25(OH)D_3$ or $25(OH)D_2$, respectively) and calcifediol (already available as $25(OH)D_3$) (Figure 3). Current guidelines on CKD-MBD management suggest to maintain 25(OH)D levels $\geq$ 30 ng/ml. However, at least in pre-dialysis CKD patients, treatment with cholecalciferol, ergocalciferol and calcifediol should be discontinued in the presence of 25(OH)D levels > 100 ng/ml and/or with persistent serum calcium levels > 10.5 mg/dl, in absence of active Vitamin D administration. It has been postulated that cholecalciferol may be more effective than ergocalciferol to achieve 25(OH)D targets [21]. However, the best treatment regimen to replenish 25(OH)D levels is still unknown and different schedules with cholecalciferol or ergocalciferol have been proposed [21].

A lower degree of PTH suppression is expected with nutritional compared to active Vitamin D administration (calcitriol) or VDRA (paracalcitol) [55]. From the early stages of CKD (stage 3b-4), calcitriol and VDRA are currently suggested to suppress PTH levels above the normal laboratory range in the absence of 25(OH)D deficiency, hypercalcemia or hyperphosphatemia [42]. A variety of VDRA are currently available on the market (doxercalciferol, paracalcitol) and other are under clinical development. It has been suggested that the adoption of selective VDRA such as paricalcitol, are expected to control PTH levels with a lower impact on calcium-phosphate load and perhaps on cardiac and vascular aging when compared to calcitriol. Despite promising experimental and observational data, inconsistent results on cardiovascular protection by VDRA vs placebo have been reported in RCTs [56]. Indeed, both the PRIMO and the OPERA trial [57, 58], failed to detect any protective action of paricalcitol against left ventricular hypertrophy (LVH) in renal patients with SHPT. In contrast, a more robust antiproteinuric effects of nutritional, and active Vitamin D on top of ACE-I and or ARBs has been repeatedly observed [21, 56]. Notably, this effect seems independent on the Vitamin D compound administered and on the specific etiology of proteinuria [21, 56].

CALCIMIMETICS

Cinacalcet is the only calcimimetics currently adopted in clinical practice. As activator of the calcium sensing receptor (CaSR), cinacalcet inhibits PTH gene expression, synthesis, and secretion [23] and is indicated for SHPT treatment in dialysis patients [42]. Its use in non-dialysis dependent patients is contraindicated due to risk of severe hypocalcemia and P overload secondary to FGF23 suppression and inhibition of PTH mediated renal excretion of P. Several trials compared the efficacy of cinacacalcet plus low doses of vitamin D vs flexible and more generous Vitamin D regimens to control SHPT in hemodialysis patients [21]. In essence, it seems that the use of cinacalcet and VDRA at escalating doses are comparable in PTH suppression. However, a substantially different biochemical profile is associated with cinalcet or VDRA use. While hypercalcemia and hyperphosphatemia is common with the use of VDRA, cinacalcet use poses the risk of hypocalcemia and is usually associated with the prescription of large doses of elemental calcium [21].

The ADVANCE trial investigated the impact of a calcimimetic plus low doses of Vitamin D based regimen vs a regimen of Vitamin D at escalating doses on coronary artery (CAC), thoracic aorta as well as mitral and aortic valve calcification [59]. Although the primary endpoint was of borderline statistical significance (p value for CAC progression attenuation: 0.07), the secondary endpoints and the subscquent *post hoc* analysis performed, suggest a protective effect of cinacalcet on vascular calcification [59]. The protective effect maybe more pronounced in the presence of cardiac valve calcification or more severe calcification at study inception as well as among patients treated with lower doses of vitamin D, as mandated by the study protocol [59-61].

The cinacalcet promise were not confirmed by the Evaluation of Cinacalcet HCl Therapy to Lower Cardiovascular Events (EVOLVE) trial. Indeed, the use of cinacalcet on top of other conventional CKD-MBD therapies was not associated with a statistically meaningful reduction in the risk of the composite endpoint of death, myocardial infarction, hospitalization for unstable angina, heart failure, or a peripheral vascular event (relative hazard in the cinacalcet group vs. the placebo group, 0.93; 95% confidence interval, 0.85 to 1.02; P = 0.11) [62]. Nevertheless, the high drop-out rate as well as the use of commercially available cinacalcet in the control group may have diluted the survival signal [63]. Furthermore, secondary and *post-hoc* analysis suggest that cinacalcet use maybe associated with improved survival in patients older than 65 years of age [64], with a reduced incidence of parathyroidectomy [62], non-atherosclerotic events [65], fracture [66] and calciphylaxis [67]. Although hypothesis generating, a survival advantage was also noted among patients receiving cinacalcet and experiencing a reduction of FGF23 levels of 30% or more at follow-up [32]. Cinacalcet appears a reasonable therapeutic choice in the presence of SHPT in dialysis patients without persistent hypocalcemia and affected by sever vascular calcification or calciphylaxis.

UNMET MEDICAL NEED AND FUTURE PERSPECTIVES

Although the desirable levels of phosphorus, calcium, vitamin D and PTH are far from being determined, current evidence suggest that the large majority of CKD patients have levels of these metabolites fall outside the recommended ranges [1, 68]. In the United States, the estimated prevalence of CKD-MBD ranges from 2 to nearly 5 million individuals [69]. In Europe, as many as 86% of patients on maintenance dialysis receive treatment for CKD-MBD [1]. Consistently, the cost burden associated with CKD-MBD is considerable and it is calculated that $52-122 billion of the annual health expenditure in the USA is due to bone mineral derangements and clinical consequences [69]. Ameliorating CKD-MBD comorbidities would therefore improve survival and hopefully reduce the associated costs. However, the many limitations in the current armamentarium and the lack of clinical data on the causal link among the metabolic, renal, and vascular abnormalities seen in patients with CKD-MBD poses a challenge to effective treatment and call for more studies in this domain [69].

Several new drugs are currently under clinical development [70] to improve patient's treatment individualization, adherence and compliance to drug regimens as well as to improve the effectiveness of therapeutic strategies. Targeted therapies, such as selective VDR and CaSR modulators as well as inhibitors of the intestinal sodium phosphate co-transporter, more potent phosphate binder and/or FGF23 antibodies, drugs that inhibits vascular calcification progression will likely be available in the nearest future [70]. However, whether these new drugs offers an increased opportunity to adequately control CKD-MBD, future efforts are required to better refine the risk assessment and more studies are warranted to validate biomarkers of CKD-MBD and demonstrate the impact of CKD-MBD correction on hard outcome.

Conclusion

The awareness of the clinical implication of CKD-MBD has generated a great interest in the pharmacologic management of this syndrome. The armamentarium has progressed and will be continue to progress in the nearest future. Current CKD-MBD therapeutic strategies rely on the careful use of dialysis, nutrition, phosphate binder, vitamin D and calcimimetics. However, a considerable number of CKD patients still experience inadequately controlled calcium, phosphate, vitamin D, PTH, FGF23 levels and/or develop renal osteodistrophy and vascular calcification. All these may contribute to explain the abysmal risk observed in this population.

The introduction of targeted therapies may promote patient adherence and likely simplify treatment regimens. However, they will also provide the prerequisite features to embark in long-term hard outcome studies to shed light on the vexing question to whether treatments for CKD-MBD reduce the risk of clinical endpoints such as cardiovascular morbidity and mortality.

References

[1] Fernandez-Martin, JL; Carrero, JJ; Benedik, M; Bos, WJ; Covic, A; Ferreira, A; Floege, J; Goldsmith, D; Gorriz, JL; Ketteler, M; Kramar, R; Locatelli, F; London, G; Martin, PY; Memmos, D; Nagy, J; Naves-Diaz, M; Pavlovic, D; Rodriguez-Garcia, M;

Rutkowski, B; Teplan, V; Tielemans, C; Verbeelen, D; Wuthrich, RP; Martinez-Camblor, P; Cabezas-Rodriguez, I; Sanchez-Alvarez, JE; Cannata-Andia, JB. Cosmos: The dialysis scenario of ckd-mbd in Europe. *Nephrol Dial Transplant*, 2012.

[2] Bellasi, A; Mandreoli, M; Baldrati, L; Corradini, M; Di Nicolo, P; Malmusi, G; Santoro, A. Chronic kidney disease progression and outcome according to serum phosphorus in mild-to-moderate kidney dysfunction. *Clin J Am Soc Nephrol*, 2011, 6, 883-891.

[3] Block, GA; Klassen, PS; Lazarus, JM; Ofsthun, N; Lowrie, EG; Chertow, GM. Mineral metabolism; mortality; and morbidity in maintenance hemodialysis. *J Am Soc Nephrol*, 2004, 15, 2208-2218.

[4] Bellasi, A; Cozzolino, M; Adragao, T; Di Iorio, B; Russo, D. Phosphate binders in moderate chronic kidney disease: Where do we stand? *J Nephrol*, 2013, 0.

[5] Moe, S; Drueke, T; Cunningham, J; Goodman, W; Martin, K; Olgaard, K; Ott, S; Sprague, S; Lameire, N; Eknoyan, G. Definition, evaluation, and classification of renal osteodystrophy: A position statement from kidney disease: Improving global outcomes (kdigo). *Kidney Int*, 2006, 69, 1945-1953.

[6] Isakova, T; Wahl, P; Vargas, GS; Gutierrez, OM; Scialla, J; Xie, H; Appleby, D; Nessel, L; Bellovich, K; Chen, J; Hamm, L; Gadegbeku, C; Horwitz, E; Townsend, RR; Anderson, CA; Lash, JP; Hsu, CY; Leonard, MB; Wolf, M. Fibroblast growth factor 23 is elevated before parathyroid hormone and phosphate in chronic kidney disease. *Kidney Int*, 2011, 79, 1370-1378.

[7] Pavik, I; Jaeger, P; Ebner, L; Wagner, CA; Petzold, K; Spichtig, D; Poster, D; Wuthrich, RP; Russmann, S; Serra, AL. Secreted klotho and fgf23 in chronic kidney disease stage 1 to 5: A sequence suggested from a cross-sectional study. *Nephrol Dial Transplant*, 2013, 28, 352-359.

[8] Fernandez-Martin, JL; Martinez-Camblor, P; Dionisi, MP; Floege, J; Ketteler, M; London, G; Locatelli, F; Gorriz, JL; Rutkowski, B; Ferreira, A; Bos, WJ; Covic, A; Rodriguez-Garcia, M; Sanchez, JE; Rodriguez-Puyol, D; Cannata-Andia, JB. Improvement of mineral and bone metabolism markers is associated with better survival in haemodialysis patients: The cosmos study. *Nephrol Dial Transplant*, 2015, 30, 1542-1551.

[9] Bellasi, A; Raggi, P. Vascular imaging in chronic kidney disease. *Curr Opin Nephrol Hypertens*, 2012, 21, 382-388.

[10] Wolf, M. Forging forward with 10 burning questions on fgf23 in kidney disease. *J Am Soc Nephrol*, 2010, 21, 1427-1435.

[11] Bellasi, A; Kestenbaum, B. Pro: Should phosphate binders be used in chronic kidney disease stage 3-4? *Nephrol Dial Transplant*, 2015.

[12] Kestenbaum, B; Bellasi, A. Con: Phosphate binders in chronic kidney disease. *Nephrol Dial Transplant*, 2015.

[13] Bellasi, A; Galassi, A; Cozzolino, M; Di Iorio, B. The evolving world of chronic kidney disease mineral bone disorder (ckd-mbd). *EMJ Neph*, 2013, 1, 20-31.

[14] Kuro-o, M. Klotho; phosphate and fgf-23 in ageing and disturbed mineral metabolism. *Nature reviews Nephrology*, 2013, 9, 650-660.

[15] Moe, SM; Zidehsarai, MP; Chambers, MA; Jackman, LA; Radcliffe, JS; Trevino, LL; Donahue, SE; Asplin, JR. Vegetarian compared with meat dietary protein source and

phosphorus homeostasis in chronic kidney disease. *Clin J Am Soc Nephrol*, 2011, 6, 257-264.

[16] Bellasi, A; Kooienga, L; Block, GA. Phosphate binders: New products and challenges. *Hemodial Int*, 2006, 10, 225-234.

[17] Mathew, S; Tustison, KS; Sugatani, T; Chaudhary, LR; Rifas, L; Hruska, KA. The mechanism of phosphorus as a cardiovascular risk factor in ckd. *Journal of the American Society of Nephrology: JASN*, 2008, 19, 1092-1105.

[18] Di Iorio, BR; Torraca, S; Sirico, ML; Di Micco, L. Urinary phosphate excretion and fibroblast growth factor 23 in chronic kidney disease. *J Ren Nutr*, 2012.

[19] Spiegel, DM; Brady, K. Calcium balance in normal individuals and in patients with chronic kidney disease on low- and high-calcium diets. *Kidney Int*, 2012, 81, 1116-1122.

[20] Hill, KM; Martin, BR; Wastney, ME; McCabe, GP; Moe, SM; Weaver, CM; Peacock, M. Oral calcium carbonate affects calcium but not phosphorus balance in stage 3-4 chronic kidney disease. *Kidney Int*, 2013, 83, 959-966.

[21] Galassi, A; Bellasi, A; Auricchio, S; Papagni, S; Cozzolino, M. Which vitamin d in ckd-mbd? The time of burning questions. *BioMed Research International*, 2013, 2013, 10.

[22] Saliba, W; El-Haddad, B: Secondary hyperparathyroidism: Pathophysiology and treatment. *Journal of the American Board of Family Medicine: JABFM*, 2009, 22, 574-581.

[23] McCann, LM; Beto, J. Roles of calcium-sensing receptor and vitamin d receptor in the pathophysiology of secondary hyperparathyroidism. *Journal of renal nutrition: the official journal of the Council on Renal Nutrition of the National Kidney Foundation*, 2010, 20, 141-150.

[24] Tentori, F; Blayney, MJ; Albert, JM; Gillespie, BW; Kerr, PG; Bommer, J; Young, EW; Akizawa, T; Akiba, T; Pisoni, RL; Robinson, BM; Port, FK. Mortality risk for dialysis patients with different levels of serum calcium, phosphorus, and pth: The dialysis outcomes and practice patterns study (dopps). *American journal of kidney diseases: the official journal of the National Kidney Foundation*, 2008, 52, 519-530.

[25] Elder, G. Pathophysiology and recent advances in the management of renal osteodystrophy. *Journal of bone and mineral research: the official journal of the American Society for Bone and Mineral Research*, 2002, 17, 2094-2105.

[26] Faul, C; Amaral, AP; Oskouei, B; Hu, MC; Sloan, A; Isakova, T; Gutierrez, OM; Aguillon-Prada, R; Lincoln, J; Hare, JM; Mundel, P; Morales, A; Scialla, J; Fischer, M; Soliman, EZ; Chen, J; Go, AS; Rosas, SE; Nessel, L; Townsend, RR; Feldman, HI; St John Sutton, M; Ojo, A; Gadegbeku, C; Di Marco, GS; Reuter, S; Kentrup, D; Tiemann, K; Brand, M; Hill, JA; Moe, OW; Kuro, OM; Kusek, JW; Keane, MG; Wolf, M. Fgf23 induces left ventricular hypertrophy. *J Clin Invest*, 2011, 121, 4393-4408.

[27] Capuano, A; Serio, V; Pota, A; Memoli, B; Andreucci, VE. Beneficial effects of better control of secondary hyperparathyroidism with paricalcitol in chronic dialysis patients. *Journal of nephrology*, 2009, 22, 59-68.

[28] Cogan, MG; Covey, CM; Arieff, AI; Wisniewski, A; Clark, OH; Lazarowitz, V; Leach, W. Central nervous system manifestations of hyperparathyroidism. *The American journal of medicine*, 1978, 65, 963-970.

[29] Mak, RH; Bettinelli, A; Turner, C; Haycock, GB; Chantler, C. The influence of hyperparathyroidism on glucose metabolism in uremia. *The Journal of clinical endocrinology and metabolism*, 1985, 60, 229-233.

[30] Tentori, F; McCullough, K; Kilpatrick, RD; Bradbury, BD; Robinson, BM; Kerr, PG; Pisoni, RL. High rates of death and hospitalization follow bone fracture among hemodialysis patients. *Kidney international*, 2014, 85, 166-173.

[31] Jamal, SA; Vandermeer, B; Raggi, P; Mendelssohn, DC; Chatterley, T; Dorgan, M; Lok, CE; Fitchett, D; Tsuyuki, RT. Effect of calcium-based versus non-calcium-based phosphate binders on mortality in patients with chronic kidney disease: An updated systematic review and meta-analysis. *Lancet*, 2013.

[32] Moe, SM; Chertow, GM; Parfrey, PS; Kubo, Y; Block, GA; Correa-Rotter, R; Drueke, TB; Herzog, CA; London, GM; Mahaffey, KW; Wheeler, DC; Stolina, M; Dehmel, B; Goodman, WG; Floege, J. Cinacalcet, fibroblast growth factor-23, and cardiovascular disease in hemodialysis: The evaluation of cinacalcet hcl therapy to lower cardiovascular events (evolve) trial. *Circulation*, 2015, 132, 27-39.

[33] Galassi, A; Cupisti, A; Santoro, A; Cozzolino, M. Phosphate balance in esrd: Diet; dialysis and binders against the low evident masked pool. *Journal of nephrology*, 2015, 28, 415-429.

[34] Kuhlmann, MK. Phosphate elimination in modalities of hemodialysis and peritoneal dialysis. *Blood purification*, 2010, 29, 137-144.

[35] Gotch, FA; Panlilio, F; Sergeyeva, O; Rosales, L; Folden, T; Kaysen, G; Levin, N. Effective diffusion volume flow rates (qe) for urea, creatinine, and inorganic phosphorous (qeu, qecr, qeip) during hemodialysis. *Seminars in dialysis*, 2003, 16, 474-476.

[36] K/doqi clinical practice guidelines for bone metabolism and disease in chronic kidney disease. *Am J Kidney Dis*, 2003, 42, S1-201.

[37] Clinical practice guidelines for nutrition in chronic renal failure. K/doqi; national kidney foundation. *American journal of kidney diseases: the official journal of the National Kidney Foundation*, 2000, 35, S1-140.

[38] Cupisti, A; Comar, F; Benini, O; Lupetti, S; D'Alessandro, C; Barsotti, G; Gianfaldoni, D. Effect of boiling on dietary phosphate and nitrogen intake. *J Ren Nutr*, 2006, 16, 36-40.

[39] Cozzolino, M; Bruschetta, E; Cusi, D; Montanari, E; Giovenzana, ME; Galassi, A. Phosphate handling in ckd-mbd from stage 3 to dialysis and the three strengths of lanthanum carbonate. *Expert opinion on pharmacotherapy*, 2012, 13, 2337-2353.

[40] Caldeira, D; Amaral, T; David, C; Sampaio, C. Educational strategies to reduce serum phosphorus in hyperphosphatemic patients with chronic kidney disease: Systematic review with meta-analysis. *Journal of renal nutrition: the official journal of the Council on Renal Nutrition of the National Kidney Foundation*, 2011, 21, 285-294.

[41] Cannata-Andia, JB; Fernandez-Martin, JL; Locatelli, F; London, G; Gorriz, JL; Floege, J; Ketteler, M; Ferreira, A; Covic, A; Rutkowski, B; Memmos, D; Bos, WJ; Teplan, V; Nagy, J; Tielemans, C; Verbeelen, D; Goldsmith, D; Kramar, R; Martin, PY; Wuthrich, RP; Pavlovic, D; Benedik, M; Sanchez, JE; Martinez-Camblor, P; Naves-Diaz, M; Carrero, JJ; Zoccali, C. Use of phosphate-binding agents is associated with a lower risk of mortality. *Kidney international*, 2013, 84, 998-1008.

[42] Kdigo clinical practice guideline for the diagnosis, evaluation, prevention, and treatment of chronic kidney disease-mineral and bone disorder (ckd-mbd). *Kidney Int Suppl*, 2009, S1-130.

[43] Zoccali, C; Mallamaci, F; Cannata-Andia, J. Phosphate binders and clinical outcomes in patients with stage 5d chronic kidney disease. *Seminars in dialysis*, 2015, 28, 587-593.

[44] Cozzolino, M; Mazzaferro, S; Brandenburg, V. The treatment of hyperphosphataemia in ckd: Calcium-based or calcium-free phosphate binders? *Nephrol Dial Transplant*, 2011, 26, 402-407.

[45] Oliveira, RB; Cancela, AL; Graciolli, FG; Dos Reis, LM; Draibe, SA; Cuppari, L; Carvalho, AB; Jorgetti, V; Canziani, ME; Moyses, RM. Early control of pth and fgf23 in normophosphatemic ckd patients: A new target in ckd-mbd therapy? *Clin J Am Soc Nephrol*, 2010, 5, 286-291.

[46] Gonzalez-Parra, E; Gonzalez-Casaus, ML; Galan, A; Martinez-Calero, A; Navas, V; Rodriguez, M; Ortiz, A. Lanthanum carbonate reduces fgf23 in chronic kidney disease stage 3 patients. *Nephrol Dial Transplant*, 2011, 26, 2567-2571.

[47] Vlassara, H; Uribarri, J; Cai, W; Goodman, S; Pyzik, R; Post, J; Grosjean, F; Woodward, M; Striker, GE. Effects of sevelamer on hba1c, inflammation, and advanced glycation end products in diabetic kidney disease. *Clinical journal of the American Society of Nephrology: CJASN*, 2012, 7, 934-942.

[48] de Francisco, AL; Leidig, M; Covic, AC; Ketteler, M; Benedyk-Lorens, E; Mircescu, GM; Scholz, C; Ponce, P; Passlick-Deetjen, J. Evaluation of calcium acetate/magnesium carbonate as a phosphate binder compared with sevelamer hydrochloride in haemodialysis patients: A controlled randomized study (calmag study) assessing efficacy and tolerability. *Nephrol Dial Transplant*, 2010, 25, 3707-3717.

[49] Galassi, A; Cozzolino, M. Magnesium: A renewed player of vascular ageing in diabetic ckd patients? *Clinical kidney journal*, 2014, 7, 93-96.

[50] Block, GA; Fishbane, S; Rodriguez, M; Smits, G; Shemesh, S; Pergola, PE; Wolf, M; Chertow, GM. A 12-week, double-blind, placebo-controlled trial of ferric citrate for the treatment of iron deficiency anemia and reduction of serum phosphate in patients with ckd stages 3-5. *American journal of kidney diseases: the official journal of the National Kidney Foundation*, 2015, 65, 728-736.

[51] Phan, O; Maillard, M; Malluche, HH; Stehle, JC; Funk, F; Burnier, M. Effects of sucroferric oxyhydroxide compared to lanthanum carbonate and sevelamer carbonate on phosphate homeostasis and vascular calcifications in a rat model of chronic kidney failure. *BioMed research international*, 2015, 2015, 515606.

[52] Daugirdas, JT; Finn, WF; Emmett, M; Chertow, GM. The phosphate binder equivalent dose. *Semin Dial*, 2011, 24, 41-49.

[53] Fissell, RB; Karaboyas, A; Bieber, BA; Sen, A; Li, Y; Lopes, AA; Akiba, T; Bommer, J; Ethier, J; Jadoul, M; Pisoni, RL; Robinson, BM; Tentori, F. Phosphate binder pill burden, patient-reported non-adherence; and mineral bone disorder markers: Findings from the dopps. *Hemodialysis international International Symposium on Home Hemodialysis*, 2015.

[54] Teng, M; Wolf, M; Lowrie, E; Ofsthun, N; Lazarus, JM; Thadhani, R. Survival of patients undergoing hemodialysis with paricalcitol or calcitriol therapy. *N Engl J Med*, 2003, 349, 446-456.

[55] Kandula, P; Dobre, M; Schold, JD; Schreiber, MJ; Jr., Mehrotra, R; Navaneethan, SD. Vitamin d supplementation in chronic kidney disease: A systematic review and meta-analysis of observational studies and randomized controlled trials. *Clin J Am Soc Nephrol*, 2011, 6, 50-62.
[56] Bellasi, A; Galassi, A; Salvi, P; Cozzolino, M. Paricalcitol and cardiorenal outcome: From the impact study to clinical practice. *Blood Purif*, 2013, 36, 12-16.
[57] Wang, AY; Fang, F; Chan, J; Wen, YY; Qing, S; Chan, IH; Lo, G; Lai, KN; Lo, WK; Lam, CW; Yu, CM. Effect of paricalcitol on left ventricular mass and function in ckd--the opera trial. *J Am Soc Nephrol*, 2014, 25, 175-186.
[58] Thadhani, R; Appelbaum, E; Pritchett, Y; Chang, Y; Wenger, J; Tamez, H; Bhan, I; Agarwal, R; Zoccali, C; Wanner, C; Lloyd-Jones, D; Cannata, J; Thompson, BT; Andress, D; Zhang, W; Packham, D; Singh, B; Zehnder, D; Shah, A; Pachika, A; Manning, WJ; Solomon, SD. Vitamin d therapy and cardiac structure and function in patients with chronic kidney disease: The primo randomized controlled trial. *JAMA*, 2012, 307, 674-684.
[59] Raggi, P; Chertow, GM; Torres, PU; Csiky, B; Naso, A; Nossuli, K; Moustafa, M; Goodman, WG; Lopez, N; Downey, G; Dehmel, B; Floege, J. The advance study: A randomized study to evaluate the effects of cinacalcet plus low-dose vitamin d on vascular calcification in patients on hemodialysis. *Nephrol Dial Transplant*, 2011, 26, 1327-1339.
[60] Urena-Torres, PA; Floege, J; Hawley, CM; Pedagogos, E; Goodman, WG; Petavy, F; Reiner, M; Raggi, P. Protocol adherence and the progression of cardiovascular calcification in the advance study. *Nephrol Dial Transplant*, 2013, 28, 146-152.
[61] Bellasi, A; Reiner, M; Petavy, F; Goodman, W; Floege, J; Raggi, P. Presence of valvular calcification predicts the response to cinacalcet: Data from the advance study. *The Journal of heart valve disease*, 2013, 22, 391-399.
[62] Chertow, GM; Block, GA; Correa-Rotter, R; Drueke, TB; Floege, J; Goodman, WG; Herzog, CA; Kubo, Y; London, GM; Mahaffey, KW; Mix, TC; Moe, SM; Trotman, ML; Wheeler, DC; Parfrey, PS. Effect of cinacalcet on cardiovascular disease in patients undergoing dialysis. *N Engl J Med*, 2012, 367, 2482-2494.
[63] Locatelli, F; Messa, P; Bellasi, A; Cozzolino, M; Di Luca, M; Garibotto, G; Gesualdo, L; Malberti, F; Massimetti, C; Mazzaferro, S; Mereu, MC; Morosetti, M; Morrone, LF; Panuccio, V; Rapisarda, F; Russo, D; Schinella, D. What can we learn from a statistically inconclusive trial? Consensus conference on the evolve study results. *G Ital Nefrol*, 2013, 30.
[64] Parfrey, PS; Drueke, TB; Block, GA; Correa-Rotter, R; Floege, J; Herzog, CA; London, GM; Mahaffey, KW; Moe, SM; Wheeler, DC; Kubo, Y; Dehmel, B; Goodman, WG; Chertow, GM. The effects of cinacalcet in older and younger patients on hemodialysis: The evaluation of cinacalcet hcl therapy to lower cardiovascular events (evolve) trial. *Clin J Am Soc Nephrol*, 2015, 10, 791-799.
[65] Wheeler, DC; London, GM; Parfrey, PS; Block, GA; Correa-Rotter, R; Dehmel, B; Drueke, TB; Floege, J; Kubo, Y; Mahaffey, KW; Goodman, WG; Moe, SM; Trotman, ML; Abdalla, S; Chertow, GM; Herzog, CA. Effects of cinacalcet on atherosclerotic and nonatherosclerotic cardiovascular events in patients receiving hemodialysis: The evaluation of cinacalcet hcl therapy to lower cardiovascular events (evolve) trial. *Journal of the American Heart Association*, 2014, 3, e001363.

[66] Moe, SM; Abdalla, S; Chertow, GM; Parfrey, PS; Block, GA; Correa-Rotter, R; Floege, J; Herzog, CA; London, GM; Mahaffey, KW; Wheeler, DC; Dehmel, B; Goodman, WG; Drueke, TB. Effects of cinacalcet on fracture events in patients receiving hemodialysis: The evolve trial. *J Am Soc Nephrol*, 2015, 26, 1466-1475.

[67] Floege, J; Kubo, Y; Floege, A; Chertow, GM; Parfrey, PS. The effect of cinacalcet on calcific uremic arteriolopathy events in patients receiving hemodialysis: The evolve trial. *Clin J Am Soc Nephrol*, 2015, 10, 800-807.

[68] Levin, A; Bakris, GL; Molitch, M; Smulders, M; Tian, J; Williams, LA; Andress, DL. Prevalence of abnormal serum vitamin d, pth, calcium, and phosphorus in patients with chronic kidney disease: Results of the study to evaluate early kidney disease. *Kidney Int*, 2007, 71, 31-38.

[69] Joy, SV. Clinical pearls and strategies to optimize patient outcomes. *J Am Acad Nurse Pract*, 2007, 19, 15-20.

[70] Cozzolino, M; Tomlinson, J; Walsh, L; Bellasi, A. Emerging drugs for secondary hyperparathyroidism. *Expert opinion on emerging drugs*, 2015, 20, 197-208.

In: Comorbidities in Chronic Kidney Disease
Editor: Luca Di Lullo

ISBN: 978-1-63485-070-4

Chapter 5

ANEMIA MANAGEMENT IN PATIENTS WITH CHRONIC KIDNEY DISEASE

Rodolfo F. Rivera*

Division of Nephrology and Dialysis, San Gerardo Hospital, Monza, Italy

ABSTRACT

Anemia refers to an absolute reduction of the total number of circulating red blood cells (RBC), result in in a reduction of hemoglobin (Hb) concentration. Anemia is a frequent complication in chronic kidney disease (CKD), and it is often accompanied by various clinical symptoms.

The primary cause of anemia in CKD patients is the reduction in the erythropoietin production, which results in a decrease of signaling molecule that stimulates red blood cell production. Other possible causes of anemia in CKD include iron deficiency, inflammation, and the accumulation of uremic toxins

This chapter focuses the discussion on the strategy of the management of anemia in patients with CKD.

Erythropoiesis-stimulating agents (ESAs) and adjuvant iron therapy represent the primary treatment for anemia in chronic kidney disease. The introduction of ESAs into clinical practice was a success story, mediating an increase in hemoglobin concentrations without the risk for recurrent blood transfusions and improving quality of life substantially.

Keywords: CKD, anemia, iron, Erythropoiesis-stimulating agents, blood transfusions

INTRODUCTION

The World Health Organization (WHO) has defined anemia as an absolute reduction of the total number of circulating red blood cells (RBC) resulting in a reduction of hemoglobin

*Corresponding author: R.F. Rivera, Division of Nephrology and Dialysis, San Gerardo Hospital, Monza, Italy. Email: rodolforivera@gmail.com.

concentration <13.0 g/dL for adult males and postmenopausal women and an Hb <12.0 g/dL for premenopausal women [1]. For practical purposes, anemia is considered when one or more of the following are decreased: hemoglobin (Hb), hematocrit (Ht), or red blood cell (RBC) count.

In general, anemia is more common in women, in particular, those in their childbearing years. In the latter decades of life, anemia tends to occur without any particular sex predilection. There has been a lower prevalence of anemia in current smokers, which has been attributed to secondary erythrocytosis.

Anemia is a frequent complication in chronic kidney disease (CKD), and it is often accompanied by various clinical symptoms, such as impaired physical capacity, decreased neurocognitive function, and poor quality of life [2]. However, male patients with CKD have a 30% greater risk of developing anemia as compared to their female counterparts. Although males have higher Hb values, they also have higher rates of advanced CKD.

One of the lesser known functions of the kidneys is the production of erythropoietin, a signaling molecule that stimulates red blood cell production, in response to decreased oxygen levels in the blood. Any disruption of this process, e.g., secondary to a functional abnormality due to CKD, has the potential to induce anemia, a condition in which the number of circulating red blood cells, and therefore the level of Hb, is lower than normal [3]. Other possible causes of anemia in CKD include iron deficiency, inflammation, and the accumulation of uremic toxins [1, 3]. Thus, the abnormal composition of blood or urine is an additional indicator of kidney damage.

Based upon the WHO anemia diagnostic criteria, nearly 90 percent of patients with a glomerular filtration rate (GFR) <25 to 30 mL/min have anemia, many with Hb levels <10 g/dL [4].

An observational study that included patients with selected comorbid conditions such as CKD, human immunodeficiency virus, rheumatoid arthritis, inflammatory bowel disease, congestive heart failure, and solid-tumor cancers, showed that among end-stage renal disease (ESRD) patients who required renal replacement therapy (RRRT), 68% had a hematocrit (Ht) less than 30 mg/dL and 51% a Ht less than 28 mg/dL [5]. Furthermore, although anemia is not as common in earlier stages of CKD, patients with stage III disease have a prevalence of concurrent anemia of 5.2%, whereas those with stage IV disease the prevalence of concurrent anemia is 44.1% [6].

Age and race are important risk factors for the development of anemia in CKD patients. There is a greater prevalence of anemia in those older than 60 years, as compared to those aged between 46 and 60 years. This is probably due to the greater CKD prevalence in older individuals, as well as the lower estimated GFR that are associated with aging. Black people have not only a 4-fold increased risk of developing CKD relative to white persons [7] but also an increased prevalence of anemia.

From a clinical point of view, anemia has also been implicated as a contributing factor in many of the symptoms associated with CKD, including fatigue expression, reduced exercise tolerance, dyspnea, with cognitive impairment, sleep disturbances, increase in CKD rate progression, cardiovascular consequences, such as left ventricular hypertrophy (LVH) and left ventricular systolic dysfunction [8]. It is also associated with an increased risk of morbidity and mortality, principally due to cardiac disease and stroke [9–11], and with an increased risk of hospitalization, hospital length of stay, and mortality in patients with predialysis CKD [12, 13]. On the other hands, direct healthcare costs are higher in CKD patients with anemia than in those without [3], and quality of life issues (e.g., fatigue, reduced productivity) are common. For all those reasons anemia deserves to be treated as one of the major complications or CKD.

DIAGNOSIS AND EVALUATION OF ANEMIA IN CKD

Anemia is an initial laboratory sign of an underlying clinical problem in patients with or without CKD, for which is necessary a complete blood count, that include total RBC count, Ht, and Hb concentration.

In patients with CKD but stable kidney function, the onset or the progression of anemia may predict a new clinical problem which could be the expression of a blood loss or interference with red cell production.

For this reason, anemia should be evaluated independently of CKD stage in order to identify any reversible process contributing to the anemia. There is a large list of causes and approach to the diagnosis that can be found in a standard textbook of medicine or hematology useful for the clinical general practitioner. However, the causes of acquired anemia are myriad and too many to follow all steps of internistic guideline. A comprehensive list of this causes and diagnostic approach is desirable for CKD patients. The most commonly encountered reversible cause of chronic anemia or worsening anemia in CKD patients, other than anemia directly related to CKD, is iron deficiency anemia.

CKD patients show a gradual decrease in Hb levels that usually is related to the decline in the GFR, suggesting the need for regular monitoring of the Hb concentration. As renal function declines in patients with more advanced CKD stages, the incidence and prevalence of anemia increases. Therefore, in order to identify CKD patients at high risk for therapeutic intervention, Hb concentration monitoring should be more frequent in proportion to CKD stages.

The frequency of Hb monitoring, regardless of CKD stage, should be influenced by both the Hb level and rate of decline in Hb level. Monthly monitoring of Hb concentration is recommended in patients undergoing dialysis replacement therapy (HD hemodialysis or PD: peritoneal dialysis). It is important to remember that for HD patients Hb monitoring is traditionally performed prior to a midweek HD session, while this is not essential in PD patients. As in all patients, Hb testing should be performed whenever clinically indicated, such as after a major surgical procedure, hospitalization, or bleeding episode.

Initial evaluation of the anemia in CKD, regardless of age and CKD stage, should include the following tests: Complete blood count (CBC), that should include Hb concentration, red cell indices, white blood cell count and differential, and platelet count; Absolute reticulocyte count; Serum ferritin level; Serum transferrin saturation (TSAT); Serum vitamin B12 and folate levels.

Complete blood count (CBC): CBC gives important information about the kinds, numbers and form of blood cells as well as red blood cells, white blood cells and platelets. CBS also provides information about both the severity of anemia and adequacy of bone marrow function. Since anemia of CKD is hypoproliferative, and in general, normochromic and normocytic, from the morphological point of view it is indistinguishable from the anemia of chronic disease [14]. Detection of macrocytosis may suggest folate or vitamin B12 deficiencies, whereas the presence of microcytosis is associated with iron deficiency or inherited disorders of Hb formation. Iron deficiency, especially if longstanding, is associated with hypochromia and macrocytosis with leukopenia or thrombocytopenia suggests a generalized disorder of hematopoiesis caused by toxins (e.g., alcohol), nutritional deficit (vitamin B12 or folate deficiency), or myelodysplasia. In the presence of one or more of these findings, further diagnostic evaluation are indicated. Abnormalities of the white blood cell count and differential or platelet count are not typical of CKD anemia. These alteration require investigation for other diseases. In CKD patients who have active blood loss or hemolysis, reticulocyte count may be high.

Hemoglobin(Hb) and hematocrit (Ht) concentration: Hb or Ht target in CKD or ESRD patients, would be defined as that value that is clinically optimal for each patient, based upon their special circumstances, such as general level of function and employment and comorbidities, such as coronary artery disease (CAD) and chronic heart failure (CHF).

Increasing evidence indicates the poor advantage, and even potential risk, with increased morbidity and mortality associated with targeting and maintaining Hb levels >13 g/dL in predialysis patients. According with most recent recommendation, clinicians should weigh the risk-benefit of erythropoietic-stimulating agents (ESA) therapy between decrease the need for transfusions against the increased risks for serious, adverse cardiovascular events. For each patient should be found minimum dosage of ESA to use sufficient to reduce the need for blood transfusions.

Although Hb target range is not provided, non-dialysis-dependent CKD (non-HD-CKD) patients should maintain Hb levels between 10.0 and 11.5 g/dL, and reduce or stop the treatment if the level exceeds this limits. For dialysis-dependent CKD (HD-CKD) patients the level of Hb should be <10 g/dL, and reduce or stop the treatment if Level, Hb or exceeds 11 g/dL [15]. According to the major randomized trials, there are non-benefits of Hb concentration between 11.5 and 13.0 g/dL, and Hb targets >13 g/dL were associated with adverse outcomes [16–19]. There is now general agreement that in patients with CKD and ESRD, an adequate Hb target for anemia improves physiologic and clinical parameters and quality of life, compared with the very low Hb levels that were common prior to the availability of ESAs [15, 20–23]. The National Kidney Foundation (NKF) Dialysis Outcomes Quality Initiative (DOQI) guidelines for the anemia of CKD were initially published in 1997, with revisions in 2001 and 2006 (20–22). The 2007 update recommended the range of 11 to 12 g/dL of Hb target in all CKD patients, while Hb levels should never exceed 13 g/dL [23]. The 2012 Kidney Disease Improving Global Outcomes (KDIGO) guidelines [24] recommended that HD-CKD patients should maintain Hb concentrations ≥10 g/dL. In patients with Hb <10 g/dL, therapy should be individualized based upon the rate of fall in Hb concentration, the response to iron therapy, risk of transfusion, the risks related to ESA therapy, and the presence of symptoms. In no HD-CKD patients, KDIGO suggests initiating therapy when the Hb concentration is <10 g/dL.

Iron Status: Adequate iron stores are essential to optimize the effects of ESA, such as recombinant human erythropoietin (EPO) or darbepoietin alfa. In fact, decreased iron stores or decreased availability of iron represent the most common cause for resistance to the effect of these agents. An ideal test for iron status in CKD patients would accurately indicate whether the patient has sufficient amount of iron available to support achievement and maintenance of Hb target, and an excessive amount of body iron.

Unfortunately, no test exists with accomplishes either of these goals and which is practical to administer. Currently, the two best test of iron status are the serum ferritin and the present transferrin saturation (TSAT).

Serum ferritin is the most widely used test for the assessment of storage iron, for which the ‘gold standard’ remains examination of a bone marrow aspiration stained for iron [25]. However, serum ferritin values have to be interpreted with caution in CKD patients since it may be affected by inflammation or malnutrition, especially in dialysis patients in whom subclinical inflammation may be present [26]. Serum ferritin values <30 mg/L is indicative of severe iron deficiency and are highly predictive of absent iron stores in bone marrow [27, 28].

According to NKF-KDOQI Clinical Practice Guidelines for Anemia in CKD, the recommended serum ferritin target to iron therapy in HD-CKD patients should be >200 ng/mL, while in non-HD-CKD patients >100 ng/mL. HD-CKD patients with a ferritin target up to 400-ng/mL showed a final ESA doses 28% lower than those in the lower (200-ng/mL) ferritin group, suggesting that higher ferritin target is well tolerated and reduce reduces the requirements for ESA [29].

There is no current evidence available to support treating most patients with serum ferritin levels greater than 500 ng/mL. A therapeutic response to iron therapy in a patient with a ferritin level greater than 500 ng/mL is unlikely.

The percent TSAT (serum iron multiplied by 100 and divided by total iron binding capacity: TIBC) reflects iron that is readily available for erythropoiesis. The TIBC measures circulating transferring. The tranferrin molecule contains two binding sites for transporting iron from storage sites to red progenitor cells. A TSAT of 50% indicate that half of the binding sites are activated by iron.

The distinction between absolute and functional iron deficiency is essential to understanding what constitutes adequate TSAT & circulating ferritin concentrations in ESA-treated CKD patients. In normal subjects, iron deficiency is considered “absolute” when iron store is depleted (circulating ferritin levels <12 ng/mL, and iron delivery is impaired as indicated by TSAT below 16%). Absolute iron deficiency in CKD patients has been defined as a circulating ferritin values <100 ng/mL and TSAT levels lower than 20%. Differently, functional iron deficiency results when there is a need for a greater amount of iron to support hemoglobin synthesis than can be released from iron stores. This clinical situation can be observed in a chronic pharmacological stimulation with ESA in CKD patients with adequate iron stores, and it is characterized by a reduction in TSAT percent despite normal or elevated circulating levels of ferretin [27, 28]. A TSAT lower than 20% in HD-CKD patients has been traditionally considered to be an indicator of iron deficiency.

A common clinical problem is distinguishing between functional iron deficiency and inflammatory iron block, since the TSAT could be above the 20% and circulating ferritin could be 100 to 700 ng/mL in both clinical situations. During functional iron deficiency, ESA treatment induces a decrease in circulating ferritin levels, which however remain elevated (generally more than 100 ng/mL). In contrast, inflammatory process is characterized by an abrupt increase of serum ferritin levels, that is associated with a sudden drop in the TSAT. Measurement of high sensitivity C-reactive protein (CRP) may be indicated if occult inflammation is a concern. In this situation, no further intravenous (IV) iron should be administrated until the inflammatory condition has resolved.

Reticulocyte count can be obtained with automated CBC testing, and may be high in patients who have active blood loss or hemolysis, and may be low in hypoproliferative erythropoiesis with anemia.

Other tests of iron status, such as percentage of hypochromic red blood cells and reticulocyte Hb content may be used instead of, or in addition to, TSAT and ferritin levels if available.

Hepcidin is a recently discovered peptide hormone regarded as the key regulator of iron entry into the plasma [30], is up-regulated by inflammation and increased iron stores and down-regulated by iron depletion. Hepcidin blocks iron release from the macrophages, limiting iron availability for erythropoiesis. Elevated serum levels of the bioactive hepcidin isoform, have been consistently reported in HD-CKD patients [31, 32] however, determination of circulating hepcidin levels has not been shown to be clinically useful or superior to more standard iron status tests in patients with CKD [33].

Folate and vitamin B12 deficiency are uncommon but important causes of treatable anemia, typically associated with macrocytic red blood cell (RBC) indices. The prevalence of vitamin B12 and folate deficiency in HD-CKD patients is about 10%, and limited data are available in non-HD-CKD patients. Nonetheless, since these deficiencies are easily correctable, and in the case of vitamin B12 may indicate other underlying disease processes, assessment of folate and vitamin B12 levels are generally considered standard components of anemia evaluation, especially in the presence of macrocytosis.

USE OF IRON TO TREAT ANEMIA IN CKD

Iron is an essential mineral for heme synthesis, and adequate amounts of it are required for the production of new erythrocytes. Erythropoietic stimulation during anemia treatment in CKD patients, induces a greater utilization of iron available to satisfy the increased demands of the bone marrow. Under these conditions, the amount of iron usable could become inadequate [34]. Therefore, iron supplementation in CKD patients with anemia is used to assure adequate iron stores for erythropoiesis, correct iron deficiency, and, prevent iron deficiency from developing in those patients receiving ESA treatment. Correction of iron deficiency with oral or intravenous iron supplementation can reduce the severity of anemia through the improvement of erythropoietic response to ESA treatment [35, 36].

Iron supplementation, particularly with intravenous iron, can increase erythropoiesis and raise Hb levels even when TSAT and ferritin circulating values are not indicative of absolute iron deficiency, and when bone marrow studies reveal adequate iron stores [37–39].

Due to the limited diagnostic utility of serum ferritin and TSAT test to estimate body iron stores, prescription of iron therapy in patients with CKD is complicated, which makes it difficult to predicting a Hb response to iron supplementation [40].

The prescription of iron therapy should be based on an assessment that an increase in Hb level is desirable in order to avoid transfusion or reduce the symptoms of anemia related. In addition, the potential adverse effects of iron supplementation should be considered taking into account appropriately outweighed by the expected treatment benefit.

Iron supplementation could be in the form of oral or intravenous (IV) while the use of intramuscular iron has largely been abandoned. Each administration route has its own potential advantages and disadvantages.

Oral iron is less expensive, readily available, and does not require IV access, a particular concern in non-dependent-HD CKD patients. Despite oral route is generally well tolerated and it is not associated with severe adverse effects, gastrointestinal side effects such as nausea, dyspepsia and diarrhea are common and may limit adherence [41]. In addition, variable gastrointestinal tract absorption associated with gastrointestinal intolerance, can affect the treatment efficacy, penalizing the choice of this route of administration.

IV iron avoids concerns about medication adherence and efficacy in treating iron deficiency, but requires IV access and has been associated with infrequent but severe adverse reactions. The most dangerous adverse reaction to IV iron treatment is anaphylaxis, which is the most serious expression of hypersensitivity reactions (HSR) [42]. HSR are quite rare but they could be fatal if not managed promptly [43]. They used to be more common with older formulations of high molecular weight iron dextran (HMW-ID) than with newer preparations [44–46]. Similar to iron dextran, new iron molecules with large molecular-weight have been developed. Given the reduced amount of free iron released following administration, they may have an improved safety profile. However, post-marketing data are still inadequate to draw definitive conclusions and new molecules may be object of over reporting.

The optimum route of iron administration in CKD patients is still controversial. IV iron is more effective than oral iron in HD patients in replenishing iron stores, achieving a sustained Hb response and reducing the need for red blood cell transfusions [47], and reducing the required dosage of ESA [48–51]. In non-dialysis dependent CKD patients there is no widely accepted consensus on whether IV or oral iron should be used as first-line therapy in CKD-related anemia. Despite the potential benefits of oral iron, that include the low cost and the easy administration, its use is limited by poor gastrointestinal adsorption and high rate of adverse events [41, 52–54].

Oral iron is typically prescribed to provide approximately 200□mg of elemental iron daily. Oral administration should be given between meals (e.g., 2 hours before or 1 hour after a meal). For patients who have difficulty tolerating oral iron supplements, it is possible prescribe smaller, more frequent doses; start with a lower dose and increase slowly to the target dose; try a different form or preparation; or take at bedtime. Dosage of oral iron expressed in terms of elemental iron are shown in Table 1.

Table 1. Approximate Elemental Iron Content of Various Oral Iron Preparations

Drug	Elemental Iron
Ferric pyrophosphate	120 mg/g
Ferrous gluconate	120 mg/g
Ferrous sulfate	200 mg/g
Ferrous sulfate, dried	300 mg/g
Ferrous fumarate	330 mg/g
Ferrous carbonate, anhydrous	480 mg/g
Carbonyl iron	1000 mg/g

In same CKD patients, daily smaller doses of oral iron may be useful and better tolerated. Although ferrous sulfate is commonly available and inexpensive, other oral iron preparations may also be used; there is not significant evidence to suggest that other oral iron formulations are more effective or associated with fewer adverse side effects than ferrous sulfate. If the goals of iron supplementation are not met with a 1–3 month course of oral iron, it is appropriate to consider IV iron supplementation.

IV iron may be provided as a single large dose or as repeated smaller doses depending on the specific IV iron preparation. It is common practice to provide an initial course of IV iron amounting to approximately 1000 mg; this may be repeated if an initial dose fails to increase Hb level and/or allow a decrease in ESA dose and if the TSAT remains ≤30% and serum ferritin remains ≤500 ng/ml (≤500□ìg/l) [55].

Iron dextran (ID) formulations carry a black box warning about fatal anaphylactic reactions, likely because of antibodies to the iron-carbohydrate or ID complex or the dextran component, particularly with high-molecular-weight ID (HMW-ID). The introduction of low-molecular-weight ID (LMW-ID) substantially reduces the risk of anaphylaxis. With ID therapy, test doses are required, along with an observation period for antibody reactions. Newer IV irons ferric gluconate and iron sucrose, that do not contain dextran, have a better safety profile. Chertow et al. [56] compared absolute rates of life-threatening HSR reported by the FDA from 2001 to 2003. For four different parenteral iron preparations (iron sucrose, ferric gluconate, LMW-ID, and HMW-ID), HSR were 0.6, 0.9, 3.3, and 11.3 per million patients, respectively. Ferumoxytol is the newest IV iron formulation to enter in the market [57]. It is a superparamagnetic iron oxide nanoparticle coated with a low molecular weight semi-synthetic carbohydrate. It helps to isolate the bioactive iron from plasma components until the iron-carbohydrate complex enters the reticuloendothelial system macrophages of the liver, spleen and bone marrow. The iron is released from the iron-carbohydrate complex within vesicles in the macrophages. Iron then either enters the intracellular storage iron pool (e.g., ferritin) or is transferred to plasma transferrin for transport to erythroid precursor cells for incorporation into hemoglobin. Dosage of IV iron, expressed in terms of elemental iron are shown in Table 2.

Table 2. IV Iron Products: A Comparison

Drug - Name - Manufacture	Concentration	Post-dose Observation Needed
HMW-ID (DexFerrum),	50 mg/mL	60 min after test dose, 30 min after actual dose
LMW-ID (InFed)	50 mg/mL	60 min after test dose, 30 min after actual dose
Ferric gluconate (Ferlixit),	12.5 mg/mL	30 min
Iron sucrose (Venofer),	20 mg/mL	30 min
Ferumoxytol (Feraheme),	30 mg/mL	30 min
Ferric carboxymaltose (Ferinject)	50 mg/mL	30 min

HMW-ID: high-molecular-weight iron dextran; LMW-ID: low-molecular-weight iron dextran;

USE OF ERYTHROPOIETIC-STIMULATING AGENTS TO TREAT ANEMIA IN CKD

The main cause of anemia in CKD is a loss of kidney endogenous erythropoietin (EPO) production capacity, but more recently other conditions able to aggravate this effect have been proposed, such as a derangement in oxygen sensing [58]. The introduction of recombinant human erythropoietin (rHuEPO) into clinical practice in the 1980s was a major innovation in the treatment of the anemia of patients with CKD. The development of rHuEPO was aimed at replacing the insufficient EPO production related to CKD progression. Thus, the rHuEPO therapy was considered as a useful therapy for dialysis dependent CKD patients, whose hemoglobin dropped to extremely low levels, making them transfusion-dependent.

The immediate improvement in symptoms of anemia with the administration of rHuEPO in CKD patients was associated with reduced need for blood transfusions, resulting in risk of transmission of blood-borne viral diseases, such as hepatitis B and C, less allosensitization, predispose to long waiting times or failure to receive a kidney transplant, transplant rejection, and reduced risk of hemosiderosis [59]. In many observational studies, the gradually increased and often the normalization of Hb values, showed an inversely proportional association to certain intermediate outcomes such as left ventricular hypertrophy [8], as well as patient outcomes hard as cardiovascular events hospitalization [60], and death [61].

At the beginning, the use of rHuEPO has been limited to dialysis patients with the most serious forms of anemia. In the following years, its use has been extended to the majority of dialysis patients with renal anemia, and, later, also in anemic patients with CKD 4-5 in countries where the high cost of rHuEPO did not limit number of patients who can benefit from this treatment. In this period, Hb targets also increased progressively, often into the range of normal values. The idea of a complete correction of anemia was based on improving outcomes in the medium and long term reported in observational studies [8, 59-61]. The US Normal Hematocrit Trial by Besarab et al. [16] was the first of a series of randomized controlled trials (RCTs) which cast serious doubt on the assumption that full anemia correction should be achieved in the majority of dialysis patients. Patients who achieve a normal Hb showed a greater number of myocardial infarcts, primary events and deaths than those in which was partially corrected anemia with epoetin. The study was stopped early due to inability to prove the primary hypothesis.

The double-blind Canada-Europe trial by Parfrey et al. [62] in CKD 5HD patients without symptomatic heart disease (18% with diabetic nephropathy) failed to demonstrate a beneficial effect on left ventricular volume and mass index in the full anemia correction regime using epoetin-alfa (Hb target = 13.5–14.5 g/dL), compared to partial correction one (Hb target = 9.5–11.5 g/dL).

In the CREATE study by Drueke et al. [63] in 3-5 stage CKD patients, was not demonstrate a superiority of full anemia correction (Hb target = 13.0–15.0 g/dL) in terms of cardiovascular events, as compared to partial correction of anemia (Hb target = 10.5–11.5 g/dL), when starting ESA therapy at an earlier stage than end-stage renal disease (ESRD) using epoetin-beta. Dialysis therapy was required in significantly more patients in the high Hb group than in the low Hb group. However the rate of fall of GFR in the two groups during the 3 year study was similar. Also the US CHOIR study by Singh et al. [64] was prematurely stopped after an interim analysis with a median study duration of 16 months. This study failed to demonstrate a superiority of full anemia correction (Hb targets = 13.5 g/dL) by ESA administration in terms of cardiovascular events and death, as compared to partial treatment of anemia (Hb targets = 11.3 g/dL), in patients with CKD 3–4 patients not yet on dialysis using epoetin alfa.

Finally, the international trial of darbepoetin-alfa in type 2 diabetes and CKD (TREAT) by Pfeffer et al. [65] that examined cardiovascular and kidney outcomes in CKD 3–4 patients, was not found significant differences neither in cardiovascular event and death nor in ESRD, in patients with full anemia correction (Hb targets = 12.5 g/dL) compared partial treatment of anemia (Hb targets = 10.6 g/dL),

Assessment of ESAs in CKD using meta-analysis is problematic because of the heterogeneity of patients entered, the different quality and research designs of the RCTs performed, and differences in definitions of endpoints. The most recent meta-analysis [66] concluded that higher Hb concentrations in CKD increases risk for stroke, hypertension, and vascular access thrombosis, and may perhaps increase risk for death, serious cardiovascular events or ESRD.

According to the interpretations of the combined results of the recent major RCTs, the target Hb values exceeding ≤11.5 g/dL in adult CKD patients can cause more harm than benefit. The update of the 2006 KDOQI anemia guideline in 2007, had already led to the recommendation to limit upper the target Hb to 12 g/dL, and do not exceed 13 g/dL [23].

Regarding the initiation of therapy ESA, dose adjustments ESA and rates of change, the objective is a rate of increase in Hb concentrations of 1.0 to 2.0 g/dL per month [22]. The Hb rate of increase varies greatly as a function of individual ESA responsiveness. Poor responders are more likely in female, in patients with history of cardiovascular disease, iron deficiency and inflammation, and overweight [26]. The response also depends on initial dose, dosing frequency, and route of administration. However, the last two concerns epoetin-alfa, epoetin-beta, and darbepoetin but not CERA (continuous erythropoietin receptor activator [methoxy polyethylene glycol-epoetin-beta]). Table 3 compares the different erythropoietin-stimulating agents.

Epoetin-alfa or epoetin-beta dosing usually starts at 20 to 50 IU/kg body weight three times a week. Darbepoetin-alfa dosing usually starts at 0.45 mg/kg body weight once weekly by subcutaneous (SC) or IV administration, or 0.75 mg/kg body weight once every 2 weeks by SC administration. CERA dosing starts at 0.6 mg/kg body weight once every 2 weeks by SC or IV administration for CKD ND and CKD 5D patients, respectively, or 1.2 mg/kg body weight once every 4 weeks by SC administration for CKD ND patients. Higher baseline Hb concentrations require lower initial ESA doses, except for CERA for which there is no initial dose change.

However, ESA requirements should be evaluate or reevaluate each time a patients with CKD is hospitalized. ESA responsiveness may be modified profoundly during Disease states such as severe infections or postsurgery.

Red Cell Transfusion to Treat Anemia in CKD

After the addition of ESAs to available treatments for anemia in CKD patients, there has been a marked decline in transfusion events in this population. Current anemia management guidelines recommend reaching the Hb target using the lowest possible ESA dosages to avoid the need for red blood cell transfusions [22]. Although transfusions provides a rapid primary benefits of maintaining a sufficient oxygen carrying capacity improving anemia-related symptoms, and are considerably safer than in the past, transfusion-related risks persist.

Risks associated with blood transfusion include transfusion errors, volume and iron overload, hyperkalemia, citrate toxicity (leading to metabolic alkalosis and hypocalcemia), hypothermia, coagulopathy and immunologically-mediated transfusion reactions, all of which are uncommon. The most significant current risk of mortality from blood transfusion currently to administrative error, resulting in hemolysis (one in 60,000) and death (one in 600,000) [73].

The development of antibodies to human leukocytes antigen (HLA), can affect a patient's ability to receive organ transplants [68]. The risk of HLA sensitization after blood transfusion has changed over time probably, at least in part, due to changes in blood transfusion practices and the use of more precise methods to measure allosensitization. HLA sensitization was associated with several factors such as previous pregnancies and previous transplantation. Available data suggest that men have a much lower risk of HLA sensitization following transfusion than women, and women with multiple pregnancies have a much greater risk of HLA sensitization than nulliparous women. However, more recent data from the US Renal Data System (USRDS) 2010 Annual Report [69], have challenged this assumption, suggesting that males receiving previous blood transfusions may also be at increased risk.

One of the most easily identifiable cause of transfusion-related morbidity and mortality in the United States is the transfusion-related acute lung injury (TRALI) [67]. However, because of the varied criteria used to diagnose this syndrome, the true incidence is not known. Estimated incidence of TRALI is 8 cases per 100000 units of blood components transfused. Risk factors for TRALI are age and illness severity, and the risk for development of TRALI increases with the number of units transfused. TRALI is characterized by pulmonary edema, hypoxemia, respiratory distress, and radiographic evidence of new bilateral pulmonary infiltrates occurring within minutes to 6 hours after transfusion. Fever, tachycardia, cyanosis, hypotension, and frothy sputum may also be present.

Table 3. Comparison between erythropoietin-stimulating agents

	Brand	Half-life	FDA approval
Erythtopoietin alpha	Epogen Procrit Eprex	IV: 4-13 hs SC: 13-37 hs	Approved
Erythtopoietin beta	NeoRecormon	IV: 4-12 hs SC: 8-22 hs	Approved in Europe
Darbepoietin	Aranesp	IV: 23-39 hs SC: 21-144 hs	Approved
C.E.R.A.	Mircera	IV: 4-13 hs SC: 21-144 hs	Approved

C.E.R.A.= methoxy polyethylene glycol-epoetin-beta

Table 4. Clinical indications for red cell transfusion in Chronic Kidney Diseases patients

Acute clinical situations	Chronic clinical situations
Acute severe hemorrhage	Chronic anemia and ESAs are ineffective (hemoglobinopathies, bone marrow failure, ESA resistance)
Unstable coronary artery disease	
When rapid preoperative anemia correction is required	

ESA, erythropoiesis-stimulating agent.

Risks of transfusion transmitted viral infections are extremely low, currently estimated to be approximately one in 1.4 x 106 to 2.4 x 106 units for human immunodeficiency virus (HIV), one in 872,000 to 1.7 x 106 for hepatitis C virus (HCV), and one in 58,000 to 149,000 for hepatitis B virus (HBV) [70]. Rigorous predonation screening has led to a rapid decline in prevalence of HIV and HCV in first time blood donors, with HIV decreasing from 0.03% (1991-1992) to 0.02% (1993-1996) and HCV decreasing from 0.63% (1992) to 0.40% (1996), despite an increase in prevalence in the general population for both HIV (0.3% in 1992) and HCV (1.8% in 1988-1994) [71]. The introduction of nucleic acid amplification testing (NAT) for HIV and HCV in 1999, further reduced the window period between a potential blood donor infection and detectability by screening tests at time of donation [72].

Certain urgent clinical situations as well as acute severe hemorrhage and unstable coronary artery disease, red cell transfusion may be needed for the immediate correction of anemia. Also urgent situation where surgery is required, transfusion may also be given to achieve rapid preoperative correction of Hb. In stable CKD patients, transufion should be considered when ESAs are ineffective in the treatment of chronic anemia (hemoglobinopathies, bone marrow failure, ESA resistance). In all these situations, the Hb threshold for transfusion is uncertain but the treatment should be considered when the Hb is <7 g/dL (Table 4).

Conclusion

Anemia is a frequent complication in CKD, and it is often accompanied by various clinical symptoms, morbidity, and prognosis associated with reduced kidney function determining poor quality of life.

Anemia might begin to develop in the early stages of CKD, with a reduction of 20 to 50 percent of normal kidney function, and tends to worsen as CKD progresses.

The etiology of CKD-related anemia is multifactorial. The main cause is the deficiency in the production of erythropoietin, with the consequent reduction of red blood cells by the bone marrow, inducing a deprivation of oxygen levels in the blood that causing anemia. Other common causes of CKD-related anemia include blood loss from hemodialysis and low levels of iron, vitamin B12 and folic acid.

In all CKD patients, complete blood count, hemoglobin and hematocrit concentration, mean corpuscular volume, reticulocyte count, vitamin B_{12}, folic acid, and iron status (determination of ferritin, and TSAT) should be measured as part of anemia workup. Inflammatory markers determination, as well as high sensitivity C-reactive protein may help in etiological framework.

Iron deficiency, should be treated and its causes established. It is possible to supplementary iron orally or intravenously, while it is not recommended the use of intramuscular via. Since each administration route presents potential advantages and limitation, a careful evaluation should be performed in any patient to be treated.

If Hb is less than 11 g/dL, ESA therapy initiation should be discussed with the patient with focus on potential risks and benefits. It appears from available data that higher Hb targets are not beneficial and potentially harmful. Current K-DOQI guidelines advise for a Hb target of 11 to 12 g/dL without exceeding 13 g/dL. Laboratory testing should be repeated monthly until ESA dose is stable. Hb level and iron markers should be followed every 3 months during stable ESA treatment.

Red blood cells transfusion in CKD patients should be avoided as much as possible. It is well known that transfusions may induce the formation of antibodies HLA that can reduce the success of future kidney transplantation. In addition, transfusions may cause hyper volemia and symptoms of congestive heart failure, particularly in elderly patients. The K-DOQI guidelines state that no single Hb level should justify or require transfusion. Risks and benefits of transfusion therapy should be considered in individualized patients.

REFERENCES

[1] Nutritional anaemias. Report of a WHO scientific group. *World Health Organ Tech Rep Ser.*, 1968, 405, 5–37.

[2] Astor, BC; Muntner, P; Levin, A; Eustace, JA; Coresh, J. Association of kidney function with anemia: the Third National Health and Nutrition Examination Survey (1988-1994). *Arch Intern Med.*, 2002 Jun 24, 162(12), 1401–8.

[3] Smith, RE. The clinical and economic burden of anemia. *Am J Manag Care.*, 2010 Mar, 16 Suppl Issues, S59–66.

[4] Kazmi, WH; Kausz, AT; Khan, S; Abichandani, R; Ruthazer, R; Obrador, GT; et al. Anemia: an early complication of chronic renal insufficiency. *Am J Kidney Dis Off J Natl Kidney Found.*, 2001 Oct, 38(4), 803–12.

[5] Obrador, GT; Ruthazer, R; Arora, P; Kausz, AT; Pereira, BJG. Prevalence of and Factors Associated with Suboptimal Care before Initiation of Dialysis in the United States. *J Am Soc Nephrol.*, 1999 Aug 1, 10(8), 1793–800.

[6] Centers for Disease Control and Prevention (CDC). Prevalence of chronic kidney disease and associated risk factors--United States; 1999-2004. *MMWR Morb Mortal Wkly Rep.*, 2007 Mar 2, 56(8), 161–5.

[7] National Kidney Disease Education Program (NKDEP) [Internet]. [cited 2015 Oct 11]. Available from: http://www.niddk.nih.gov/health-information/health-communication-programs/nkdep/Pages/default.aspx.

[8] Levin, A; Thompson, CR; Ethier, J; Carlisle, EJ; Tobe, S; Mendelssohn, D; et al. Left ventricular mass index increase in early renal disease: impact of decline in hemoglobin. *Am J Kidney Dis Off J Natl Kidney Found.*, 1999 Jul, 34(1), 125–34.

[9] Jurkovitz, CT; Abramson, JL; Vaccarino, LV; Weintraub, WS; McClellan, WM. Association of high serum creatinine and anemia increases the risk of coronary events:

results from the prospective community-based atherosclerosis risk in communities (ARIC) study. *J Am Soc Nephrol JASN.*, 2003 Nov, 14(11), 2919–25.

[10] Sarnak, MJ; Tighiouart, H; Manjunath, G; MacLeod, B; Griffith, J; Salem, D; et al. Anemia as a risk factor for cardiovascular disease in The Atherosclerosis Risk in Communities (ARIC) study. *J Am Coll Cardiol.*, 2002 Jul 3, 40(1), 27–33.

[11] Abramson, JL; Jurkovitz, CT; Vaccarino, V; Weintraub, WS; McClellan, W. Chronic kidney disease, anemia, and incident stroke in a middle-aged, community-based population: the ARIC Study. *Kidney Int.*, 2003 Aug, 64(2), 610–5.

[12] Xia, H; Ebben, J; Ma, JZ; Collins, AJ. Hematocrit levels and hospitalization risks in hemodialysis patients. *J Am Soc Nephrol JASN.*, 1999 Jun, 10(6), 1309–16.

[13] Collins, AJ; Li, S; St Peter, W; Ebben, J; Roberts, T; Ma, JZ; et al. Death, hospitalization, and economic associations among incident hemodialysis patients with hematocrit values of 36 to 39%. *J Am Soc Nephrol JASN.*, 2001 Nov, 12(11), 2465–73.

[14] Weiss, G; Goodnough, LT. Anemia of chronic disease. *N Engl J Med.*, 2005 Mar 10, 352(10), 1011–23.

[15] Research C for DE and. Drug Safety and Availability - FDA Drug Safety Communication: Modified dosing recommendations to improve the safe use of Erythropoiesis-Stimulating Agents (ESAs) in chronic kidney disease [Internet]. [cited 2015 Oct 11]. Available from: http://www.fda.gov/Drugs/DrugSafety/ucm259639.htm.

[16] Besarab, A; Bolton, WK; Browne, JK; Egrie, JC; Nissenson, AR; Okamoto, DM; et al. The effects of normal as compared with low hematocrit values in patients with cardiac disease who are receiving hemodialysis and epoetin. *N Engl J Med.*, 1998 Aug 27, 339(9), 584–90.

[17] Pfeffer, MA; Burdmann, EA; Chen, CY; Cooper, ME; de Zeeuw, D; Eckardt, KU; et al. A trial of darbepoetin alfa in type 2 diabetes and chronic kidney disease. *N Engl J Med.*, 2009 Nov 19, 361(21), 2019–32.

[18] Phrommintikul, A; Haas, SJ; Elsik, M; Krum, H. Mortality and target haemoglobin concentrations in anaemic patients with chronic kidney disease treated with erythropoietin: a meta-analysis. *Lancet Lond Engl.*, 2007 Feb 3, 369(9559), 381–8.

[19] Strippoli, GFM; Craig, JC; Manno, C; Schena, FP. Hemoglobin targets for the anemia of chronic kidney disease: a meta-analysis of randomized, controlled trials. *J Am Soc Nephrol JASN.*, 2004 Dec, 15(12), 3154–65.

[20] NKF-DOQI clinical practice guidelines for the treatment of anemia of chronic renal failure. National Kidney Foundation-Dialysis Outcomes Quality Initiative. *Am J Kidney Dis Off J Natl Kidney Found.*, 1997 Oct, 30(4 Suppl 3), S192–240.

[21] IV. NKF-K/DOQI Clinical Practice Guidelines for Anemia of Chronic Kidney Disease: update 2000. *Am J Kidney Dis Off J Natl Kidney Found.*, 2001 Jan, 37(1 Suppl 1), S182–238.

[22] KDOQI, National Kidney Foundation. KDOQI Clinical Practice Guidelines and Clinical Practice Recommendations for Anemia in Chronic Kidney Disease. *Am J Kidney Dis Off J Natl Kidney Found.*, 2006 May, 47(5 Suppl 3), S11–145.

[23] KDOQI. KDOQI Clinical Practice Guideline and Clinical Practice Recommendations for anemia in chronic kidney disease: 2007 update of hemoglobin target. *Am J Kidney Dis Off J Natl Kidney Found.*, 2007 Sep, 50(3), 471–530.

[24] Chapter 1: Diagnosis and evaluation of anemia in CKD. *Kidney Int*, Suppl. 2012 Aug, 2(4), 288–91.

[25] Lipschitz, DA; Cook, JD; Finch, CA. A clinical evaluation of serum ferritin as an index of iron stores. *N Engl J Med.*, 1974 May 30, 290(22), 1213–6.

[26] Rambod, M; Kovesdy, CP; Kalantar-Zadeh, K. Combined high serum ferritin and low iron saturation in hemodialysis patients: the role of inflammation. *Clin J Am Soc Nephrol CJASN.*, 2008 Nov, 3(6), 1691–701.

[27] Kalantar-Zadeh, K; Höffken, B; Wünsch, H; Fink, H; Kleiner, M; Luft, FC. Diagnosis of iron deficiency anemia in renal failure patients during the post-erythropoietin era. *Am J Kidney Dis Off J Natl Kidney Found.*, 1995 Aug, 26(2), 292–9.

[28] Fernández-Rodríguez, AM; Guindeo-Casasús, MC; Molero-Labarta, T; Domínguez-Cabrera, C; Hortal-Casc n, L; Pérez-Borges, P; et al. Diagnosis of iron deficiency in chronic renal failure. *Am J Kidney Dis Off J Natl Kidney Found.*, 1999 Sep, 34(3), 508–13.

[29] DeVita, MV; Frumkin, D; Mittal, S; Kamran, A; Fishbane, S; Michelis, MF. Targeting higher ferritin concentrations with intravenous iron dextran lowers erythropoietin requirement in hemodialysis patients. *Clin Nephrol.*, 2003 Nov, 60(5), 335–40.

[30] Nicolas, G; Viatte, L; Bennoun, M; Beaumont, C; Kahn, A; Vaulont, S. Hepcidin, a new iron regulatory peptide. *Blood Cells Mol Dis.*, 2002 Dec, 29(3), 327–35.

[31] Zaritsky, J; Young, B; Gales, B; Wang, HJ; Rastogi, A; Westerman, M; et al. Reduction of Serum Hepcidin by Hemodialysis in Pediatric and Adult Patients. *Clin J Am Soc Nephrol.*, 2010 Jun 1, 5(6), 1010–4.

[32] Kato, A; Tsuji, T; Luo, J; Sakao, Y; Yasuda, H; Hishida, A. Association of prohepcidin and hepcidin-25 with erythropoietin response and ferritin in hemodialysis patients. *Am J Nephrol.*, 2008, 28(1), 115–21.

[33] Tessitore, N; Girelli, D; Campostrini, N; Bedogna, V; Pietro Solero, G; Castagna, A; et al. Hepcidin is not useful as a biomarker for iron needs in haemodialysis patients on maintenance erythropoiesis-stimulating agents. *Nephrol Dial Transplant Off Publ Eur Dial Transpl Assoc - Eur Ren Assoc.*, 2010 Dec, 25(12), 3996–4002.

[34] Macdougall, IC. Monitoring of iron status and iron supplementation in patients treated with erythropoietin. *Curr Opin Nephrol Hypertens.*, 1994 Nov, 3(6), 620–5.

[35] Mircescu, G; Gârneata, L; Capusa, C; Ursea, N. Intravenous iron supplementation for the treatment of anaemia in pre-dialyzed chronic renal failure patients. *Nephrol Dial Transplant Off Publ Eur Dial Transpl Assoc - Eur Ren Assoc.*, 2006 Jan, 21(1), 120–4.

[36] Silverberg, DS; Iaina, A; Peer, G; Kaplan, E; Levi, BA; Frank, N; et al. Intravenous iron supplementation for the treatment of the anemia of moderate to severe chronic renal failure patients not receiving dialysis. *Am J Kidney Dis Off J Natl Kidney Found.*, 1996 Feb, 27(2), 234–8.

[37] Spinowitz, BS; Kausz, AT; Baptista, J; Noble, SD; Sothinathan, R; Bernardo, MV; et al. Ferumoxytol for treating iron deficiency anemia in CKD. *J Am Soc Nephrol JASN.*, 2008 Aug, 19(8), 1599–605.

[38] Silverberg, DS; Blum, M; Agbaria, Z; Deutsch, V; Irony, M; Schwartz, D; et al. The effect of i.v. iron alone or in combination with low-dose erythropoietin in the rapid correction of anemia of chronic renal failure in the predialysis period. *Clin Nephrol.*, 2001 Mar, 55(3), 212–9.

[39] Stancu, S; Bârsan, L; Stanciu, A; Mircescu, G. Can the response to iron therapy be predicted in anemic nondialysis patients with chronic kidney disease? *Clin J Am Soc Nephrol CJASN.*, 2010 Mar, 5(3), 409–16.

[40] Tessitore, N; Solero, GP; Lippi, G; Bassi, A; Faccini, GB; Bedogna, V; et al. The role of iron status markers in predicting response to intravenous iron in haemodialysis patients on maintenance erythropoietin. *Nephrol Dial Transplant Off Publ Eur Dial Transpl Assoc - Eur Ren Assoc.*, 2001 Jul, 16(7), 1416–23.

[41] Macdougall, IC. Strategies for iron supplementation: oral versus intravenous. *Kidney Int Suppl.*, 1999 Mar, 69, S61–6.

[42] Rampton, D; Folkersen, J; Fishbane, S; Hedenus, M; Howaldt, S; Locatelli, F; et al. Hypersensitivity reactions to intravenous iron: guidance for risk minimization and management. *Haematologica.*, 2014 Nov, 99(11), 1671–6.

[43] Behera, V; Chauhan, R; Sinha, S; Nair, V. Anaphylactic Shock Secondary to Intravenous Iron Sucrose in Chronic Kidney Disease. *Indian J Hematol Blood Transfus Off J Indian Soc Hematol Blood Transfus.*, 2015 Sep, 31(3), 391–3.

[44] Bailie, GR; Verhoef, JJ. Differences in the reporting rates of serious allergic adverse events from intravenous iron by country and population. *Clin Adv Hematol Oncol HO.*, 2012 Feb, 10(2), 101–8.

[45] Bircher, AJ; Auerbach, M. Hypersensitivity from intravenous iron products. *Immunol Allergy Clin North Am.*, 2014 Aug, 34(3), 707–23, x – xi.

[46] Auerbach, M; Adamson, J; Bircher, A; Breymann, C; Fishbane S; Gafter-Gvili A; et al. On the safety of intravenous iron; evidence trumps conjecture. *Haematologica.*, 2015 May, 100(5), e214–5.

[47] Litton, E; Xiao, J; Ho, KM. Safety and efficacy of intravenous iron therapy in reducing requirement for allogeneic blood transfusion: systematic review and meta-analysis of randomised clinical trials. *BMJ.*, 2013, 347, f4822.

[48] Allegra, V; Mengozzi, G; Vasile, A. Iron deficiency in maintenance hemodialysis patients: assessment of diagnosis criteria and of three different iron treatments. *Nephron.*, 1991, 57(2), 175–82.

[49] Macdougall, IC; Tucker, B; Thompson, J; Tomson, CR; Baker, LR; Raine, AE. A randomized controlled study of iron supplementation in patients treated with erythropoietin. *Kidney Int.*, 1996 Nov, 50(5), 1694–9.

[50] Albaramki, J; Hodson, EM; Craig, JC; Webster, AC. Parenteral versus oral iron therapy for adults and children with chronic kidney disease. *Cochrane Database Syst Rev.*, 2012, 1, CD007857.

[51] Susantitaphong, P; Alqahtani, F; Jaber, BL. Efficacy and safety of intravenous iron therapy for functional iron deficiency anemia in hemodialysis patients: a meta-analysis. *Am J Nephrol.*, 2014, 39(2), 130–41.

[52] Van Wyck, DB; Roppolo, M; Martinez, CO; Mazey, RM; McMurray, S. United States Iron Sucrose (Venofer) Clinical Trials Group. A randomized, controlled trial comparing IV iron sucrose to oral iron in anemic patients with nondialysis-dependent CKD. *Kidney Int.*, 2005 Dec, 68(6), 2846–56.

[53] Charytan, C; Qunibi, W; Bailie, GR. Venofer Clinical Studies Group. Comparison of intravenous iron sucrose to oral iron in the treatment of anemic patients with chronic kidney disease not on dialysis. *Nephron Clin Pract.*, 2005, 100(3), c55–62.

[54] Agarwal, R; Rizkala, AR; Bastani, B; Kaskas, MO; Leehey, DJ; Besarab, A. A randomized controlled trial of oral versus intravenous iron in chronic kidney disease. *Am J Nephrol.*, 2006, 26(5), 445–54.

[55] KDIGO Clinical Practice Guideline for Anemia in Chronic Kidney Disease. Chapter 2: Use of iron to treat anemia in CKD. *Kidney Int Suppl.*, 2012 Aug, 2(4), 292–8.

[56] Chertow, GM; Mason, PD; Vaage-Nilsen, O; Ahlmén, J. Update on adverse drug events associated with parenteral iron. *Nephrol Dial Transplant Off Publ Eur Dial Transpl Assoc - Eur Ren Assoc.*, 2006 Feb, 21(2), 378–82.

[57] Auerbach, M; Ballard, H. Clinical use of intravenous iron: administration, efficacy, and safety. *Hematol Educ Program Am Soc Hematol Am Soc Hematol Educ Program.*, 2010, 2010, 338–47.

[58] Bernhardt, WM; Wiesener, MS; Scigalla, P; Chou, J; Schmieder, RE; Günzler, V; et al. Inhibition of prolyl hydroxylases increases erythropoietin production in ESRD. *J Am Soc Nephrol JASN.*, 2010 Dec, 21(12), 2151–6.

[59] Goodnough, LT; Brecher, ME; Kanter, MH; AuBuchon, JP. Transfusion medicine. First of two parts--blood transfusion. *N Engl J Med.*, 1999 Feb 11, 340(6), 438–47.

[60] Harnett, JD; Foley, RN; Kent, GM; Barre, PE; Murray, D; Parfrey, PS. Congestive heart failure in dialysis patients: prevalence, incidence, prognosis and risk factors. *Kidney Int.*, 1995 Mar, 47(3), 884–90.

[61] Collins, AJ. Influence of target hemoglobin in dialysis patients on morbidity and mortality. *Kidney Int Suppl.*, 2002 May, (80), 44–8.

[62] Parfrey, PS; Foley, RN; Wittreich, BH; Sullivan, DJ; Zagari, MJ; Frei, D. Double-blind comparison of full and partial anemia correction in incident hemodialysis patients without symptomatic heart disease. *J Am Soc Nephrol JASN.*, 2005 Jul, 16(7), 2180–9.

[63] Drüeke, TB; Locatelli, F; Clyne, N; Eckardt, KU; Macdougall, IC; Tsakiris, D; et al. Normalization of hemoglobin level in patients with chronic kidney disease and anemia. *N Engl J Med.*, 2006 Nov 16, 355(20), 2071–84.

[64] Singh, AK; Szczech, L; Tang, KL; Barnhart, H; Sapp, S; Wolfson, M; et al. Correction of anemia with epoetin alfa in chronic kidney disease. *N Engl J Med.*, 2006 Nov 16, 355(20), 2085–98.

[65] Pfeffer, MA; Burdmann, EA; Chen, CY; Cooper, ME; de Zeeuw, D; Eckardt, KU; et al. A trial of darbepoetin alfa in type 2 diabetes and chronic kidney disease. *N Engl J Med.*, 2009 Nov 19, 361(21), 2019–32.

[66] Palmer, SC; Navaneethan, SD; Craig, JC; Johnson, DW; Tonelli, M; Garg, AX; et al. Meta-analysis: erythropoiesis-stimulating agents in patients with chronic kidney disease. *Ann Intern Med.*, 2010 Jul 6, 153(1), 23–33.

[67] Looney, MR; Gropper, MA; Matthay, MA. Transfusion-related acute lung injury: a review. *Chest.*, 2004 Jul, 126(1), 249–58.

[68] Opelz, G; Graver, B; Mickey, MR; Terasaki, PI. Lymphocytotoxic antibody responses to transfusions in potential kidney transplant recipients. *Transplantation.*, 1981 Sep, 32(3), 177–83.

[69] Collins, AJ; Foley, RN; Chavers, B; Gilbertson, D; Herzog, C; Johansen, K; et al. 'United States Renal Data System 2011 Annual Data Report: Atlas of chronic kidney disease & end-stage renal disease in the United States. *Am J Kidney Dis Off J Natl Kidney Found.*, 2012 Jan, 59(1 Suppl 1), A7, e1–420.

[70] Goodnough, LT; Brecher, ME; Kanter, MH; AuBuchon, JP. Transfusion medicine. First of two parts--blood transfusion. *N Engl J Med.*, 1999 Feb 11, 340(6), 438–47.

[71] Glynn, SA; Kleinman, SH; Schreiber, GB; Busch, MP; Wright, DJ; Smith, JW; et al. Trends in incidence and prevalence of major transfusion-transmissible viral infections

in US blood donors, 1991 to 1996. Retrovirus Epidemiology Donor Study (REDS). *JAMA.*, 2000 Jul 12, 284(2), 229–35.

[72] Dodd, RY; Notari, EP; Stramer, SL. Current prevalence and incidence of infectious disease markers and estimated window-period risk in the American Red Cross blood donor population. *Transfusion (Paris).* 2002 Aug, 42(8), 975–9.

[73] Linden, JV; Tourault, MA; Scribner, CL. Decrease in frequency of transfusion fatalities. *Transfusion (Paris).*, 1997 Feb, 37(2), 243–4.

In: Comorbidities in Chronic Kidney Disease
Editor: Luca Di Lullo

ISBN: 978-1-63485-070-4

Chapter 6

CORONARY ARTERY DISEASE AND CHRONIC KIDNEY DISEASE

Agnès Rafecas and José A. Barrabés*
Acute Cardiac Care Unit, Cardiology Service,
Hospital Universitari Vall d'Hebron,
Universitat Autònoma de Barcelona, Barcelona, Spain

ABSTRACT

There is a wealth of data demonstrating a close association between chronic kidney disease (CKD) and cardiovascular disease, particularly coronary artery disease (CAD). About one half of deaths in patients with end-stage renal disease (ESRD) are of cardiovascular causes. The association between CKD and ischemic heart disease can be explained in part because both conditions are related to the traditional risk factors for atherosclerotic vascular disease. However, CKD might also have a casual role in the development and progression of CAD, with several mechanisms potentially involved. Among CAD patients, those with CKD have systematically a worse prognosis than those without CKD irrespective of the clinical presentation or the treatments applied. Current therapy is based on small trials and observational data and by extrapolating the strategies that have proven useful in the general population, although many treatments that have shown to improve the prognosis of CAD patients are underused in those with renal impairment.

Keywords: coronary artery disease, atherosclerosis, chronic kidney disease, coronary revascularization

* Correspondence to: José A. Barrabés, MD, Acute Cardiac Care Unit, Cardiology Service, Hospital Universitari Vall d'Hebron, Pg. Vall d'Hebron, 119-129, 08035 Barcelona, Spain. Tel/Fax +34 932746002. E-mail: jabarrabes@vhebron.net.

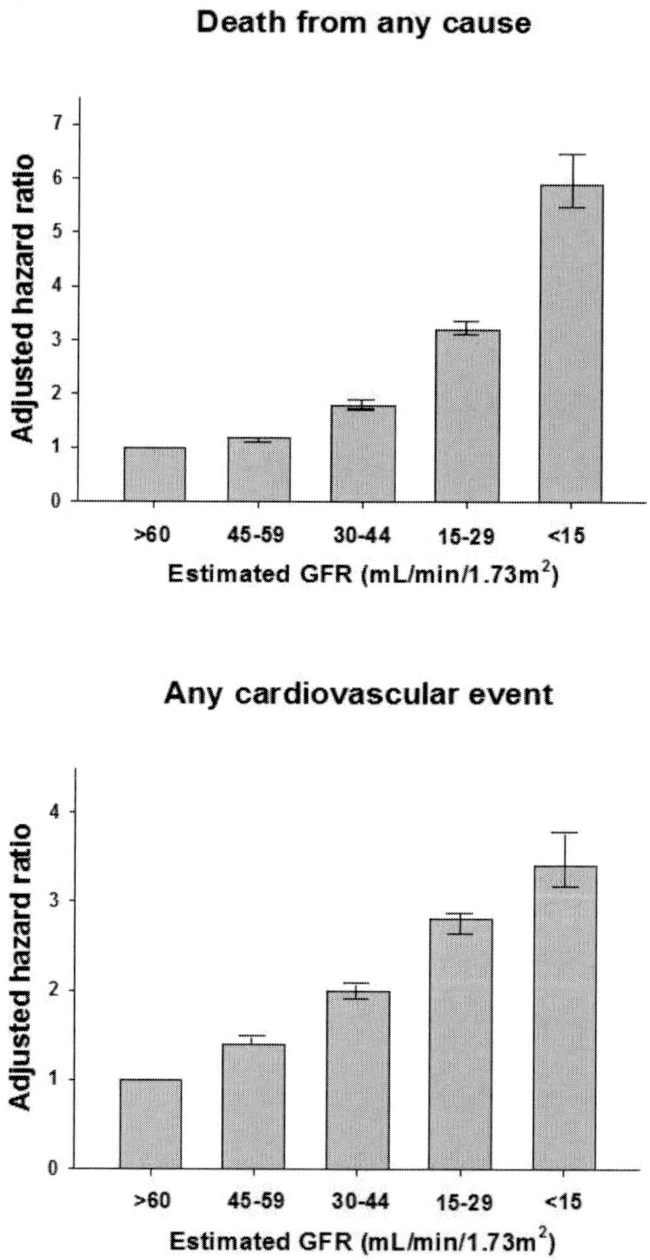

Figure 1. Adjusted hazard ratios for death from any cause and cardiovascular events among 1.120,295 ambulatory adults, according to the estimated glomerular filtration rate (adapted from Go et al. [3]).

EPIDEMIOLOGY

There is a wealth of data demonstrating a close association between chronic kidney disease (CKD) and cardiovascular disease, particularly coronary artery disease (CAD). About one half of deaths in patients with end-stage renal disease (ESRD) are of cardiovascular causes [1, 2], but less severe forms of CKD also increase cardiovascular risk, and patients with CKD are more likely to die of cardiovascular disease than to develop ESRD [1, 2]. In the largest study performed so far, Go et al. assessed the association between estimated glomerular filtration rate (GFR) and the risk of death, cardiovascular events, and hospitalization in 1.120,295 adults followed up for a median of 2.84 (interquartile range 1.65-4.01) years [3]. The risk of all these events increased sharply as GFR decreased (Figure 1). As compared with subjects with an estimated GFR ≥60 mL/min/1.73 m^2, the adjusted risk of cardiovascular events, defined as hospitalization for coronary disease, heart failure, stroke, or peripheral arterial disease, ranged from a 43% increase in subjects with an estimated GFR of 45-59 ≥mL/1.73 m^2 to a 343% increase with an estimated GFR of <15 mL/1.73 m^2 [3]. A large meta-analysis of population cohorts obtained similar results [4]. The association between CKD and cardiovascular disease has been reported not only in the general population but also in patients with hypertension [5], with other cardiovascular risk factors or stable cardiovascular disease [6] or with diabetes mellitus and macroalbuminuria [7].

Table 1. Estimation of cardiovascular risk according to the 2012 European Guidelines on cardiovascular disease prevention in clinical practice [18]

1. Very high risk. Subjects with any of the following:
   - Documented CVD by invasive or non-invasive testing, previous myocardial infarction, acute coronary syndrome, coronary revascularization and other arterial revascularization procedures, ischemic stroke, peripheral artery disease.
   - Diabetes mellitus (type 1 or type 2) with one or more cardiovascular risk factors and/or target organ damage (such as microalbuminuria).
   - Severe CKD (glomerular filtration rate <30 mL/min/1.73 m^2).
   - A calculated SCORE ≥10% for 10-year risk of fatal CVD.
2. High risk. Subjects with any of the following:
   - Markedly elevated single risk factors such as familial dyslipidemias and severe hypertension.
   - Diabetes mellitus (type 1 or type 2) but without cardiovascular risk factors or target organ damage.
   - Moderate CKD (glomerular filtration rate 30-59 mL/min/1.73 m^2).
   - A calculated SCORE ≥5% and <10% for 10-year risk of fatal CVD.
3. Moderate risk:
   - A calculated SCORE ≥1% and <5% at 10 years (further modulated by factors such as a family history of premature coronary artery disease, abdominal obesity, physical activity pattern, high density lipoprotein-cholesterol, triglycerides, hs-C-reactive protein, lipoprotein(a), fibrinogen, homocysteine, apolipoprotein-B, and social class).
4. Low risk:
   - A calculated SCORE <1% at 10 years without none of those qualifiers.

CVD, cardiovascular disease; CKD, chronic kidney disease.

Macro- and microalbuminuria have also been related to an increased cardiovascular risk even at levels of albumin excretion in the normal range [8, 9]. A large meta-analysis reported the existence of a lineal association between urine albumin excretion and total or cardiovascular mortality that was independent in part of GFR [4]. In this study, as compared to an albumin-to-creatinine ratio of 5 mg/g, hazard ratios for all-cause mortality at albumin-to-creatinine ratios of 10, 30, and 300 mg/g were 1.20 (95% CI 1.15-1.26), 1.63 (1.50-1.77), and 2.22 (1.97-2.51), respectively, and similar results were observed for cardiovascular mortality [4].

Pathophysiology

The association between CKD and ischemic heart disease can be explained in part because both conditions are related to the traditional risk factors for atherosclerotic vascular disease. However, CKD might also have a casual role in the development and progression of CAD, with several mechanisms potentially involved [9, 10]. First, microalbuminuria and GFR deterioration have been related to impaired flow-mediated vasodilatation and to increased levels of biochemical markers of endothelial damage or of asymmetric dimethylarginine and other nitric oxide synthase inhibitors, suggesting that CKD may induce endothelial dysfunction [11-13]. Second, chronic inflammation, as a consequence in part of increased oxidative stress, is frequent in CKD patients [9, 14] and could enhance the atherosclerotic process. Finally, CKD is also related to activation of the renin-angiotensin system and of the sympathetic nervous system, which may favor the progression of CAD through their causing hypertension or by direct effects on the coronary vasculature [9, 15]. A distinct feature of CAD in CKD patients is the high propensity to vascular calcification, which affects both the intima and the media, occurs typically in advanced stages of the disease and has a complex pathophysiology, related to the disease itself and to its therapy [9, 16].

Due to the strength of the epidemiological association between CKD and CAD and the biological plausibility of a cause-effect relationship, CKD is nowadays considered as a risk factor for cardiovascular events [17, 18] (Table 1).

Diagnosis

The diagnosis of CAD in patients with CKD is challenging, both in the acute setting and in stable conditions. A significant proportion of CKD patients with severe CAD are asymptomatic or have atypical symptoms [19], possibly due to autonomic dysfunction but also to the frequent association between CKD and advanced age or diabetes [20]. In addition, interpretation of the ECG is more difficult in these patients due to frequent confounders such as left ventricular hypertrophy, ST-segment deviation, T-wave changes or intraventricular conduction delays [21], that also complicate the interpretation of exercise ECG in these patients.

Among biomarkers, high-sensitivity troponins are of paramount importance for the evaluation of chest pain of suspected cardiac origin [22]. However, troponins are chronically elevated in CKD, for which reason considering higher cut-off values or looking at the change in troponin values among serial determinations has been proposed in these patients [23]. On the other hand, and despite these shortcomings for the diagnosis of acute myocardial infarction, cardiac troponins predict CAD, other structural heart disease and worse cardiac outcomes in CKD patients in the absence of suspected myocardial ischemia [24]. Copeptin, natriuretic peptides, and other biomarkers have shown some usefulness in the diagnostic or prognostic assessment of patients with suspected myocardial ischemia but their use is not routinely recommended in this clinical setting [22].

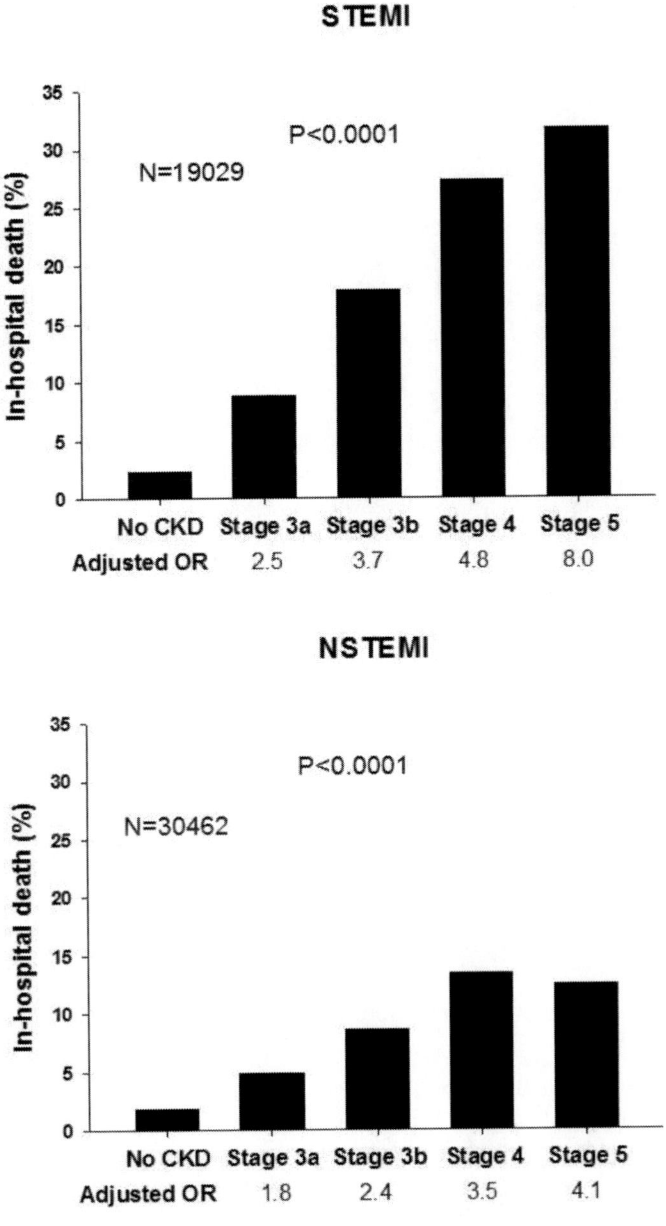

Figure 2. Crude rates and adjusted odds ratios (OR) for in-hospital death by chronic kidney disease (CKD) stages in patients hospitalized with ST-segment elevation myocardial infarction (STEMI) and non-ST-segment elevation myocardial infarction (NSTEMI) (adapted from Fox et al. [33]).

Stress imaging is preferred over exercise ECG for the non-invasive evaluation of ischemia [25, 26]. Because patients with CKD frequently have a reduced exercise capacity [27], pharmacological stress is often required. Stress single photon emission computed tomography or dobutamine echocardiography are the two techniques more widely used. Both are able to detect stress-induced ischemia and to assess global and regional ventricular function. The sensitivity and specificity of these techniques for the detection of significant CAD in CKD patients are variable and below the figures reported in the general population, particularly in ESRD [25, 26]. De Lima et al. compared the accuracy of these techniques for the detection of ischemia and the prediction of adverse events in 126 high-risk patients evaluated for renal transplant and observed that the sensitivity of both tests for CAD detection was below 75% and that their results were poorly related to cardiac events [28]. However, in a meta-analysis of 12 studies involving 913 patients with ESRD, inducible ischemia detected by either of these two techniques was a strong predictor of cardiac events and mortality [29] and in another recent meta-analysis of 52 studies including 7,401 potential kidney transplant recipients, these tests were as good as coronary angiography for predicting cardiovascular mortality and major cardiac adverse events [30]. Current AHA/ACC guidelines recommend that noninvasive stress testing may be considered in kidney transplantation candidates with no active cardiac conditions based on the presence of multiple CAD risk factors regardless of functional status [26].

Other imaging techniques have less value in CKD patients. There are limited data on computed tomographic angiography, but this technique is especially useful to rule out CAD in patients with a low pre-test probability, which is not the case in CKD patients, in whom, on the other hand, assessment of coronary lesions is often hampered by coronary calcification [25]. Cardiac magnetic resonance imaging is frequently contraindicated these patients due to the risk of gadolinium-associated systemic fibrosis.

Prognosis

Among CAD patients, those with CKD have systematically a worse prognosis than those without CKD irrespective of the clinical presentation or the treatments applied. Earlier reports showed very high in-hospital mortality in acute myocardial infarction patients with stage 5 CKD [31] and subsequent studies showed a graded rise in complications across increasing CKD strata, with patients with mild renal dysfunction also being at higher risk [32-34] (Figure 2). Similar results were obtained for non-ST-segment elevation acute coronary syndromes (NSTE-ACS) [33-35], and plasma creatinine level is one of the key components of the GRACE score for prediction of outcomes in patients admitted with acute coronary syndromes (ACS) [36].

Although the reasons for the worse prognosis in CKD patients are not fully understood, it is likely that more frequent comorbidities, a more extensive CAD, a more conservative management, both pharmacological and interventional, and an increased risk of bleeding and other complications contribute significantly [37]. Similarly to the acute setting, CKD confers a worse prognosis in patients with stable CAD [38, 39].

Pharmacologic Management

Since most randomized trials have excluded patients with severe CKD, there is limited evidence on the pharmacologic management of CAD in this population. Current therapy is based on small trials and observational data and by extrapolating the strategies that have proven useful in the general population [37], although many treatments that have shown to improve the prognosis of CAD patients are underused in those with renal impairment [33, 37].

a) Anti-ischemic drugs

Optimal medical treatment is especially important in CKD patients, in whom adequate revascularization is often not possible due to the presence of extensive CAD or to an increased risk of the procedure.

Beta blockers reduce myocardial oxygen demand and, by decreasing heart rate and prolonging diastole, also increase coronary perfusion and oxygen supply and are first-line antianginal drugs in stable CAD [40]. Among beta blockers, atenolol, nadolol, timolol and sotalol are water-soluble and have a predominant renal elimination, while metoprolol, propranolol, labetalol, carvedilol and nebivolol are lipid-soluble and metabolized mainly by the liver, for which reason they may be preferable in the presence of significant renal dysfunction. Bisoprolol has a combined route of elimination (50% renal, 50% hepatic), and esmolol is rapidly metabolized in red blood cells.

Calcium channel blockers are also first-line antianginal drugs [40]. These drugs, especially the dihydropyridine subfamily (e.g., nifedipine, amlodipine, or nicardipine), are potent vasodilators, and the non-dihydropyridines verapamil and diltiazem have negative inotropic and chronotropic effects that reduce oxygen consumption, contributing to angina relief. Their metabolism and elimination are greatly hepatic, so they can be used safely in CKD, although close surveillance is advised in severe renal impairment.

Nitrates induce systemic venodilation, which reduces preload, and coronary artery dilatation. Sublingual nitroglycerin gives a rapid relief of angina and is safe in CKD patients, although it can induce hypotension in patients with volume depletion, such as during or after hemodialysis. Long-acting nitrates have a good profile in CKD and there is no need for dose adjustment.

Ivabradine inhibits the If current in the sinoatrial node, reducing heart rate and improving angina. It can be used instead of or in association with beta blockers but should be avoided in patients receiving verapamil or diltiazem. Since there are limited data on the safety and efficacy of ivabradine in patients with advanced CKD, it should be used with caution in this population. Ranolazine does not have hemodynamic effects and improves angina by inhibiting the late phase of the inward sodium current. Ranolazine is metabolized in the liver and cleared by the kidney, so careful dose titration is advisable in patients with moderate renal dysfunction and is contraindicated in patients with severe renal impairment.

Nicorandil is a vasodilator drug acting as a nitrate and as a potassium channel opener. It is metabolized and mainly eliminated by the kidney but it can be used without restrictions in CKD. Trimetazidine, also a metabolic modulator, is a less proven, second- or third-line anti-ischemic drug. It is contraindicated in severe CKD and should be used with caution in moderate renal dysfunction. Trimetazidine could be useful in the prevention of contrast-induced nephropathy among patients with mild to moderate renal insufficiency.

b) Antiplatelet agents

Antiplatelet agents are mainstay in the treatment of CAD both in stable phases of the disease, when they are normally used in monotherapy, and following an ACS or percutaneous coronary intervention (PCI), when they are used in combination. CKD is of important concern when choosing an antiplatelet regimen, as it increases both thrombotic and bleeding risks [41]. A recent meta-analysis –using mainly post-hoc analyses of CKD subpopulations– of 36 trials of patients with ACS, PCI, stable or no cardiovascular disease suggested that the increased bleeding risk of aggressive antiplatelet regimens might outweigh their antithrombotic benefit in CKD patients [42]. The European Society of Cardiology Guidelines for the management of ACS without persistent ST-elevation recommend systematically assessing bleeding risk [22]. Renal function is a major determinant of one of the most used bleeding risk scores, the Can Rapid risk stratification of Unstable angina patients Suppress ADverse outcomes with Early implementation of the ACC/AHA guidelines (CRUSADE). This score ranges from 1 to 96 points, of which different degrees of renal impairment give 7 to 39, being the factor that scores the most [43]. Dose adjustment of antithrombotic drugs in CKD patients according to the abovementioned guidelines [22] is summarized in Table 2.

Table 2. Recommendations for the use of antithrombotic drugs in CKD (adapted from the 2011 European Society of Cardiology Guidelines for the management of acute coronary syndromes without persistent ST elevation [22])

Drug	Dose-adjustment	Particular recommendations
Antiplatelet agents		
Aspirin	No	Safe
Clopidogrel	No	Safe
Prasugrel	No	No experience in ESRD or dialysis
Ticagrelor	No	No experience in ESRD or dialysis
Abciximab	No	Careful evaluation of hemorrhagic risk needed
Eptifibatide	If GFR 30-49 mL/min, reduce infusion dose to 1.0 μg/kg/min (bolus 180 μg/kg unchanged)	Contraindicated if GFR <30 mL/min
Tirofiban	If GFR <30 mL/min: 50% of the bolus and infusion doses	
Anticoagulants		
UFH	No	Safe
Enoxaparin	If GFR <30 mL/min: dose reduction to 1.0 mg/kg/24h	Consider monitoring of anti-Xa activity
Fondaparinux	No	Drug of choice if GFR 30-60 mL/min. Contraindicated if GFR <20 mL/min.
Bivalirudin	No dose reduction (1.75 mg/kg/h) if GFR 30-59 ml/min. If GFR <30 mL/min reduce infusion dose to 1 mg/kg/h. In hemodialysis 0.25 mg/kg/h.	Contraindicated in GFR <30 ml/min

CKD, chronic kidney disease; ESRD, end-stage renal disease, GFR, glomerular filtration rate, UFH, unfractioned heparin.

Aspirin is the most frequently used antiplatelet agent. Data from observational registries and small trials suggest that it reduces ischemic complications without a significant excess of major bleeding across the spectrum of CKD severity [41, 44, 45].

Clopidogrel added to aspirin reduces the risk of ischemic events during the first year after an ACS. In a subanalysis of the Clopidogrel in Unstable Angina to Prevent Recurrent Events (CURE) trial, clopidogrel reduced ischemic events in all three tertiles of GFR, with an increase in bleeding that was not related to renal function [46].

Prasugrel is a more potent P2Y12 receptor antagonist. Levels of its active metabolite decrease significantly in ESRD, although with similar platelet inhibition [41]. In a large randomized clinical trial, prasugrel reduced ischemic events as compared with clopidogrel in ACS patients treated with PCI, at the cost of increasing bleeding [47]. The fact that this trial had a small proportion of CKD patients complicates the extrapolation of the results to the CKD population. In another study that compared the effect of prasugrel and clopidogrel in medically treated ACS patients, no treatment interactions for ischemic or bleeding events were observed with renal function [48].

Ticagrelor is another potent P2Y12 inhibitor that, as compared to clopidogrel, reduced ischemic events and mortality and increased non-coronary bypass surgery-related bleeding in ACS patients in the PLATO trial, which did not include patients on dialysis [49]. In this trial, 21% of patients had CKD and the reduction of events by ticagrelor was of greater magnitude in these patients than in those with normal renal function, although no statistically significant interactions for any treatment effects with renal function were detected [50].

Glycoprotein IIb/IIIa inhibitors added to double antiplatelet therapy provide some additional protection against thrombotic events but increase significantly the risk of bleeding in the general ACS population, so they should be used very cautiously, and at reduced doses when indicated, in CKD patients [22].

c) Anticoagulants and thrombolytics

Along with antiplatelet drugs, anticoagulants are essential in the treatment of ACS since they reduce significantly the rates of ischemic events. Unfractionated heparin (UHF) binds to endothelial cells and is cleared by macrophages, being theoretically the ideal anticoagulant for CKD because no dose adjustment is necessary. Nevertheless, continuous intravenous administration and frequent TTPa controls make it less applicable in daily practice.

Enoxaparin has a primarily renal clearance, so dose adjustment is necessary in severe renal dysfunction [22]. It has shown some benefit over UHF in reducing ischemic events in ACS patients presenting with and without ST elevation. Information on CKD patients is limited because most studies excluded those with severe renal dysfunction. Some studies did not find any significant interaction between the treatment applied and renal function for ischemic and bleeding events [51], whereas in others the benefit of enoxaparin over UFH appeared to be restricted to patients with normal renal function [52].

Fondaparinux is a synthetic heparin that inhibits factor Xa, has renal excretion and is contraindicated if GFR <20 mL/min. The OASIS-5 trial, that excluded patients with creatinine values ≥3 mg/dL, demonstrated non-inferiority of fondaparinux vs. enoxaparin in NSTE-ACS patients with less bleeding. A subgroup analysis showed that the benefit of fondaparinux on the composite endpoint was significant only in patients with GFR <58 mL/min [53], so it is an attractive choice for patients with moderate CKD.

Bivalirudin is a synthetic thrombin inhibitor with significant renal clearance and is contraindicated in ESRD [41]. It has shown similar antithrombotic efficacy with reduced bleeding as compared to the combination of heparin plus GPIIb/IIIa blockade in ACS patients with and without ST elevation treated with PCI. In a substudy of the ACUITY trial, these results were confirmed in patients with mild and moderate CKD [54].

Thrombolysis still has a role in the treatment of ST-elevation myocardial infarction when primary PCI is not readily available. Despite the increased bleeding risk in CKD, renal impairment is not a contraindication to thrombolysis. Among fibrinolytic agents, those fibrin-specific (alteplase, reteplase or tenecteplase) are preferred and there is no need for dose-adjustment in renal dysfunction [55].

d) Other drugs for secondary prevention

Studies have consistently shown that CAD patients with CKD, especially those with ESRD, are undertreated, receiving less often secondary prevention therapies such as aspirin, statins, angiotensin converting enzyme inhibitors and beta blockers [56, 57].

A post-hoc, pooled analysis of two large randomized trials comparing carvedilol vs. placebo in patients with heart failure (a large proportion of ischemic etiology) showed that, in the subset with mild to moderate CKD, carvedilol reduced all-cause and cardiovascular mortality and re-hospitalization rates [58]. Whether this therapy is similarly beneficial in patients with more advanced CKD remains to be elucidated, although a small trial that randomized patients with dilated cardiomyopathy (68% with ischemic heart disease) and ESRD on dialysis to receive carvedilol or placebo reported a significant improvement in functional class and left ventricle ejection fraction at one year in the carvedilol group [59].

Most trials that have evaluated the efficacy of angiotensin converting enzyme inhibitors or angiotensin receptor blockers for primary or secondary prevention of cardiovascular events excluded patients with CKD. Some small studies with fosinopril demonstrated efficacy for primary prevention. The HOPE trial, that excluded patients with serum creatinine >2.3 mg/dL, demonstrated that ramipril reduced the composite endpoint of cardiovascular death, stroke and myocardial infarction in a population with previous vascular disease. A post-hoc analysis in CKD patients was consistent with the overall results [6]. There is little information as to whether angiotensin receptor blockers can be protective in patients with CAD and CKD [57].

Many studies have demonstrated that aggressive LDL-cholesterol reduction reduces adverse outcomes in patients with or at risk of CAD. However, two randomized, placebo-controlled trials performed on ESRD patients on dialysis failed to show a reduction of ischemic events with atorvastatin [60] or rosuvastatin [61]. In contrast, a post-hoc analysis in stage 3 CKD patients from three trials comparing pravastatin with placebo (two of them in patients with previous myocardial infarction) demonstrated a significant reduction of cardiovascular events by the statin [62]. Registry data also support a protective effect of statins in CAD patients [63]. Finally, the SHARP trial randomized 9,270 CKD patients (including 3,023 on dialysis) without known history of myocardial infarction or coronary revascularization to simvastatin plus ezetimibe versus placebo and demonstrated a 17% reduction of atherosclerotic events after a median of 4.9 years of follow-up with the active therapy [64]. Importantly, this benefit was consistent across different GFR categories and in patients with or without dialysis therapy [64].

Coronary Revascularization

Many questions remain unanswered regarding the expected benefit of coronary revascularization in all CKD categories as well as its optimal timing, mode and technical approach. Again, these patients have frequently been excluded from randomized clinical trials. Nevertheless, although both coronary artery bypass surgery (CABG) and PCI are associated with an increased short-term rate of complications [65, 66], population studies suggest that CKD patients benefit from revascularization [67, 68]. However, coronary angiography and revascularization (either PCI or CABG) are underused after an acute myocardial infarction in patients with renal impairment [69], especially in those with severe CKD [70].

The current European Society of Cardiology Guidelines on myocardial revascularization [71] give some specific recommendations for CKD patients that are summarized in Table 3.

a) Revascularization in different clinical settings

Mild-to-moderate CKD is not associated with an increased incidence of restenosis after PCI in patients with stable CAD [72]. The benefits of coronary angiography and revascularization in these patients have not been demonstrated in the general population or in the subset with CKD. A subanalysis of CKD patients (most with moderate renal impairment) with stable CAD included in the Clinical Outcomes Utilizing Revascularization and Aggressive Drug Evaluation (COURAGE) trial showed that, similarly to the general study cohort, PCI added to optimal medical treatment did not offer any advantage in survival, protection from infarction or angina relief over medical therapy alone [73]. Considering these results and the risk of contrast-induced nephropathy, the decision of performing a coronary angiography has to be carefully considered in stable CAD patients with renal dysfunction.

There has been some controversy regarding the indication of an invasive management in NSTE-ACS patients with CKD, favored by the lack of randomized studies. A national registry including 23,262 patients with non-ST elevation myocardial infarction, 24.4% with moderate-to-severe CKD, reported that an early revascularization strategy was associated with lower 1-year mortality in patients with normal renal function or mild-to-moderate renal dysfunction but not in those with severe renal impairment or hemodialysis [70]. However, a recent meta-analysis of 7 studies with 23,234 NSTE-ACS patients with CKD showed that early revascularization was associated with an improved 1-year survival in all CKD stages, including dialysis patients [68]. These results suggest that, in NSTE-ACS patients with CKD, the indication of an invasive strategy should not differ from that in patients with normal renal function.

No specific trials have evaluated the effect of primary PCI for ST-elevation myocardial infarction in CKD patients. A report from the GRACE Registry showed that, in patients with moderate renal dysfunction, primary PCI was associated with mortality reduction at 6 months, which was not observed with thrombolysis or in severe renal dysfunction [74]. Despite their higher risk [31-34, 74], the indications of primary PCI in CKD patients are the same than in the general population [55].

b) Percutaneous vs. surgical revascularization

In patients with single-vessel disease (excluding the left main artery), PCI is in general preferable over CABG, but the decision about the best method of revascularization in those with multivessel disease is sometimes difficult and should be discussed by a multidisciplinary team including all the professionals involved [71]. In CKD patients, the decision can even be more challenging and a nephrologist should take part on it. Although no randomized trials have evaluated the best revascularization strategy in CKD, some observational studies have addressed this issue. In a regional registry of CAD patients undergoing coronary angiography, CABG was associated with a better survival in patients with normal renal function and in those with CKD, while PCI was advantageous compared to medical treatment in dialysis patients, although not in non-dialysis CKD [67]. A subanalysis of CKD patients included in the Arterial Revascularization Therapies Study (ARTS) trial, that assigned patients with multivessel disease to PCI or CABG, showed no differences in mortality, myocardial infarction or stroke at 3 years, but higher repeat revascularization rate for PCI [75]. In a single-center report, in patients with non-dialysis CKD and multivessel CAD, CABG led to better survival than PCI with drug-eluting stents, but CABG patients had a higher short-term risk of requiring permanent hemodialysis [65]. The analysis of a large registry database also including patients with single-vessel disease led to similar results, with lower incidence of ESRD throughout follow-up after PCI, but lower risks of death or combined death and ESRD after CABG [76]. A recent propensity-score analysis of a regional database of CKD patients with multivessel disease also showed that CABG was related to an increased survival and less coronary events compared to multivessel PCI [77].

Table 3. Recommendations for revascularization in patients with moderate or severe CKD according to the European Society of Cardiology guidelines on myocardial revascularization [71]

• CABG should be considered over PCI in patients with multivessel CAD and symptoms/ischemia whose surgical risk profile is acceptable and life expectancy is beyond 1 year (class IIa recommendation, level of evidence B). • PCI should be considered over CABG in patients with multivessel CAD and symptoms/ischemia whose surgical risk profile is high or life expectancy is less than 1 year (IIa, B). • It should be considered to delay CABG after coronary angiography until the effect of contrast media on renal function has subsided (IIa, B). • Off-pump CABG may be considered rather than on-pump CABG (IIb, B). • New-generation drug-eluting stents are recommended over bare metal stents (I, B).

CABG, coronary artery bypass surgery;
CAD, coronary artery disease;
CKD, chronic kidney disease;
PCI, percutaneous coronary intervention.

In the ESRD subpopulation, a registry with a 5-year follow-up showed no differences among CABG and PCI with respect to total mortality, but cardiac and sudden death were more frequent after PCI [78]. A meta-analysis of retrospective studies concluded that, despite being associated with an increased short-term mortality, CABG was superior to PCI in long-term survival and was related to lesser myocardial infarctions and repeat revascularization procedures [79].

The European Society of Cardiology Guidelines on myocardial revascularization recommend CABG over PCI in CKD patients with symptomatic multivessel CAD when the surgical risk is acceptable and life expectancy is >1 year [71].

c) Technical issues

In experienced hands the radial approach is the preferred method of access for coronary angiography since it reduces the incidence of bleeding events and mortality as compared with the femoral approach, at least in ACS patients [71, 80, 81] and might reduce as well the risk of acute kidney injury [82]. However, permanent damage of the radial artery can occur and may compromise the future creation of an arteriovenous fistula, which represents a concern in ESRD patients [37]. Iodinated contrast quantity must be reduced to the minimum.

As compared with bare metal stents, drug-eluting stents reduce the rate of restenosis but require a more prolonged duration of dual antiplatelet therapy. Some observational studies suggested that drug-eluting stents are associated with a better survival and fewer major adverse cardiovascular events in CKD patients than bare metal stents [83], but other studies did not find survival differences [84]. In a large cohort of patients older than 65 years, drug-eluting stents were associated with lower 30-month mortality in all CKD stages, lower 30-month myocardial infarction rate in all groups except long-term dialysis patients, and similar rates of revascularization and bleeding than bare metal stents [85]. Recently, Tomai et al. compared in a randomized trial the efficacy of a second-generation drug-eluting stent and a bare metal stent in 215 CKD patients with multivessel CAD (n = 512 vessels). The primary endpoint of ischemia-driven coronary revascularization at 1 year was significantly reduced by drug-eluting stents in a consistent manner across all CKD stages, including dialysis [86]. Thus, new-generation drug-eluting stents are recommended over bare metal stents in CKD patients [71].

In a CABG registry, no differences were observed in hospital mortality between on-pump versus off-pump CABG among patients without CKD, whereas off-pump surgery was associated with higher survival in those with renal dysfunction. Off-pump CABG was also related to a lesser incidence of postoperative renal replacement therapy, especially among the patients with poorer renal function [87]. In a recent randomized trial in which 24% of the patients had CKD with GFR 15-60 ml/min/1.73m^2, off-pump CABG was associated with significantly reduced rates of acute kidney injury than on-pump CABG, but long-term renal function was similar in both groups [88]. The current European Revascularization guidelines suggest that off-pump CABG may be considered over on-pump surgery in CKD patients [71].

CKD is associated with a worse outcome after any cardiac surgery, including CABG, as it increases the risks of bleeding and acute kidney injury. Renal dysfunction is one of the factors considered in the scores to calculate surgical risk (including euroSCORE). Ideally, surgery and postoperative management of these patients should be performed in centers experienced in complex cases, with all the facilities for renal replacement therapy and by a working team that includes nephrologists.

References

[1] Tonelli M, Wiebe N, Culleton B, House A, Rabbat C, Fok M, McAlister F, Garg AX. Chronic kidney disease and mortality risk: a systematic review. *J Am Soc Nephrol.* 2006;17:2034-47.

[2] United States Renal Data System. 2014 Annual Data Report. http://www.usrds.org/adr.aspx.

[3] Go AS, Chertow GM, Fan D, McCulloch CE, Hsu CY. Chronic kidney disease and the risks of death, cardiovascular events, and hospitalization. *N Engl J Med.* 2004;351:1296-305.

[4] Matsushita K, van der Velde M, Astor BC, Woodward M, Levey AS, de Jong PE, Coresh J, Gansevoort RT. Association of estimated glomerular filtration rate and albuminuria with all-cause and cardiovascular mortality in general population cohorts: a collaborative meta-analysis. *Lancet. 2010*; 375:2073-81.

[5] Ruilope LM, Salvetti A, Jamerson K, Hansson L, Warnold I, Wedel H, Zanchetti A. Renal function and intensive lowering of blood pressure in hypertensive participants of the hypertension optimal treatment (HOT) study. *J Am Soc Nephrol.* 2001;12:218-25.

[6] Mann JF, Gerstein HC, Pogue J, Bosch J, Yusuf S. Renal insufficiency as a predictor of cardiovascular outcomes and the impact of ramipril: the HOPE randomized trial. *Ann Intern Med.* 2001;134:629-36.

[7] de Zeeuw D, Remuzzi G, Parving HH, Keane WF, Zhang Z, Shahinfar S, Snapinn S, Cooper ME, Mitch WE, Brenner BM. Albuminuria, a therapeutic target for cardiovascular protection in type 2 diabetic patients with nephropathy. *Circulation.* 2004;110:921-7.

[8] Mann JF, Yi QL, Gerstein HC. Albuminuria as a predictor of cardiovascular and renal outcomes in people with known atherosclerotic cardiovascular disease. *Kidney Int Suppl.* 2004;92:S59-62.

[9] Schiffrin EL, Lipman ML, Mann JF. Chronic kidney disease: effects on the cardiovascular system. *Circulation.* 2007;116:85-97.

[10] Hajhosseiny R, Khavandi K, Goldsmith DJ. Cardiovascular disease in chronic kidney disease: untying the Gordian knot. *Int J Clin Pract.* 2013;67:14-31.

[11] Vallance P, Leone A, Calver A, Collier J, Moncada S. Accumulation of an endogenous inhibitor of nitric oxide synthesis in chronic renal failure. *Lancet.* 1992;339:572-5.

[12] Stehouwer CD, Henry RM, Dekker JM, Nijpels G, Heine RJ, Bouter LM. Microalbuminuria is associated with impaired brachial artery, flow-mediated vasodilation in elderly individuals without and with diabetes: further evidence for a link between microalbuminuria and endothelial dysfunction--the Hoorn Study. *Kidney Int Suppl.* 2004;92:S42-4.

[13] Stam F, van Guldener C, Becker A, Dekker JM, Heine RJ, Bouter LM, Stehouwer CD. Endothelial dysfunction contributes to renal function-associated cardiovascular

mortality in a population with mild renal insufficiency: the Hoorn study. *J Am Soc Nephrol.* 2006;17:537-45.

[14] Jofré R, Rodriguez-Benitez P, López-Gómez JM, Pérez-Garcia R. Inflammatory syndrome in patients on hemodialysis. *J Am Soc Nephrol.* 2006;17(Suppl 3):S274-80.

[15] Converse RL Jr, Jacobsen TN, Toto RD, Jost CM, Cosentino F, Fouad-Tarazi F, Victor RG. Sympathetic overactivity in patients with chronic renal failure. *N Engl J Med.* 1992;327:1912-8.

[16] Ketteler M, Schlieper G, Floege J. Calcification and cardiovascular health: new insights into an old phenomenon. *Hypertension.* 2006;47:1027-34.

[17] Catapano AL, Reiner Z, De Backer G, Graham I, Taskinen MR, Wiklund O, Agewall S, Alegria E, Chapman M, Durrington P, Erdine S, Halcox J, Hobbs R, Kjekshus J, Filardi PP, Riccardi G, Storey RF, Wood D; European Society of Cardiology (ESC); European Atherosclerosis Society (EAS). ESC/EAS Guidelines for the management of dyslipidaemias The Task Force for the management of dyslipidaemias of the European Society of Cardiology (ESC) and the European Atherosclerosis Society (EAS). *Atherosclerosis.* 2011;217:3-46.

[18] Perk J, De Backer G, Gohlke H, Graham I, Reiner Z, Verschuren M, Albus C, Benlian P, Boysen G, Cifkova R, Deaton C, Ebrahim S, Fisher M, Germano G, Hobbs R, Hoes A, Karadeniz S, Mezzani A, Prescott E, Ryden L, Scherer M, Syvänne M, Scholte op Reimer WJ, Vrints C, Wood D, Zamorano JL, Zannad F; European Association for Cardiovascular Prevention & Rehabilitation (EACPR); ESC Committee for Practice Guidelines (CPG). European Guidelines on cardiovascular disease prevention in clinical practice (version 2012). The Fifth Joint Task Force of the European Society of Cardiology and Other Societies on Cardiovascular Disease Prevention in Clinical Practice (constituted by representatives of nine societies and by invited experts). *Eur Heart J.* 2012;33:1635-701 [Erratum in: *Eur Heart J.* 2012;33:2126].

[19] Braun WE, Phillips DF, Vidt DG, Novick AC, Nakamoto S, Popowniak KL, Paganini E, Magnusson M, Pohl M, Steinmuller DR, et al. Coronary artery disease in 100 diabetics with end-stage renal failure. *Transplant Proc.* 1984;16:603-7.

[20] Canto JG, Fincher C, Kiefe CI, Allison JJ, Li Q, Funkhouser E, Centor RM, Selker HP, Weissman NW. Atypical presentations among Medicare beneficiaries with unstable angina pectoris. *Am J Cardiol.* 2002;90:248-53.

[21] Abe S, Yoshizawa M, Nakanishi N, Yazawa T, Yokota K, Honda M, Sloman G. Electrocardiographic abnormalities in patients receiving hemodialysis. *Am Heart J.* 1996;131:1137-44.

[22] Hamm CW, Bassand JP, Agewall S, Bax J, Boersma E, Bueno H, Caso P, Dudek D, Gielen S, Huber K, Ohman M, Petrie MC, Sonntag F, Uva MS, Storey RF, Wijns W, Zahger D; ESC Committee for Practice Guidelines. ESC Guidelines for the management of acute coronary syndromes in patients presenting without persistent ST-segment elevation: The Task Force for the management of acute coronary syndromes (ACS) in patients presenting without persistent ST-segment elevation of the European Society of Cardiology (ESC). *Eur Heart J.* 2011;32:2999-3054.

[23] Parikh RH, Seliger SL, deFilippi CR. Use and interpretation of high sensitivity cardiac troponins in patients with chronic kidney disease with and without acute myocardial infarction. *Clin Biochem.* 2015;48:247-53.

[24] deFilippi C, Wasserman S, Rosanio S, Tiblier E, Sperger H, Tocchi M, Christenson R, Uretsky B, Smiley M, Gold J, Muniz H, Badalamenti J, Herzog C, Henrich W. Cardiac troponin T and C-reactive protein for predicting prognosis, coronary atherosclerosis, and cardiomyopathy in patients undergoing long-term hemodialysis. *JAMA.* 2003;290:353-9.
[25] Karthikeyan V, Ananthasubramaniam K. Coronary risk assessment and management options in chronic kidney disease patients prior to kidney transplantation. *Curr Cardiol Rev. 2009*;5:177-86.
[26] Lentine KL, Costa SP, Weir MR, Robb JF, Fleisher LA, Kasiske BL, Carithers RL, Ragosta M, Bolton K, Auerbach AD, Eagle KA; American Heart Association Council on the Kidney in Cardiovascular Disease and Council on Peripheral Vascular Disease; American Heart Association; American College of Cardiology Foundation. Cardiac disease evaluation and management among kidney and liver transplantation candidates: a scientific statement from the American Heart Association and the American College of Cardiology Foundation: endorsed by the American Society of Transplant Surgeons, American Society of Transplantation, and National Kidney Foundation. *Circulation.* 2012;126:617-63.
[27] Ting SM, Hamborg T, McGregor G, Oxborough D, Lim K, Koganti S, Aldridge N, Imray C, Bland R, Fletcher S, Krishnan NS, Higgins RM, Townend J, Banerjee P, Zehnder D. Reduced cardiovascular reserve in chronic kidney failure: a matched cohort study. *Am J Kidney Dis.* 2015;66:274-84.
[28] De Lima JJ, Sabbaga E, Vieira ML, de Paula FJ, Ianhez LE, Krieger EM, Ramires JA. Coronary angiography is the best predictor of events in renal transplant candidates compared with noninvasive testing. *Hypertension.* 2003;42:263-8.
[29] Rabbat CG, Treleaven DJ, Russell JD, Ludwin D, Cook DJ. Prognostic value of myocardial perfusion studies in patients with end-stage renal disease assessed for kidney or kidney-pancreas transplantation: a meta-analysis. *J Am Soc Nephrol.* 2003;14:431-9.
[30] Wang LW, Masson P, Turner RM, Lord SW, Baines LA, Craig JC, Webster AC. Prognostic value of cardiac tests in potential kidney transplant recipients: a systematic review. *Transplantation.* 2015;99: 731-45.
[31] Herzog CA, Ma JZ, Collins AJ. Poor long-term survival after acute myocardial infarction among patients on long-term dialysis. *N Engl J Med.* 1998;339:799-805.
[32] Beattie JN, Soman SS, Sandberg KR, Yee J, Borzak S, Garg M, McCullough PA. Determinants of mortality after myocardial infarction in patients with advanced renal dysfunction. *Am J Kidney Dis.* 2001;37:1191-200. Erratum in: *Am J Kidney Dis* 2001;38:701.
[33] Fox CS, Muntner P, Chen AY, Alexander KP, Roe MT, Cannon CP, Saucedo JF, Kontos MC, Wiviott SD. Use of evidence-based therapies in short-term outcomes of ST-segment elevation myocardial infarction and non-ST-segment elevation myocardial infarction in patients with chronic kidney disease: a report from the National Cardiovascular Data Acute Coronary Treatment and Intervention Outcomes Network registry. *Circulation* 2010;121:357-365.
[34] Marenzi G, Cabiati A, Assanelli E. Chronic kidney disease in acute coronary syndromes. *World J Nephrol.* 2012;1:134-45.

[35] Santopinto JJ, Fox KA, Goldberg RJ, Budaj A, Piñero G, Avezum A, Gulba D, Esteban J, Gore JM, Johnson J, Gurfinkel EP; GRACE Investigators. Creatinine clearance and adverse hospital outcomes in patients with acute coronary syndromes: findings from the global registry of acute coronary events (GRACE). *Heart.* 2003;89:1003-8.

[36] Granger CB, Goldberg RJ, Dabbous O, Pieper KS, Eagle KA, Cannon CP, Van De Werf F, Avezum A, Goodman SG, Flather MD, Fox KA; Global Registry of Acute Coronary Events Investigators. Predictors of hospital mortality in the global registry of acute coronary events. *Arch Intern Med.* 2003;163:2345-53.

[37] Marenzi G, Cosentino N, Guastoni C. How to balance risks and benefits in the management of CKD patients with coronary artery disease. *J Nephrol.* 2015;28:403-13.

[38] Sedlis SP, Jurkovitz CT, Hartigan PM, Goldfarb DS, Lorin JD, Dada M, Maron DJ, Spertus JA, Mancini GB, Teo KK, O'Rourke RA, Boden WE, Weintraub WS; COURAGE Study Investigators. Optimal medical therapy with or without percutaneous coronary intervention for patients with stable coronary artery disease and chronic kidney disease. *Am J Cardiol.* 2009;104:1647-53.

[39] Mohandas R, Segal MS, Huo T, Handberg EM, Petersen JW, Johnson BD, Sopko G, Bairey Merz CN, Pepine CJ. Renal function and coronary microvascular dysfunction in women with symptoms/signs of ischemia. *PLoS One.* 2015;10:e0125374.

[40] Montalescot G, Sechtem U, Achenbach S, et al. 2013 ESC guidelines on the management of stable coronary artery disease: the Task Force on the management of stable coronary artery disease of the European Society of Cardiology. *Eur Heart J.* 2013;34:2949-3003.

[41] Basra SS, Tsai P, Lakkis NM. Safety and efficacy of antiplatelet and antithrombotic therapy in acute coronary syndrome patients with chronic kidney disease. *J Am Coll Cardiol.* 2011;58:2263-9.

[42] Palmer SC, Di Micco L, Razavian M, Craig JC, Perkovic V, Pellegrini F, Copetti M, Graziano G, Tognoni G, Jardine M, Webster A, Nicolucci A, Zoungas S, Strippoli GF. Effects of antiplatelet therapy on mortality and cardiovascular and bleeding outcomes in persons with chronic kidney disease: a systematic review and meta-analysis. *Ann Intern Med.* 2012;156:445-59.

[43] Subherwal S, Bach RG, Chen AY, Gage BF, Rao SV, Newby LK, Wang TY, Gibler WB, Ohman EM, Roe MT, Pollack CV Jr., Peterson ED, Alexander KP. Baseline risk of major bleeding in non-ST-segment-elevation myocardial infarction: the CRUSADE (Can Rapid risk stratification of Unstable angina patients Suppress ADverse outcomes with Early implementation of the ACC/AHA Guidelines) Bleeding Score. *Circulation.* 2009;119:1873-82.

[44] Berger AK, Duval S, Krumholz HM. Aspirin, beta-blocker, and angiotensin-converting enzyme inhibitor therapy in patients with end-stage renal disease and an acute myocardial infarction. *J Am Coll Cardiol.* 2003;42:201-8.

[45] Baigent C, Landray M, Leaper C, Altmann P, Armitage J, Baxter A, Cairns HS, Collins R, Foley RN, Frighi V, Kourellias K, Ratcliffe PJ, Rogerson M, Scoble JE, Tomson CR, Warwick G, Wheeler DC. First United Kingdom Heart and Renal Protection (UK-HARP-I) study: biochemical efficacy and safety of simvastatin and safety of low-dose aspirin in chronic kidney disease. *Am J Kidney Dis.* 2005;45:473-84.

[46] Keltai M, Tonelli M, Mann JF, Sitkei E, Lewis BS, Hawken S, Mehta SR, Yusuf S; CURE Trail Investigators. Renal function and outcomes in acute coronary syndrome: impact of clopidogrel. *Eur J Cardiovasc Prev Rehabil.* 2007;14:312-8.

[47] Wiviott SD, Braunwald E, McCabe CH, Montalescot G, Ruzyllo W, Gottlieb S, Neumann FJ, Ardissino D, De Servi S, Murphy SA, Riesmeyer J, Weerakkody G, Gibson CM, Antman EM; TRITON-TIMI 38 Investigators. Prasugrel versus clopidogrel in patients with acute coronary syndromes. *N Engl J Med.* 2007;357:2001-15.

[48] Melloni C, Cornel JH, Hafley G, Neely ML, Clemmensen P, Zamoryakhin D, Prabhakaran D, White HD, Fox KA, Ohman EM, Armstrong PW, Roe MT. Impact of chronic kidney disease on long-term ischemic and bleeding outcomes in medically managed patients with acute coronary syndromes: Insights from the TRILOGY ACS Trial. *Eur Heart J Acute Cardiovasc Care.* 2015, Jul 30.

[49] Wallentin L, Becker RC, Budaj A, Cannon CP, Emanuelsson H, Held C, Horrow J, Husted S, James S, Katus H, Mahaffey KW, Scirica BM, Skene A, Steg PG, Storey RF, Harrington RA; PLATO Investigators, Freij A, Thorsén M. Ticagrelor versus clopidogrel in patients with acute coronary syndromes. *N Engl J Med.* 2009;361:1045-57.

[50] James S, Budaj A, Aylward P, Buck KK, Cannon CP, Cornel JH, Harrington RA, Horrow J, Katus H, Keltai M, Lewis BS, Parikh K, Storey RF, Szummer K, Wojdyla D, Wallentin L. Ticagrelor versus clopidogrel in acute coronary syndromes in relation to renal function: results from the Platelet Inhibition and Patient Outcomes (PLATO) trial. *Circulation.* 2010;122:1056-67.

[51] Spinler SA, Mahaffey KW, Gallup D, Levine GN, Ferguson JJ 3rd, Rao SV, Gallo R, Ducas J, Goodman SG, Antman E, White HD, Biasucci L, Becker RC, Col JJ, Cohen M, Harrington RA, Califf RM; SYNERGY Trial Investigators. Relationship between renal function and outcomes in high-risk patients with non-ST-segment elevation acute coronary syndromes: results from SYNERGY. *Int J Cardiol.* 2010 Sep 24;144(1):36-41.

[52] Fox KA, Antman EM, Montalescot G, Agewall S, SomaRaju B, Verheugt FW, Lopez-Sendon J, Hod H, Murphy SA, Braunwald E. The impact of renal dysfunction on outcomes in the ExTRACT-TIMI 25 trial. *J Am Coll Cardiol.* 2007;49:2249-55.

[53] Fox KA, Bassand JP, Mehta SR, Wallentin L, Theroux P, Piegas LS, Valentin V, Moccetti T, Chrolavicius S, Afzal R, Yusuf S. Influence of renal function on the efficacy and safety of fondaparinux relative to enoxaparin in non ST-segment elevation acute coronary syndromes. *Ann Intern Med.* 2007;147:304-10.

[54] Mehran R, Nikolsky E, Lansky AJ, Kirtane AJ, Kim YH, Feit F, Manoukian S, Moses JW, Ebrahimi R, Ohman EM, White HD, Pocock SJ, Dangas GD, Stone GW. Impact of chronic kidney disease on early (30-day) and late (1-year) outcomes of patients with acute coronary síndromes treated with alternative antithrombotic treatment strategies: an ACUITY (Acute Catheterization and Urgent Intervention Triage strategY) substudy. *JACC Cardiovasc Interv.* 2009;2:748-57.

[55] Steg PG, James SK, Atar D, Badano LP, Blömstrom-Lundqvist C, Borger MA, Di Mario C, Dickstein K, Ducrocq G, Fernandez-Aviles F, Gershlick AH, Giannuzzi P, Halvorsen S, Huber K, Juni P, Kastrati A, Knuuti J, Lenzen MJ, Mahaffey KW, Valgimigli M, van 't Hof A, Widimsky P, Zahger D. Task Force on the management of

ST-segment elevation acute myocardial infarction of the European Society of Cardiology (ESC). ESC Guidelines for the management of acute myocardial infarction in patients presenting with ST-segment elevation. *Eur Heart J.* 2012;33:2569-619.

[56] Shlipak MG, Heidenreich PA, Noguchi H, Chertow GM, Browner WS, McClellan MB. Association of renal insufficiency with treatment and outcomes after myocardial infarction in elderly patients. *Ann Intern Med.* 2002;137:555-62.

[57] Afsar B, Turkmen K, Covic A, Kanbay M. An update on coronary artery disease and chronic kidney disease. *Int J Nephrol.* 2014;2014:767424.

[58] Wali RK, Iyengar M, Beck GJ, Chartyan DM, Chonchol M, Lukas MA, Cooper C, Himmelfarb J, Weir MR, Berl T, Henrich WL, Cheung AK. Efficacy and safety of carvedilol in treatment of heart failure with chronic kidney disease: a meta-analysis of randomized trials. *Circ Heart Fail.* 2011;4:18-26.

[59] Cice G, Ferrara L, Di Benedetto A, Russo PE, Marinelli G, Pavese F, Iacono A. Dilated cardiomyopathy in dialysis patients—beneficial effects of carvedilol: a double-blind, placebo-controlled trial. *J Am Coll Cardiol.* 2001;2:407-11.

[60] Wanner C, Krane V, März W, Olschewski M, Mann JF, Ruf G, Ritz E; German Diabetes and Dialysis Study Investigators. Atorvastatin in patients with type 2 diabetes mellitus undergoing hemodialysis. *N Engl J Med.* 2005;3:238-48.

[61] Fellström BC, Jardine AG, Schmieder RE, Holdaas H, Bannister K, Beutler J, Chae DW, Chevaile A, Cobbe SM, Grönhagen-Riska C, De Lima JJ, Lins R, Mayer G, McMahon AW, Parving HH, Remuzzi G, Samuelsson O, Sonkodi S, Sci D, Süleymanlar G, Tsakiris D, Tesar V, Todorov V, Wiecek A, Wüthrich RP, Gottlow M, Johnsson E, Zannad F; AURORA Study Group. Rosuvastatin and cardiovascular events in patients undergoing hemodialysis. *N Engl J Med.* 2009;14:1395-407.

[62] Tonelli M, Isles C, Curhan GC, Tonkin A, Pfeffer MA, Shepherd J, Sacks FM, Furberg C, Cobbe SM, Simes J, Craven T, West M. Effect of pravastatin on cardiovascular events in people with chronic kidney disease. *Circulation.* 2004;110:1557-63.

[63] Dasari TW, Cohen DJ, Kleiman NS, Keyes MJ, Yen CH, Hanna EB, Saucedo JF. Statin therapy in patients with chronic kidney disease undergoing percutaneous coronary intervention (from the Evaluation of Drug Eluting Stents and Ischemic Events Registry. *Am J Cardiol.* 2014;113:621-5.

[64] Baigent C, Landray MJ, Reith C, Emberson J, Wheeler DC, Tomson C, Wanner C, Krane V, Cass A, Craig J, Neal B, Jiang L, Hooi LS, Levin A, Agodoa L, Gaziano M, Kasiske B, Walker R, Massy ZA, Feldt-Rasmussen B, Krairittichai U, Ophascharoensuk V, Fellström B, Holdaas H, Tesar V, Wiecek A, Grobbee D, de Zeeuw D, Grönhagen-Riska C, Dasgupta T, Lewis D, Herrington W, Mafham M, Majoni W, Wallendszus K, Grimm R, Pedersen T, Tobert J, Armitage J, Baxter A, Bray C, Chen Y, Chen Z, Hill M, Knott C, Parish S, Simpson D, Sleight P, Young A, Collins R; SHARP Investigators. The effects of lowering LDL cholesterol with simvastatin plus ezetimibe in patients with chronic kidney disease (Study of Heart and Renal Protection): a randomised placebo-controlled trial. *Lancet.* 2011;377:2181-92.

[65] Ashrith G, Lee VV, Elayda MA, Reul RM, Wilson JM. Short- and long-term outcomes of coronary artery bypass grafting or drug-eluting stent implantation for multivessel coronary artery disease in patients with chronic kidney disease. *Am J Cardiol.* 2010;106:348-53.

[66] Gupta T, Paul N, Kolte D, Harikrishnan P, Khera S, Aronow WS, Mujib M, Palaniswamy C, Sule S, Jain D, Ahmed A, Cooper HA, Frishman WH, Bhatt DL, Fonarow GC, Panza JA. Associtation of chronic renal insufficiency with in-hospital outcomes after percutaneous coronary intervention. *J Am Heart Assoc.* 2015;4:e002069.

[67] Hemmelgarn BR, Southern D, Culleton BF, Mitchell LB, Knudtson ML, Ghali WA. Survival after coronary revascularization among patients with kidney disease. *Circulation.* 2004;110:1890-5.

[68] Huang HD, Alam M, Hamzeh I, Virani S, Deswal A, Aguilar D, Rogers P, Kougias P, Birnbaum Y, Paniagua D, Kar B, Ballantyne C, Bozkurt B, Jneid H. Patients with severe chronic kidney disease benefit from early revascularization after acute coronary syndrome. *Int J Cardiol* 2013; 168:3741–3746.

[69] Charytan D, Mauri L, Agarwal A, Servoss S, Scirica B, Kuntz RE. The use of invasive cardiac procedures after acute myocardial infarction in long-term dialysis patients. *Am Heart J.* 2006;152:558-64.

[70] Szummer K, Lundman P, Jacobson SH, Schon S, Lindback J, Stenestrand U, Wallentin L, Jernberg T. Influence of renal function on the effects of early revascularization in non-ST-elevation myocardial infarction: data from the Swedish WebSystem for Enhancement and Development of Evidence-Based Care in Heart Disease Evaluated According to Recommended Therapies (SWEDEHEART). *Circulation.* 2009;120:851-8.

[71] Windecker S, Kolh P, Alfonso F, Collet JP, Cremer J, Falk V, Filippatos G, Hamm C, Head SJ, Jüni P, Kappetein AP, Kastrati A, Knuuti J, Landmesser U, Laufer G, Neumann FJ, Richter DJ, Schauerte P, Sousa Uva M, Stefanini GG, Taggart DP, Torracca L, Valgimigli M, Wijns W, Witkowski A. 2014 ESC/EACTS Guidelines on myocardial revascularization: The Task Force on Myocardial Revascularization of the European Society of Cardiology and the European Association for Cardio-Thoracic Surgery, developed with the special contribution of the European Associtation of Percutaneous Cardiovascular Interventions. *Eur Heart J.* 2014;35:2541-619.

[72] Best PJ, Berger PB, Davis BR, Grines CL, Sadeghi HM, Williams BA, Willerson JT, Granett JR, Holmes DR Jr; PRESTO Investigators. Impact of mild or moderate chronic kidney disease on the frequency of restenosis: results from the PRESTO trial. *J Am Coll Cardiol.* 2004;44:1786-91.

[73] Sedlis SP, Jurkovitz CT, Hartigan PM, Goldfarb DS, Lorin JD, Dada M, Maron DJ, Spertus JA, Mancini GB, Teo KK, O'Rourke RA, Boden WE, Weintraub WS. Optimal medical therapy with or without percutaneous coronary intervention for patients with stable coronary artery disease and chronic kidney disease. *Am J Cardiol.* 2009;104:1647-53.

[74] Medi C, Montalescot G, Budaj A, Fox KA, López-Sendón J, FitzGerald G, Brieger DB; GRACE Investigators. Reperfusion in patients with renal dysfunction after presentation with ST-segment elevation or left bundle branch block: GRACE (Global Registry of Acute Coronary Events). *JACC Cardiovasc Interv.* 2009;2:26-33.

[75] Ix JH, Mercado N, Shlipak MG, Lemos PA, Boersma E, Lindeboom W, O'Neill WW, Wijns W, Serruys PW. Association of chronic kidney disease with clinical outcomes after coronary revascularization: the Arterial Revascularization Therapies Study (ARTS). *Am Heart J.* 2005;149:512-9.

[76] Charytan DM, Li S, Liu J, Herzog CA. Risks of death and end-stage renal disease after surgical compared with percutaneous coronary revascularization in elderly patients with chronic kidney disease. *Circulation*. 2012;126:S164-9.
[77] Chang TI, Leong TK, Kazi DS, Lee HS, Hlatky MA, Go AS. Comparative effectiveness of coronary artery bypass grafting and percutaneous coronary intervention for multivessel coronary disease in a community-based population with chronic kidney disease. *Am Heart J*. 2013;165:800-8.
[78] Marui A, Kimura T, Nishiwaki N, Mitsudo K, Komiya T, Hanyu M, Shiomi H, Tanaka S, Sakata R. Percutaneous coronary intervention versus coronary artery bypass grafting in patients with end-stage renal disease requiring dialysis (5-year outcomes of the CREDO-Kyoto PCI/CABG Registry Cohort-2). *Am J Cardiol*. 2014;114:555-61.
[79] Zheng H, Xue S, Lian F, Huang RT, Hu ZL, Wang YY. Meta-analysis of clinical studies comparing coronary artery bypass grafting with percutaneous coronary intervention in patients with end-stage renal disease. *Eur J Cardiothorac Surg*. 2013;43:459-67.
[80] Jolly SS, Yusuf S, Cairns J, Niemelä K, Xavier D, Widimsky P, Budaj A, Niemelä M, Valentin V, Lewis BS, Avezum A, Steg PG, Rao SV, Gao P, Afzal R, Joyner CD, Chrolavicius S, Mehta SR; RIVAL trial group. Radial versus femoral access for coronary angiography and intervention in patients with acute coronary syndromes (RIVAL): a randomised, parallel group, multicentre trial. *Lancet*. 2011 23;377:1409-20. Erratum in: Lancet. 2011;377:1408. *Lancet*. 2011;378:30.
[81] Valgimigli M, Gagnor A, Calabró P, Frigoli E, Leonardi S, Zaro T, Rubartelli P, Briguori C, Andò G, Repetto A, Limbruno U, Cortese B, Sganzerla P, Lupi A, Galli M, Colangelo S, Ierna S, Ausiello A, Presbitero P, Sardella G, Varbella F, Esposito G, Santarelli A, Tresoldi S, Nazzaro M, Zingarelli A, de Cesare N, Rigattieri S, Tosi P, Palmieri C, Brugaletta S, Rao SV, Heg D, Rothenbühler M, Vranckx P, Jüni P; MATRIX Investigators. Radial versus femoral access in patients with acute coronary syndromes undergoing invasive management: a randomised multicentre trial. *Lancet*. 2015;385:2465-76.
[82] Kooiman J, Seth M, Dixon S, Wohns D, LaLonde T, Rao SV, Gurm HS. Risk of acute kidney injury after percutaneous coronary interventions using radial versus femoral vascular access: insights from the Blue Cross Blue Shield of Michigan Cardiovascular Consortium. *Circ Cardiovasc Interv*. 2014;7:190-8.
[83] Shenoy C, Boura J, Orshaw P, Harjai KJ. Drug-eluting stents in patients with chronic kidney disease: a prospective registry study. *PLoS One*. 2010;5:e15070.
[84] Green SM, Selzer F, Mulukutla SR, Tadajweski EJ, Green JA, Wilensky RL, Laskey WK, Cohen HA, Rao SV, Weisbord SD, Lee JS, Reis SE, Kip KE, Kelsey SF, Williams DO, Marroquin OC. Comparison of bare-metal and drug-eluting stents in patients with chronic kidney disease (from the NHLBI Dynamic Registry). *Am J Cardiol*. 2011;108:1658-64.
[85] Tsai TT, Messenger JC, Brennan JM, Patel UD, Dai D, Piana RN, Anstrom KJ, Eisenstein EL, Dokholyan RS, Peterson ED, Douglas PS. Safety and efficacy of drug-eluting stents in older patients with chronic kidney disease: a report from the linked CathPCI Registry-CMS claims database. *J Am Coll Cardiol*. 2011;58:1859-69.
[86] Tomai F, Ribichini F, De Luca L, Petrolini A, Ghini AS, Weltert L, Spaccarotella C, Proietti I, Trani C, Nudi F, Pighi M, Vassanelli C. Randomized comparison of Xience

V and Multi-Link Vision coronary stents in the same multivessel patient with chronic kidney disease (RENAL-DES) study. *Circulation.* 2014;129:1104-12.

[87] Chawla LS, Zhao Y, Lough FC, Schroeder E, Seneff MG, Brennan JM. Off-pump vs. on-pump coronary artery bypass grafting outcomes stratified by preoperative renal function. *J Am Soc Nephrol.* 2012; 23:1389-97.

[88] Garg AX, Deveraux PJ, Yusuf S, Cuerden MS, Parikh CR, Coca SG, Walsh M, Novick R, Cook RJ, Jain AR, Pan X, Noiseux N, Vik K, Stolf NA, Ritchie A, Favaloro RR, Parvathanemi S, Whitlock RP, Ou Y, Lawrence M, Lamy A. Kidney function after off-pump or on-pump coronary artery bypass graft surgery: a randomized clinical trial. *JAMA.* 2014;311:2191-8.

In: Comorbidities in Chronic Kidney Disease
Editor: Luca Di Lullo
ISBN: 978-1-63485-070-4

Chapter 7

ARRHYTHMIAS AND SUDDEN CARDIAC DEATH IN CHRONIC KIDNEY DISEASE

Rodolfo F. Rivera*
Division of Nephrology and Dialysis,
San Gerardo Hospital, Monza, Italy

ABSTRACT

Patients with chronic kidney disease (CKD) have a marked increase in the risk of cardiovascular mortality, and the risk of sudden cardiac death (SCD) increases as renal function declines.

In the general population, coronary artery disease (CAD) associated risk factors are the major determinants of occurrence of SCD. However current evidence suggests that in CKD patients, these factors has a lesser important role. Complex relationships between CKD-specific risk factors, structural heart disease, and ventricular arrhythmias (VA) contribute to the high risk of SCD. In dialysis patients, the occurrence of VA and SCD could be exacerbated by electrolyte shifts, divalent ion abnormalities, sympathetic over activity, in addition to inflammation and perhaps iron deposition.

The proportion of individuals with CKD is growing, the incidence of cardiovascular disease is high, the risk of cardiac death in these patients is high, and survival of CKD patients after cardiac arrest is poor.

Primary and secondary prevention of cardiac arrest could reduce cardiovascular mortality in patients with CKD.

Keywords: CKD, cardiovascular mortality, cardiac arrhythmias, sudden cardiac death

* Correspondence to: R.F. Rivera, Division of Nephrology and Dialysis, San Gerardo Hospital, Monza, Italy. Email: rodolforivera@gmail.com.

Introduction

Cardiovascular diseases (CVD) continue to be the leading cause of death for both men and women worldwide and account for approximately 50% of the highly premature mortality observed in chronic kidney disease (CKD) patients. CKD affects approximately 13% of the adult population in the United States and the prevalence at any stage continues to rise as the population ages, and obesity, hypertension, and diabetes increase in prevalence.

These patients are exposed to substantial hemodynamic stress and metabolic perturbations, which predispose them to cardiomyopathy, atherosclerosis, and arteriosclerosis. A clinical and a complex pathophysiology overlap between CKD and CVD is increasingly being recognized. Heart and kidney disease are very common, frequently coexist, significantly increase morbidity and mortality and lead to increase the complexity and cost of care. Recently, the Acute Dialysis Quality Initiative (ADQI) Working Group convened a consensus conference to develop a classification scheme for the Cardio-Renal Syndrome (CRS) for five discrete subtypes [1]. These CRS subtypes likely share pathophysiologic mechanisms, however they also have distinguishing clinical features, in terms of precipitating events, risk identification, natural history, and outcomes (Figure 1).

The elevated risk of CV morbidity and mortality in patients with CRS often precedes progression to end-stage renal disease (ESRD) and dialysis [2–4]. For this reason, a good knowledge of the heart-kidney interaction stratified for different subtypes of CRS is fundamental not only to understand the phenomena associated with morbidity and mortality but also to optimizing health resource utilization. Mortality attributed to sudden cardiac death (SCD) is about 14-fold increased among dialysis patients when compared to non-renal subjects with cardiovascular history, and this finding had always been considered as a complications of atherosclerotic disease [5].

Many authors have tried to identify factors associated with the risk of SCD in CKD patients.

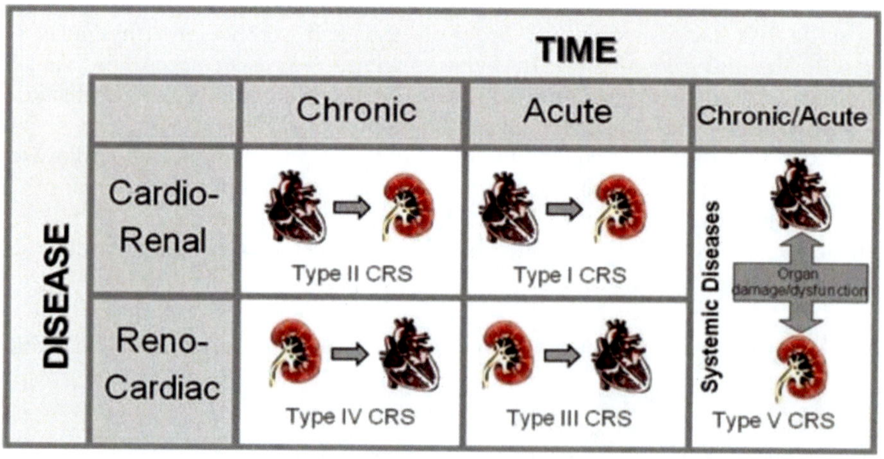

Figure 1. Cardiorenal Syndrome Classification [1].

Since a considerable proportion of cardiac deaths are not directly linked to myocardial infarction (MI), stroke, or chronic heart failure (CHF), other risk factors than traditional ones are under investigation [5, 6]. Kidney dysfunction has recently been considered as an independent risk factor for SCD, which has been adjudicated as a distinct endpoint in various cohort studies and clinical trials. This review examines recent data on the epidemiology, pathophysiology, and mechanisms of SCD among CKD patients and examines current evidence regarding the use of pharmacologic and non-pharmacologic (device-based) therapies for the management of SCD risk.

EPIDEMIOLOGY

Incidence of Cardiac Sudden Death in General Population

SCD is a sudden, unexpected death caused by loss of heart function (sudden cardiac arrest). In general, SCD events are defined as those that either are preceded by a witnessed collapse, occur within one hour of an acute change in clinical condition, or occur not more than twenty-four hours since the deceased individual was known to be in his or her usual state of health [7, 8]. It is the largest cause of natural death in the U.S., causing more than 300,000 adult deaths each year. SCD is responsible for half of all heart disease deaths.

Although major advances in cardiopulmonary resuscitation and post-critical care in recent years, survival to hospital discharge after cardiac arrest remains poor. In the general population, SCD was recently estimated to be about 8% of the out-of-hospital cardiac arrests that were treated by emergency medical services personnel [9]. Unfortunately, the majority of SCDs occur at home, where the event happens in the absence of relatives or other witnesses.

A correct *clinical* identification of patients at high risk is crucial for rational management, given the demonstrated effectiveness of implantable cardioverter-defibrillators (ICD) on the reduction of SCD.

Approximately 50% of all coronary artery disease (CAD) deaths are sudden and unexpected, often occurring shortly after the onset of symptoms [10]. Since CAD is the dominant cause of both sudden and non-sudden cardiac deaths in the U.S. and Europe, the fraction of total cardiac deaths that are sudden is similar to the fraction of CAD deaths that are sudden. In addition, it is quite interesting that the age-adjusted decline in CAD mortality in the U.S. during the last decades has not changed the number of coronary deaths that are sudden and unexpected [11, 12]. Furthermore, the decreasing age-adjusted mortality does not imply a decrease in absolute numbers of SCD because of the growth and aging of the population, as well as the increasing prevalence of chronic heart disease [13, 14].

Based on the results of multiple clinical trials, systolic left ventricular dysfunction expressed reduction in Left Ventricular Ejection Fraction (LVEF) using New York Heart Association functional classification (NYHA) is an important diagnostic risk factor for SCD. This is currently the only recommended diagnostic and clinical criterion to identify higher risk patients that would benefit from prophylactic cardioverter-defibrillators (ICDs) for the primary prevention of SCD [15]. However, the systematic implementation of prophylactic ICD recommendations results in a substantial number of inappropriate ICD implantations, while failing to prevent the majority of SCD occurring in the general population.

Current international guidelines consider LVEF $\leq$35% as a criterion for ICD implantation as the primary preventive measure in patients with Non-ischemic CHF. However, it is interesting that, although LVEF is considered a major risk factor for SCD, several other events occur in patients with LVEF >35% [17]. In addition, the relative risk of SCD is significantly higher in patients with LVEF ≤35% than in those with LVEF >35%. The absolute number of SCD cases is higher among patients with more preserved LVEF, considering that these patients represent a much larger subgroup.

Data from The Maastricht Circulatory Arrest Registry indicate that, among patients for whom EF was measured before an SCD episode, 52% had EF > 30% and 32% had EF > 40% [18]. The authors found that CHF was seen in only a minority of the SCD population. Most SCD victims did not know they had heart disease or did not exhibit any of the variables consistent with poor left ventricular function. Interestingly, it was found that CAD, more specifically previous MI, is frequently associated with SCD and the median time interval between previous MI and SCD was many years (9.0) with a wide variation.

To address this public health dilemma, intermediate or other vulnerable subgroups of the population need to be identified effectively so that preventive and management strategies can be evaluated. In addition, an understanding of the mechanisms underlying SCD in well-defined subgroups may help to provide additional insight into this condition across the entire population.

Incidence of SCD in CKD Patients

In CKD patients, the definition of SCD could be problematic. The high comorbidity and large amount of time in health-care facilities that characterize these patients gives a particular difficult to predict fatal events. Deaths in CKD patients are frequently unobserved, and the exact timing is unknown. Other possible non-cardiac causes of sudden death, as well as cerebrovascular event, may contribute to global mortality in CKD patients.

According to the US Renal Data System [19, 20], approximately 22% of all deaths are caused by SCD, and the incidence increases with age: 2% per year for ages 20 to 44 years, 3.7% per year for ages 45 to 64 years, and 7% per year for ages 65 years and older.

These circumstances make CKD patients unique, so they should have a special consideration.

To facilitate communication between disciplines and interpretation of preexisting literature, a commonly accepted definitions of SCD for CKD patients should be adopted. In this context, sudden death occurring in the setting of missed hemodialysis treatment should not be considered SCD. For this reason it may be useful to differentiate the SCD occurs in dialysis patients than that observed in non dialysis-dependent CKD patients.

a) SCD in non dialysis-dependent CKD patients:

Non-dialysis-dependent CKD patients have an increased risk of SCD, the prognosis from cardiac arrest is worse than the general population and the likelihood of survival decreases with a GFR decline. However, few studies have evaluated the association between less severe reductions in kidney function and SCD incidence and the benefit of prophylactic ICD therapy in CKD patients. In the Multicenter Automatic Defibrillator Implantation Trial-II (MADIT-II) [21], that included patients with a previous MI and a LVEF of ≤35% treated only with optimal medical therapy, the risk for SCD was 17% higher for every 10 ml/min/1.73 m^2

decrement in the estimated GFR (eGFR) [22]. In a similar way, the Comparison of Medical Therapy, Pacing, and Defibrillation in Heart Failure trial [23], that confirmed a benefit of cardiac resynchronization therapy in reducing death and hospitalization in patients with advanced CHF, renal dysfunction was associated with a 67% greater risk of SCD during the follow-up period [24]. In this setting, however, it is difficult to discern whether CKD is just a marker of CHF severity or an independent predictor of SCD risk.

Two recent observational studies have demonstrated an association between moderate kidney dysfunction and SCD risk in peoples with cardiovascular disease. In the first one, examining more than 2,700 postmenopausal women with CAD participating at The Heart and Estrogen Replacement Study, the rate of SCD was higher in those patients with lower kidney function, and the presence of CHF and CAD mediate only part of this association [25, 26].

The second study included a large cohort of CKD patients from the Duke Databank for Cardiovascular Disease [25, 26] has clearly shown that reductions in the eGFR in CKD stage III-IV are associated with a progressive increase in risk of SCD in patients with CAD.

Despite these findings, the majority of these participants had a history of CAD, CHF or systolic dysfunction, making it difficult to understand whether chronic kidney dysfunction was just a marker of CVD or an independent predictor of risk for SCD.

In a community-based study that included more than 4,400 ambulatory older adults, impaired kidney function was associated with increased risk of SCD [27]. In this study, the incidence of SCD events increased both across cystatin C tertiles: 0.1% (per year), 0.25% and 0.32%, and creatinine-based eGFR tertiles: 0.15% per year, 0.22% and 0.27%. After adjusting for multiple variables including CHF and MI, cystatin C tertiles retained an independent risk of SCD. Elevated cystatin C concentration also captures a state of preclinical kidney disease that is highly prevalent among ambulatory older patients. A preclinical state of kidney disease refers to a specific condition that precedes the development of overt, clinical disease and is associated with adverse health consequences [28].

Further analysis from this study showed that in patients without CKD (eGFR $\geq$60 ml/min per 1.73 m^2) and elevated cystatin C levels (cystatin C $\geq$1.0 mg/L) there was a substantially increased risk for SCD events during the follow-up period. After multivariate adjustment, SCD risk is twice as likely in the preclinical kidney disease group compared with the normal kidney function referent group (creatinine-based eGFR $\geq$60 ml/min per 1.73 m^2 and cystatin C <1.0 mg/L). These findings suggest that even mild reductions in kidney function, evidenced by higher cystatin C levels, increase risk of SCD, especially within susceptible populations such as the elderly without any clinical evidence of CHF, CAD or systolic dysfunction.

b) SCD in dialysis-dependent CKD patients:

The majority of cardiovascular-related death in advanced CKD are attributable to SCD events, and three-quarters of dialysis patients who have a cardiac arrest do not survive, despite the specialized care of Emergency Medical Services [29]. In a case-control study encompassing 43,200 HD patients, sudden cardiac arrest were 4.5 events per 100,000 dialysis treatments during the three year study period [30].

In the USRDS database [31], the cause of death attributed to arrhythmic mechanisms is noted in the Centers for Medicare and Medicaid Services (CMS) death notification by either cardiac arrest/cause unknown or arrhythmia. Based upon this definition, arrhythmias may therefore be responsible for 56% of all cardiac deaths or 25% of all-cause mortality in peritoneal dialysis patients, and 65% of all cardiac deaths or 27% of all-cause mortality in hemodialysis patients. Using a more comprehensive death notification form for annual data collection, including causes, context and location of death, and excluding deaths from sepsis, malignancy, hyperkaliemia and withdrawal from dialysis, the USRDS Cardiovascular Special Studies Center (CVSSV) [31] has been estimated that 29.7% of deaths in prevalent dialysis patients are related to SCD.

The overall best current estimate is that SCD is responsible for 27 ± 2% of all-cause mortality in dialysis patients. Similar findings on the relative contribution (22 to 26%) of sudden death to all-cause mortality in dialysis patients have been reported in multiple studies including HEMO [32], 4D trial [33], the CHOICE cohort [34], and the Dialysis Outcomes and Practice Patterns Study (DOPPS) [35].

The CVSSC [31] has also estimated that there was a slow, steady decline in the overall cardiac mortality rate between 2002 and 2011 in the US dialysis population (from 6.9% to 5.4% per year). The recent increase in the use of "evidence-based therapies" (such as beta-blockers) in dialysis patients could explain this phenomenon [36].

It is noteworthy that there is also an enhanced risk of SCD in the first hemodialysis session of the week. Compared with the average risk of SCD, there is a 50% increased frequency of SCD on the firth hemodialysis session after the long weekend interval [37]. In addition, one study [38] reported that the SCD risk is increased threefold in the twelve hour period before the end of the long weekend interval and 1.7 times increased in the twelve hours starting with the dialysis procedure following this long interval (Figure 2).

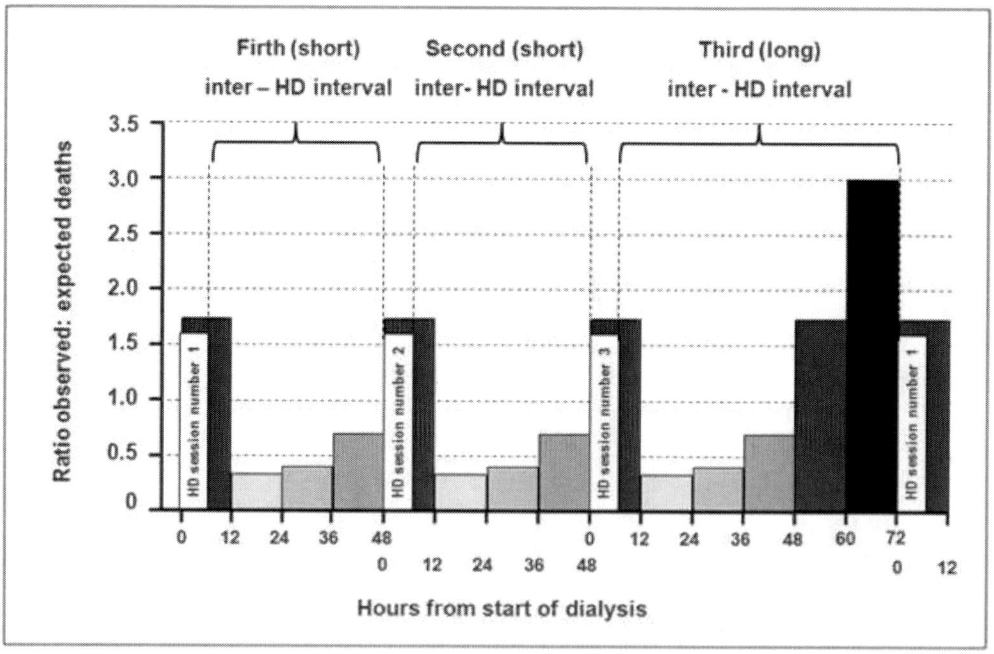

Figure 2. Timing of sudden cardiac death in hemodialysis patients. Graphical representation of the three hemodialysis sessions during the week. There are two short inter-HD intervals during the week and one long inter-HD interval during the weekend. Ratio of actual to expected number of occurrences of sudden death for each 12 h interval beginning with the start of hemodialysis. (Modified from Bleyer AJ, et al. Characteristics of sudden death in hemodialysis patients. Kidney Int. 2006; 69(12):2268–73).

A high incidence of SCD over a five year longitudinal follow-up with a rate of 4.9% per year, was also observed in a prospective cohort study [39] of Chinese patients receiving chronic peritoneal dialysis (PD). This observation is not surprising, given that PD patients are similarly subjected to kidney disease or uremia-related risk factors as in hemodialysis patients.

Finally, the strong association between advanced CKD and SCD extends to the pediatric population as well. In a retrospective analysis that included nearly 1400 deaths among patients who started CKD treatment aged 0–30 years from the USRDS, cardiac arrests and arrhythmias comprised the majority of cardiac-related deaths, which occurred at a rate >2% per year [40]. These findings suggest the existence of other mechanisms different to atherosclerotic disease and CHF are responsible for triggering fatal arrhythmias in advanced CKD population.

RISK FACTORS AND HYPOTHESIZED MECHANISMS OF SCD IN CKD

Pathophysiology of SCD in CKD is complex and is probable the interaction between transient events and underlying substrate. In CKD patients, cardiomyopathy frequently occurs as a consequence of elevated ventricular pressure and volume. This adverse condition, which is likely exacerbated by rapid electrolytes shifts, divalent ion abnormalities, diabetes and sympathetic overactivity, predisposes CKD patients to electrical instability, ventricular arrhythmias, conduction abnormalities and SCD followed by hemodynamic collapse. Inflammation, iron deposition, impaired baroreflex effectiveness and sensitivity, as well as obstructive sleep apnea might also contribute to the risk of SCD. An understanding of mechanisms inciting these events may help clarify the interaction between a triggering event and underlying substrate (Figure 3).

1. *Uremic Cardiomyopathy:* Left ventricular hypertrophy (LVH) has been shown to be a major predictor of SCD independent of left ventricular systolic function in several clinical conditions, such as essential hypertension and ischemic heart disease [41]. LVH is common in CKD patients and increases as GFR falls [42]. At start dialysis, LVH is present in almost 75% of patients, it's evolves after dialysis initiated towards left ventricular dilation [43, 44] and is associated with the subsequent development of CHF [45]. Hypertension, anemia, volume overload and other risk factors can partly explained the progression of cardiac hypertrophy [46]. LVH has been reported to be a predictor of cardiac death in dialysis patients independent of hypertension [47] and its progression has been clearly linked to risk of SCD through increasing arrhythmogenesis or by prolongation the time of ventricular depolarization and repolarization. In addition, regression of LVH with therapy has been reported to improve survival [48]. The molecular basis of LVH in uremic patients includes activation of growth factors, proto-oncogenes, plasma noradrenalin, cytokines and angiotensin II. These factors regulate intracellular process that accelerate cardiac hypertrophy, myocardial fibrosis and apoptosis [49]. Both LVH and cardiac fibrosis

has been implicated in increasing risk for sustained ventricular arrhythmias and the predisposition to SCD [50, 51].

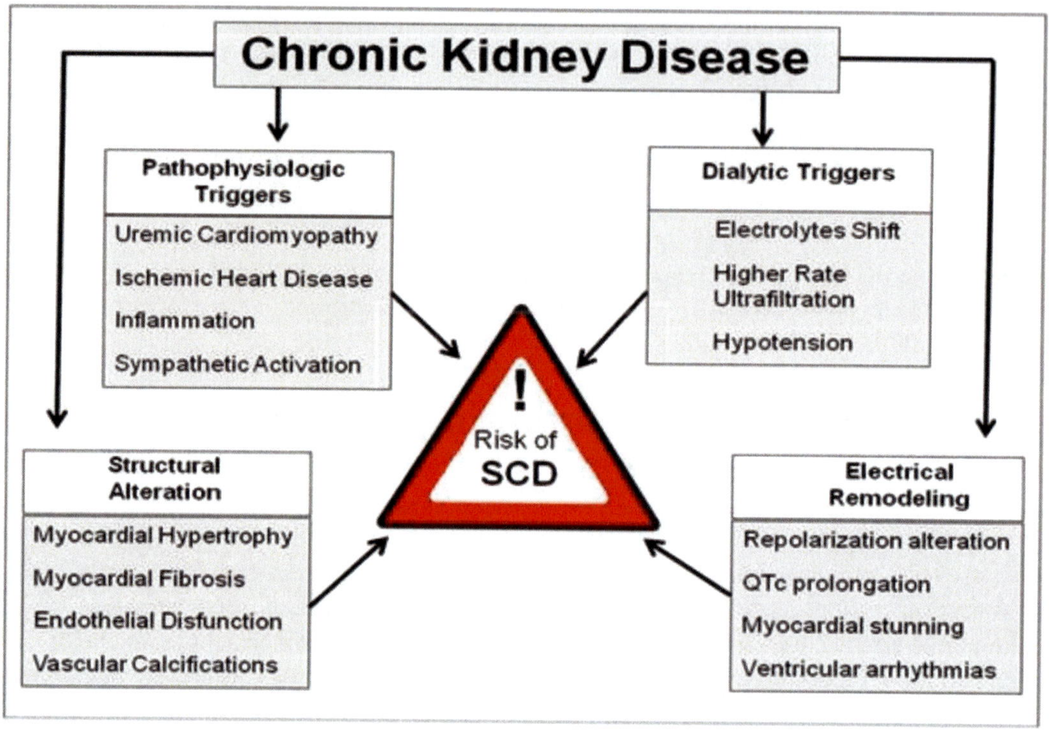

Figure 3. Risk Factors and hypothesized mechanisms of sudden cardiac death in chronic kidney disease. Pathophysiology risk factors and hypothesized mechanisms of sudden cardiac death in chronic kidney disease patients: the interaction between transient events and underlying substrate.

The stimulus provided by dialysis treatment to ventricular arrhythmias is a well-known phenomenon. In the first large survey on the dialysis population conducted in 1988 by the "*Gruppo Emodialisi e Patologia Cardiovascolare*" [52], the incidence of ventricular arrhythmias was reported in 76% of cases. Dialysis treatment was reported as the most important arrhythmogenic factor not only during the dialysis session but also several hours after the end of the treatment.

2. *Ischemic Heart Disease:* In hemodialysis patients, CAD probably induces an arrhythmogenic effect, and the severity of coronary stenosis is associated with the persistence of ventricular arrhythmias during and after the treatment [34, 47]. In addition, the number of premature ventricular complexes (PVC) during and after hemodialysis session is higher in patients with CAD than in those without CAD [34, 53].

A number of cardiac biomarkers were identified as predictors of outcomes in CKD patients. Cardiac troponins T and I (cTnT and cTnI) are the preferred markers for the diagnosis of myocardial injury for all patients, including those with CKD, and are preferred to the MB isoenzyme of creatine kinase (CK-MB) because of their superior specificity and sensitivity for myocardial injury [54]. According with the data from a meta-analysis of three studies that included CKD patients, the risk of cardiac mortality, acute MI, ischemia, revascularization, ventricular arrhythmias, CHF, and a composite of these outcomes increased with elevated cTnT [55]. High cTnI levels were associated with higher risk of short-term cardiac outcomes among dialysis patients in three studies. Stably increased serum troponin levels also predict worse long-term cardiovascular outcomes and poor survival in asymptomatic CKD patients in the absence of AMI [56].

Others markers of coronary ischemia as well as brain natriuretic peptide (BNP), inflammatory markers, adhesion molecules, and asymmetric dimethylarginine (ADMA), can detect CKD patients at high risk of SCD [57].

Recently, prospective studies on CVD outcomes in CKD patients using new cardiac biomarkers of HDL dysfunction and/or oxidative stress, have appeared in the literature: paraoxonase-1 (PON-1) [58] and ischemia modified albumin (IMA) [59]. PON-1 is an enzyme (calcium-dependent esterase associated with HDL subfractions that contain apo A-I and clusterin, conferring protection against oxidative damage of various cells and lipoproteins. Low levels serum of PON-1have been reported in HD and non-HD dependent CKD patients [60, 61], and its levels significant increase after HD treatment [62].

In the presence of myocardial ischemia, structural changes take place in the N-terminus of albumin, reducing its binding capacity for transitional metals. The effect is caused by albumin circulating through the ischemic capillary as a CVD, especially in acute coronary syndromes [63]. IMA is thus considered as a CVD-related biomarker that is sensitive to myocardium ischemia [64]. Recent studies have shown significantly higher IMA levels in CKD patients compared to controls and further increased levels after HD treatment [65].

Despite the great attention paid to the roles of PON-1 and IMA as a cardiac biomarkers, the actual association to CKD is unknown.

3. *Inflammation:* Inflammation has been found to be associated with SCD independently of traditional cardiovascular risk factors [34]. Levels of proinflammatory cytokines increase as renal function deteriorates [66]. Highest levels C-reactive protein (CRP) and cytokines (such as IL-6 and platelet-activating factor, PDF) have been associated with ventricular arrhythmias through the modulation of ion channel function [34, 67, 68] and the aggravation of sympathetic tone. CRP and IL-6 were also associated with a doubled risk of SCD. In addition, a decrease in serum albumin level was associated with increased risk of SCD compared with the lowest level [34]. Pathogenic mechanisms are not known, however premature atherosclerosis and cytokine-induced plaque instability may induce a direct effect on the myocardium and the electrical conduction system [34]. Myocardial fibrosis associated with the inflammatory process, could affect ventricular conduction causing a delay in repolarization that could lead to ventricular arrhythmias [14, 34]. This condition might cause SCD.

In CKD patients it has been shown that high levels of inflammatory mediators induce the production of reactive oxygen species resulting in an accelerated vascular atherosclerosis and arterial calcification [41]. The accumulation of asymmetric dimethyl-arginine inhibits nitric oxide synthesis in endothelial cells, inducing endothelial dysfunction, vasoconstriction, and atherosclerosis [66].

Elevated levels of serum homocysteine (Hcy) have been implicated in cardiac pathological conditions including CAD, CHF, acute MI, arrhythmogenesis and CHF. However, the underlying mechanisms are unknown. Hcy is an agonist of the N-methyl-D-aspartate receptor that are present in cardiac tissue. The activation of this receptor increase intracellular Ca++ leading to an increased cell excitability. In addition, Hyc induce oxidative stress in myocardial cells and activate matrix metalloproteinases that degrade cell membrane proteins. In HD patients, hyper-Hcy is commonly found and is associated with atherothrombotic events and incident cardiovascular mortality [69].

4. *Electrolyte shifts, divalent ions abnormalities, QT interval and ventricular arrhythmias:* The rapid shift between extracellular and intracellular electrolytes concentration during an HD session, which depends on the electrochemical gradient, leads to a cellular membrane polarization exposing it to an electrical instability. Calcium (Ca++) and Potassium (K+) plays an important role in maintaining the electrical potential across the cellular membrane, and it was the subjects of interventional studies.

The heart rate-corrected QT (QTc) interval is a recognized ECG marker of the ventricular repolarization, and its prolongation has been associated with increased risk of arrhythmias. CKD can be associated with prolonged QT interval, which increase the risk of torsade de pointes; these conditions can be a cause of SCD [70]. The QTc in HD patients is associated with several manifestations of uremic cardiomyopathy including increased LVH, left ventricular dilatation, and reduced left ventricular ejection fraction [45, 70]. In addition, more premature ventricular complexes (PVCs) occur during hemodialysis in patients with LVH compared with those without LVH [47].

In patients with CKD, especially in those undergoing dialysis treatment, prolonged QT interval usually results from inappropriate myocardial depolarization and repolarization due to lengthening of action potential duration that secondary occurs in LVH and intercardiomyocytic fibrosis [71]. A prolongation of QT interval [72, 73], an increase of QT dispersion [74], and an alteration of the capacity to adapt QT interval to heart rate changes (QTc) have been reported during HD session [75].

Three Italian studies [76–78] showed a direct link between K+ concentration and QT interval prolongation. In these studies, complex arrhythmias were observed more frequently during and after HD session in those with a decreasing potassium profile compared with individuals whose potassium levels were kept constant. Data from patients treated at Fresenius Medical Care North America-affiliated centers [37, 79] showed that dialysis with a K+ dialyzate concentration of 0 mmol/L or 1 mmol/L was a significant risk factor for SCD [79]. Using this prescription, cardiac arrests were more frequent than in controls (17.1% vs 8.8%; $p < 0.0001$), and were prevalently observed during HD sessions carried out on a Monday compared with a Wednesday and Friday.

Calcium homeostasis during HD session can affect left ventricular relaxation. In HD patients, prolongation of QTc interval was inversely correlated with intradialytic variation of Ca++, suggesting that greatest reduction in Ca++ are associated with greatest increases of Qtc prolongation at the end of HD session [80]. These findings were confirmed by others [81]. In addition, hypocalcemia observed after HD session correlated with prolonged QTc interval and SCD even in patients without cardiovascular manifestations [73].

Greater QTc interval dispersion was associated with an increase of total and cardiovascular mortality in both hemodialysis and in peritoneal dialysis patients [82]. Intradialytic serum magnesium variations do not show an important role in QTc dispersion [83].

Hyperphosphatemia usually develops as kidney function deteriorates and is a common problem among patients with CKD [84]. Hyperphosphatemia causes secondary hyperparathyroidism, smooth muscle proliferation, vascular calcification, and coronary atherosclerosis [70]. Hyperphosphatemia-induced myocardial calcification could alter microcirculatory hemodynamics, raise extravascular resistance and threaten myocardial perfusion [85]. Hyperphosphatemia and elevated Ca++ x PO_4 product were correlated with an increase in the risk of death related to CAD and SCD in a linear manner [86]. In addition, SCD was also related to parathyroid hormone levels in a nonlinear fashion (U-shaped relationship) [86].

5. *Rapid fluid removal during hemodialysis:* Ultrafiltration (UF), also referred to as convection, is the fluid flow through the membrane, forced by a difference in pressure on the two sides of the dialyzer (pressure gradient). Thus, UF plays a key role to maintain circulating blood volume controlling the patient's weight, but simultaneously it is associated with non-physiological fluid shifts and hemodynamic instability. Consequently, UF may contribute to an acute reduction of circulating volume, hypotension, tissue ischemia, maladaptive cardiac structural changes, arrhythmia, and SCD [87]. Thus, researchers are investigating the associations between UF rate and both, all-cause and cardiovascular mortality in HD patients. Despite obvious biological plausibility, the association between UF rate and CV mortality has been poorly studied. One of the first evidence in this regard showing a small increase in all-cause mortality without increase in cardiac mortality in patients undergoing a UF rate higher than 10 mL/h/kg [88]. Subsequent data suggest that the cut point of 10 mL/h/kg may have been too low to observe a true UF rate associated CV mortality [89]. Using data from the HEMO study that included more than 1800 HD patients treated three times per week, UF rate were categorized as ≤10 ml/h/kg, 10–13 ml/h/kg, and >13 ml/h/kg [87]. Compared to UF rates ≤10 ml/h/kg, UF rates >13 ml/h/kg were significantly associated with increased all-cause and CV mortality with adjusted hazard ratios (HR) of 1.59 and 1.71, respectively. UF rate between 10 and 13 ml/kg/h was not significantly associated with greater all-cause mortality and CV mortality. Only among patients with CHF there was a significant association between this UF rate category and all-cause mortality. Secondary analysis also showed that UF rate >13 ml/h/kg was significantly associated with a greater HR for the composite outcome of CV hospitalization and CV mortality, whereas UF rate 10–13 ml/h/kg was not. According to this data, higher UF rates are associated with greater CV mortality. During dialysis, fluid is removed directly from the vascular space. When dialytic removal exceeds resorption from other compartments, circulating volume is reduced and transient myocardial ischaemia can result. This transient ischemia could result in *myocardial stunning*, which is an ischemia mediated temporary reduction in cardiac function, i.e., regional wall motion abnormalities. Intradialytic recurrent myocardial stunning may over time lead to

irreversible fibrotic changes and CHF, arrhythmias and SCD [90]. Following seventy HD patients without severe left ventricular dysfunction, McIntyre et al. [91] observed a significant reduction in cardiac systolic function in more than 60% of patients. Interestingly, the only predictor in multivariate analysis were UF and intradialytic hypotension. Even in pediatric patients without arteriosclerosis epicardial or small vessels disease exhibited regional wall motion abnormalities during HD treatment [92]. Thus, it appears that across the spectrum of age and CV risk profile, significant cardiac dysfunction occurs in a majority of HD patients.

6. *Others factors:* There are others factors able to influence the onset of SCD. In CKD patients, iron overload has been associated with elevated rates of hospitalization and mortality [93]. Iron can promote the production of reactive oxygen species and free radicals resulting in intercardiomyocytic fibrosis [94]. High iron saturation was an independent risk factor for prolonged QTc dispersion in patients undergoing peritoneal dialysis [95] suggesting that iron overload could increases the risk of SCD due to conduction abnormalities in CKD patients.

Patients with CKD are characterized by a tonic elevation of sympathetic tone. This factor largely contributes to their increased CV risk [96, 97]. Augmented sympathetic activity is also seen during HD sessions, and usually subside following bilateral nephrectomy, suggesting that this mechanisms is volume independent [96–98]. Sympathetic over-activity is usually secondary to an afferent signal of renal sensory nerves activating the sympathetic nervous system, resulting in enhanced sympathetic and norepinephrine release. The latter response could aggravate hypertension, ventricular hypertrophy, and heart failure, as well as result in increased risk of SCD [97].

Impaired arterial baroreflex sensitivity (BRS) is associated with an increased risk of ventricular arrhythmia and SCD [99]. The baroreflex effectiveness index (BEI), a novel index reflecting the number of times the baroreflex is active in controlling the heart rate in response to blood fluctuations, is associated with prognosis in CKD. In stage 4-5 CKD patients with hypertension, both BRS and BEI were reduced compared with age-matched healthy controls [99]. In a subsequent paper, the same authors have documented that reduced BEI was an independent predictor of all-cause mortality, while reduced BRS was an independent predictor of SCD [100]. However both BRS and BEI are useful markers that provide prognostic information that may have clinical implication for CKD patients with CV diseases.

Therapeutic Strategies to Prevent SCD

There are few trials designed specifically to evaluate the efficacy of therapeutics and interventions for SCD in CKD population. The approach to reducing the risk of SCD in this group of patients is based on data obtained from other high-risk populations and subgroup analysis of clinical trials (Figure 4).

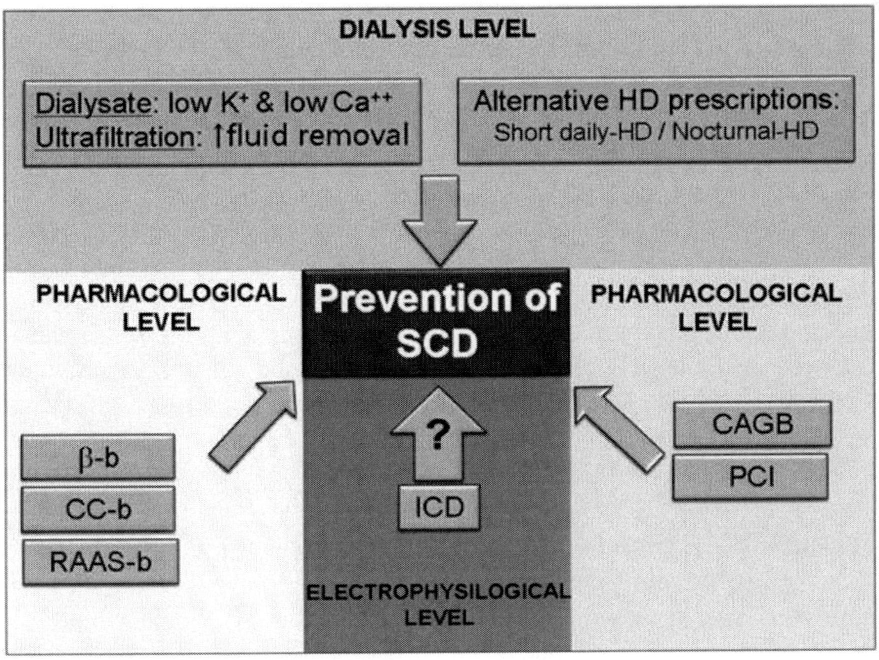

Figure 4. Levels of intervention for the prevention and treatment of SCD.

Pharmacological Drugs

a) Beta-blockers (b): b are antiarrhythmic and anti-ischemic agents that reduce not only the risk of hospitalization and death but also the risk of SCD [101]. However, the majority of randomized clinical trials (RCT) providing this evidence have excluded subjects with CKD. In a retrospective study, HD patients using b had a lower rate of SCD [102]. Similarly, after multivariate analysis adjusting for comorbidities, blood results and dialysis parameters, the Dialysis Outcomes and Practice Patterns Study (DOPPS) found that b were associated with lower risk of SCD [35]. In a recent meta-analysis that evaluate the efficacy of b in CKD patients with CHF, there was a 34% relative reduction in cardiovascular mortality in treated patients compared with placebo [103]. There is limited data about the effect of b therapy in patients with CKD without CHF. Adequate powered prospective RCT assessing the effects of b in both advanced CKD and dialysis patients are necessary.
b) Calcium channel blockers (CCb): CCb may have potential cardioprotective effects by preventing coronary artery spasm, normalizing intracellular Ca++ concentration, limiting the injury after cardiac arrest and preventing fatal arrhythmia [104]. Despite CCb may be beneficial for patients with CKD because they decrease blood pressure, uraemic calcinosis and pressure induced calcium entry into vessel walls [105], there are limited data about the effects of this drugs on SCD. In a retrospective study [106] the administration of CCb was with a significant reduction in mortality of 67% in HD patients. After adjustment for case mix factors, tunneled catheters and concomitant medications, CCb treatment was associated with a significant survival advantage at twenty-four hours after cardiac arrest in outpatient hemodialysis clinics [107]. The

authors also found an association between β-b and angiotensin-converting enzyme inhibitor/angiotensin II receptor blocker treatment with improved survival.

This data, therefore, suggests that dihydropyridine CCb may have a protective role in increasing survival post-cardiac arrest.

c) Digoxin: Digoxin increases the strength and efficiency of myocardial contractions, and is useful in the treatment of CHF and control cardiac rate and rhythm through the inhibition membrane sodium-potassium ATPase activity and reduction of sympathetic tone. The basic clinical facts about digoxin for non-CKD patients come from two venerable RCT [108, 109]. These studies show that the addition of digoxin did not improve survival and it increased the rates of other cardiovascular death, presumably from ventricular arrhythmias and fibrillation.

The role of digoxin, in HD patients would seem less controversial. The narrow therapeutic window, long half-life, and the potential for lethal arrhythmias of the drug—especially in the context of hypokalemia—are widely known. Because hemodialysis inevitably involves large potassium fluxes, digoxin and dialysis would seem to be a bad combination. In the largest study conducted to date including more than 120,000 HD patients from Fresenius Medical Care database [110], the use of digoxin and increasing digoxin levels were associated with increased mortality. In addition, the mortality risk increases with low pre-dialysis potassium. Therefore, digoxin is unlikely to be a useful preventative therapy for SCD.

d) Amiodarone: Amiodarone is a class III antiarrhythmic agent used for various types of cardiac dysrhythmias, both ventricular and atrial. It is an effective drug for prevention of SCD in the general population. A meta-analysis of fifteen RCTs [111] conducted to examining the use of amiodarone vs. placebo/control for the prevention of SCD, reported a 29% reduction of the SCD risk in treated patients. However, amiodarone therapy is neutral with respect to all-cause mortality and is associated with a two- and five-fold increased risk of pulmonary and thyroid toxicity. As a result, amiodarone is no longer the first-line agent for arrhythmia control in the general population. No RCT data exist for its use in CKD-5D specifically. Consequently, amiodarone is used in line with current guidelines for use in the general population.
e) Renin-Angiostensin-Aldosterone System (RAAS) blockers: Alterations in the RAAS comprises a fundamental abnormality in cardiorenal disorders. High aldoserone levels are reported to be an independent risk factor for SCD in non-CKD patients. The treatment with RASS blockers increase survival in patients with CHF or MI [112]. The benefits of angiotensin-converting enzyme inhibitors (ACE-i) extend to patients with mild kidney dysfunction [113]. However, no equivalent RCT data exist for patients with CKD-5D. In the Fosinopril in Dialysis Trial (FOSIDIAL) [114], there was no reduction in cardiovascular events in the treated patients group. Only after adjustments for risk factors was a trend towards benefit observed in the treatment arm. A further small open label RCT [115] investigated the effect of candesartan versus placebo in HD patients without cardiomyopathy. The study found

a protective effect in the treated group with a reduction in CV events and CV mortality compared to placebo group. However, the study was inconclusive on the effects of candesartan on SCD. In the general population, the Randomised Aldactone Evaluation Study (RALES Study) [116], reported that Spironolactone reduced SCD by 20–30%, but CKD-5D patients were not included in this trial. In this patients, clinicians are cautious about using RAAS blocker for fear of hyperkalaemia. However, in a systematic review [117] of six studies including more than 7000 CKD-5D patients with CHF, hyperkalaemia episodes were rare; mean serum potassium was 4.9 mmol/L and no patients developed an adverse event as a result of hyperkalaemia.

Many studies in HD patients are underpowered and news RCTs of RAAS blocker to evaluate the SCD risk in this population are needed.

f) Statins: Statins are known to prevent CV disease and improve lipid profiles. However, their effects in HD patients remained uncertain. A recent meta-analysis [118] including three RCT (4D, AURORA, SHARP) with, more than 7,000 HD patients, assessed the effects of statins compared to placebo in dialysis patients. This study showed that patient on dialysis treated with statins showed a modest benefit in terms of atherosclerotic CV event, but not for stroke and all-cause mortality.

Similarly, in another meta-analysis [119] of twenty-one RCT including 8,186 dialysis patients, also showed a benefit in reducing all cardiac events, but had no effect on CV deaths or all-cause mortality.

However, a Cochrane meta-analysis of 25 studies involving 8289 dialysis patients found no benefit of statin therapy on major CV events, cardiovascular mortality, all-cause mortality or myocardial infarction, despite efficacious lipid lowering [120].

In conclusion, statins had no impact on all-cause or CV mortality, while it seems the existence of an improvement for CV events in dialysis patients.

Non-Pharmacological Options

a) Implantable cardioverter defibrillator (ICD): According to the results of a meta-analysis [121] that combined the results of all three larger studies available in the general population, the first-line therapy for primary and secondary prevention of SCD is the inclusion of an ICD. However, major cardiovascular disease trials have excluded patients with CKD or did not provide adequate information on the renal function of enrollees or the effect of interventions on patients with renal disease. Since ICD therapy data in CKD patients are lacking, there is no general consensus on the use of device therapy in these patients. In non-dialysis-dependent CKD patients with CHF, ICDs appear to reduce mortality risk. A retrospective analysis from MADIT-II [22], showed a significant reduction in the risk of all-cause mortality and SCD risk in CKD patients with eGFR >35 ml/min per 1.73 m^2 treated with ICD compared with those in the conventional therapy. However, no significant difference was found in both outcomes between the two treatment groups for patients with eGFR <35 ml/min per 1.73 m^2. Similarly, Alsheikh-Ali et al. [122] who had categorized patients according to the CHF-NYHA class and the CKD stage, observed the greatest benefits of ICDs therapy in patients clinically less compromised. These data suggest that SCD risk in patients treated with ICD and conventionally treated are equivalent in advanced stages of CKD and CHF. In dialysis patients hospitalized for ventricular fibrillation/cardiac arrest who received ICD implantation within thirty days of admission, Herzog et al. [123] observed a 42% reduction in overall death risk of death, concluding that ICD therapy improve survival in dialysis patients. However, the source of this retrospective study derived from Medicare claims, and important clinical data regarding systolic function, serum K+ levels, CAD, and utilization of pharmacologic agents, were unavailable. In a study conducted on moderate to severe CKD patients with a LVEF <35%, Khan et al. [124] observed that in patients who were not receiving dialysis, ICD therapy was associated with a better rate of survival, whereas in the group receiving dialysis, ICD placement did not impact survival. Differently from Herzog et al. [123], in this smaller study, survival analysis data was adjusted for clinical confounders such as CAD, CHF, hypertension, utilization of pharmacologic agents, eGFR, sex and race. The difference observed in survival according to dialysis therapy may depend on the presence of comorbidities that do not affect ICD therapy, the number of ventricular arrhythmias that could be reduced after ICD implantation, or the defibrillation threshold that may be increased in dialysis patients.

Although better survival reached with ICD therapy is less evident in CKD patients compared to normal kidney function patients, this benefit is not to be neglected. Despite the high risk for ventricular arrhythmias and SCD in CKD patients, ICD therapy appears to be underutilized. In the study from Herzog et al. [123] only 8% of eligible patients received an ICD, and other data [36] and studies [125] have also confirmed this evidence.

In conclusion, the results of this studies and meta-analysis seems to indicate that the use of ICD therapy improves survival in CKD patients. However, prospective, randomized studies about ICD therapy in CKD patients are needed. To know more about the role of ICD therapy and confounding factors in dialysis patients, we should expect the results of the ICD2 trial [126], not available until 2017.

b) Coronary revascularization: In patients with severe CAD, revascularization procedures appear to provide benefit over medical therapy alone. However, the risk of long-term repeat revascularization, myocardial infarction, and SCD is greater in patients with CKD than in those with normal kidney function. Randomized studies [127, 128] demonstrate comparable rates of death and myocardial infarction but higher rates of repeat revascularization in non-dialysis patients undergoing percutaneous coronary intervention (PCI) with bare metal stents (BMS) compared with coronary artery bypass grafting (CABG). CKD patients undergoing maintenance dialysis have been excluded from any randomized evaluation of the comparative efficacy of coronary revascularization strategies.

A series of small retrospective studies have shown that long-term survival rates are higher in CKD patients who undergo CABG than in those who undergo PTCA [129–131]. In a large, retrospective study of the USRDS national database that compared CKD patients undergoing CABG with PTCA, a higher perioperative mortality rates in the CABG-treated patients (12.5% vs 5.4%) was observed [131]. However, surgical therapy was associated with a significant reduction of two and five years mortality, both all-cause death, and cardiac death, compared to PTCA.

Despite the introduction of drug-eluting stents (DES) in the majority of PCI procedures has resulted in a reduction of restenosis and repeat revascularization, it have failed to demonstrate any survival advantage relative to BMS in the general population [132]. A large cohort from US Medicare [133] reported a statistically significant mortality benefit associated with DES compared with BMS in dialysis patients.

This data was confirmed by a meta-analysis [134], where a significant reduction in repeat revascularization and a trend toward reduced mortality was reported in DES compared with BMS treated dialysis patients.

Another exploratory meta-analysis [135] of seventeen studies evaluating CABG versus PCI concluded that existing data are inadequate to make a determination on the optimal strategy of coronary revascularization for dialysis patients. Thus, the optimal option for coronary revascularization in dialysis patients remains a matter of debate.

c) Dialysis: Dialysis treatment is a remarkable cardiac stressor, that is not stopped and with a frequency of this stimulus is three times per week. In an effort to replace one hundred and sixty-right hours of renal function every week in twelve hours, hemodialysis is associated with a series of events that affect intra-dialytic hemodynamic stability that depend on acute reduction of circulating volume such as hypotension, collapse, tissue ischemia, maladaptive cardiac structural changes, arrhythmia, and SCD [87]. Since there is a threefold increase of SCD risk in the first hemodialysis session of the week [38], it is appropriate to point out two main areas where it is possible intervene effectively: dialysate and ultrafiltration.

i. Dialysate: There is a well known link between dialysate K+ concentration and QT interval prolongation and the subsequent risk of complex arrhythmias [76–78]. For this reason, dialysate K+ concentration is one of the most important measures to considerate for reducing the risk of SCD during the dialysis treatment. In a multivariate Cox regression analysis of HD patients [136], pre-HD hyperkalaemia conferred a 2.7-fold increase of risk of SCD. The optimal pre-HD serum K+ in respect of long-term survival was found in an observational study [137] between 4.6 and 5.3 mmol/L. K+ dialyzate concentration from 0 mmol/L to 1 mmol/L, is associated with increased risk of cardiac arrest [79]. However, it has also been reported that K+ dialysate of <2 mmol/L (or <3 mmol/L if pre-HD serum K+ is <5 mmol/L) confers an increased risk of SCD [30]. Electrical conduction is also dependent on Ca++ handling. Low dialysate Ca++ levels is associated with increased QT dispersion and prolongation of QTc interval [80, 81] suggesting the predisposition to ventricular arrhythmias, even in patients without cardiovascular manifestations [73]. In a study that examined covariate-adjusted SCD risk associations with serum Ca++, dialysate Ca++, serum dialysate Ca gradient++, and low dialysate Ca++ were associated with aberrations in cardiac conduction such as QT dispersion and QTc prolongation

[138]. Thus, serum and dialysate Ca++, and serum-dialysate Ca++ gradients should be considered in determining the optimal dialysate Ca prescription.

ii. Ultrafiltration: High rates of fluid removal may result in intra-HD hypotension, myocardial stunning and injury, predisposing to arrhythmia or circulatory collapse. In DOPPS, a large UF volume (>5.7% of post-dialysis weight) increased the risk for SCD [35]. A recent observational study reported that depressed heart rate variability (HRV) is associated with fluid overload in HD patients [139], and a strict fluid management plan resulted in an increase of HRV. Thus, the axis HRV-UF may be one of the pathophysiological mechanisms by which fluid overload predisposes to arrhythmias. In patients of greater fragility, in which it is necessary to remove large volumes of fluid—such as those with pulmonary edema and large intra-dialysis weight gain, daily dialysis or nocturnal hemodialysis therapies can prevent prolonged myocardial damage by removing excessive fluid in a session. In a twenty-five article systematic review including patients undergoing daily-HD for almost three months [140], the most consistent results were a decrease in systolic or mean arterial blood pressure. Only two studies [141, 142] reported a decrease in LVMI, and there were no studies available relating mortality data. In a RCT study [143], patients treated 2.5 h for six times a week, showed more favourable survival and decreased LVMI compared with those treated 3.5 h three times a week. Similarly, in a case control study [144], patients undergoing nocturnal HD showed a survival benefit compared with patients receiving conventional after two years of follow-up (19% vs 27% of mortality). Daily dialysis and nocturnal dialysis may remove more solute than conventional HD, with less hemodynamic instability.

Conclusion

Epidemiological data show that a quarter of HD patients will die from SCD. Risk factors for SCD are poorly understood and understudied among CKD patients. In the general population, CAD-associated risk factors are the most important determinants of SCD risk, but among CKD patients, there is evidence that these factors play a much smaller role. There are many potential pathological precipitants as most patients with CKD have structurally or functionally abnormal hearts.

Prevention of SCD can be seen as a legitimate target to improve survival in this patient group. Therefore, it is important that strategies are developed to attenuate this risk.

Unfortunately trials to test the benefits of therapies in any context tend to exclude patients with CKD. In addition, there are few evidence to support the therapies used in the general population applied to HD patients. Indeed, available data for treatment in HD patients usually derived from small post hoc or observational studies.

Regarding cardio-protective medications in HD patients, no one drug therapy has been shown to reduce the risk of SCD. However, retrospectives studies indicate that β-b, CCb and RAAS blocker have been associated with survival benefit after an arrhythmic cardiac arrest.

Current evidence suggests that revascularization does not eliminate completely the risk of SCD in HD patients, and the major cause of death post-revascularization remains to be arrhythmia. The prescription to revascularize should be made on an individual basis, and additional therapies may be needed to prevent SCD. CKD patients should not be excluded from receiving ICD implantation based on the indication for device therapy from current guidelines. However, the benefits of primary prevention from ICD implant in HD patients remains to be proven. Results of the ICD2 Trial are eagerly awaited, and may shed light on this topic. Dialysis treatment remains a considerable tool that clinician can modulate in order to reduce the risk of SCD. The dialysate handling represents a determining factor: Both low potassium dialysate and extremes of serum potassium levels, as well as low calcium dialysate and large serum to dialysate calcium gradients, have been shown to increase risk of SCD It is also important to avoid excessive rates of fluid removal per HD session, as high UF volumes have been associated with SCD.

Alternative prescription from conventional HD as well as short daily-HD or nocturnal-HD may be considered, specially for patients with greater fragility or those with hemodynamic instability. Removing large amounts of fluid in patients with pulmonary edema and exaggerated intra-dialysis weight gain through short daily-HD and/or nocturnal-HD can prevent hemodynamic instability, prolonged myocardial damage, and SCD risk.

References

[1] Ronco C, McCullough P, Anker SD, Anand I, Aspromonte N, Bagshaw SM, et al. Cardio-renal syndromes: report from the consensus conference of the acute dialysis quality initiative. *Eur Heart J.* 2010 Mar;31(6):703–11.

[2] Foley RN, Murray AM, Li S, Herzog CA, McBean AM, Eggers PW, et al. Chronic kidney disease and the risk for cardiovascular disease, renal replacement, and death in the United States Medicare population, 1998 to 1999. *J Am Soc Nephrol JASN.* 2005 Feb;16(2):489–95.

[3] Muntner P, He J, Hamm L, Loria C, Whelton PK. Renal Insufficiency and Subsequent Death Resulting from Cardiovascular Disease in the United States. *J Am Soc Nephrol.* 2002 Mar 1;13(3):745–53.

[4] Parfrey PS, Foley RN. The Clinical Epidemiology of Cardiac Disease in Chronic Renal Failure. *J Am Soc Nephrol.* 1999 Jul 1;10(7):1606–15.

[5] Roberts MA, Polkinghorne KR, McDonald SP, Ierino FL. Secular trends in cardiovascular mortality rates of patients receiving dialysis compared with the general population. *Am J Kidney Dis Off J Natl Kidney Found.* 2011 Jul;58(1):64–72.

[6] Deo R, Fyr CLW, Fried LF, Newman AB, Harris TB, Angleman S, et al. Kidney dysfunction and fatal cardiovascular disease--an association independent of atherosclerotic events: results from the Health, Aging, and Body Composition (Health ABC) study. *Am Heart J.* 2008 Jan;155(1):62–8.

[7] Fishman GI, Chugh SS, Dimarco JP, Albert CM, Anderson ME, Bonow RO, et al. Sudden cardiac death prediction and prevention: report from a National Heart, Lung, and Blood Institute and Heart Rhythm Society Workshop. *Circulation.* 2010 Nov 30;122(22):2335–48.

[8] Zipes DP, Camm AJ, Borggrefe M, Buxton AE, Chaitman B, Fromer M, et al. ACC/AHA/ESC 2006 Guidelines for Management of Patients With Ventricular Arrhythmias and the Prevention of Sudden Cardiac Death: a report of the American College of Cardiology/American Heart Association Task Force and the European Society of Cardiology Committee for Practice Guidelines (writing committee to develop Guidelines for Management of Patients With Ventricular Arrhythmias and the Prevention of Sudden Cardiac Death): developed in collaboration with the European Heart Rhythm Association and the Heart Rhythm Society. *Circulation.* 2006 Sep 5;114(10):e385–484.

[9] Nichol G, Thomas E, Callaway CW, Hedges J, Powell JL, Aufderheide TP, et al. Regional variation in out-of-hospital cardiac arrest incidence and outcome. *JAMA.* 2008 Sep 24;300(12):1423–31.

[10] Kannel WB, Cupples LA, D'Agostino RB. Sudden death risk in overt coronary heart disease: the Framingham Study. *Am Heart J.* 1987 Mar;113(3):799–804.

[11] Myerburg RJ. Sudden cardiac death: exploring the limits of our knowledge. *J Cardiovasc Electrophysiol.* 2001 Mar;12(3):369–81.

[12] Huikuri HV, Castellanos A, Myerburg RJ. Sudden death due to cardiac arrhythmias. *N Engl J Med. 2001* Nov 15;345(20):1473–82.

[13] Braunwald E. Shattuck lecture--cardiovascular medicine at the turn of the millennium: triumphs, concerns, and opportunities. *N Engl J Med.* 1997 Nov 6;337(19):1360–9.

[14] Myerburg RJ, Kessler KM, Castellanos A. Sudden cardiac death. Structure, function, and time-dependence of risk. *Circulation.* 1992 Jan;85(1 Suppl):I2–10.

[15] Members WC, Epstein AE, DiMarco JP, Ellenbogen KA, Estes NAM, Freedman RA, et al. ACC/AHA/HRS 2008 Guidelines for Device-Based Therapy of Cardiac Rhythm Abnormalities A Report of the American College of Cardiology/American Heart Association Task Force on Practice Guidelines (Writing Committee to Revise the ACC/AHA/NASPE 2002 Guideline Update for Implantation of Cardiac Pacemakers and Antiarrhythmia Devices): Developed in Collaboration With the American Association for Thoracic Surgery and Society of Thoracic Surgeons. *Circulation.* 2008 May 27;117(21):e350–408.

[16] Russo AM, Stainback RF, Bailey SR, Epstein AE, Heidenreich PA, Jessup M, et al. ACCF/HRS/AHA/ASE/HFSA/SCAI/SCCT/SCMR 2013 appropriate use criteria for implantable cardioverter-defibrillators and cardiac resynchronization therapy: a report of the American College of Cardiology Foundation appropriate use criteria task force, Heart Rhythm Society, American Heart Association, American Society of Echocardiography, Heart Failure Society of America, Society for Cardiovascular Angiography and Interventions, Society of Cardiovascular Computed Tomography, and Society for Cardiovascular Magnetic Resonance. *Heart Rhythm Off J Heart Rhythm Soc.* 2013 Apr;10(4):e11–58.

[17] Goldberger JJ, Cain ME, Hohnloser SH, Kadish AH, Knight BP, Lauer MS, et al. American Heart Association/american College of Cardiology Foundation/heart Rhythm Society scientific statement on noninvasive risk stratification techniques for identifying patients at risk for sudden cardiac death: a scientific statement from the American Heart Association Council on Clinical Cardiology Committee on Electrocardiography and Arrhythmias and Council on Epidemiology and Prevention. *Heart Rhythm Off J Heart Rhythm Soc.* 2008 Oct;5(10):e1–21.

[18] Gorgels APM, Gijsbers C, de Vreede-Swagemakers J, Lousberg A, Wellens HJJ. Out-of-hospital cardiac arrest--the relevance of heart failure. The Maastricht Circulatory Arrest Registry. *Eur Heart J.* 2003 Jul;24(13):1204–9.

[19] Collins AJ, Kasiske B, Herzog C, Chen S-C, Everson S, Constantini E, et al. Excerpts from the United States Renal Data System 2003 Annual Data Report: atlas of end-stage renal disease in the United States. *Am J Kidney Dis Off J Natl Kidney Found.* 2003 Dec;42(6 Suppl 5):A5–7, S1–230.

[20] Meier P, Vogt P, Blanc E. Ventricular arrhythmias and sudden cardiac death in end-stage renal disease patients on chronic hemodialysis. *Nephron.* 2001 Mar;87(3):199–214.

[21] Moss AJ, Zareba W, Hall WJ, Klein H, Wilber DJ, Cannom DS, et al. Prophylactic implantation of a defibrillator in patients with myocardial infarction and reduced ejection fraction. *N Engl J Med.* 2002 Mar 21;346(12):877–83.

[22] Goldenberg I, Moss AJ, McNitt S, Zareba W, Andrews ML, Hall WJ, et al. Relations among renal function, risk of sudden cardiac death, and benefit of the implanted cardiac defibrillator in patients with ischemic left ventricular dysfunction. *Am J Cardiol.* 2006 Aug 15;98(4):485–90.

[23] Bristow MR, Saxon LA, Boehmer J, Krueger S, Kass DA, De Marco T, et al. Cardiac-resynchronization therapy with or without an implantable defibrillator in advanced chronic heart failure. *N Engl J Med.* 2004 May 20;350(21):2140–50.

[24] Saxon LA, Bristow MR, Boehmer J, Krueger S, Kass DA, De Marco T, et al. Predictors of sudden cardiac death and appropriate shock in the Comparison of Medical Therapy, Pacing, and Defibrillation in Heart Failure (COMPANION) Trial. *Circulation.* 2006 Dec 19;114(25):2766–72.

[25] Deo R, Lin F, Vittinghoff E, Tseng ZH, Hulley SB, Shlipak MG. Kidney dysfunction and sudden cardiac death among women with coronary heart disease. *Hypertension.* 2008 Jun;51(6):1578–82.

[26] Pun PH, Smarz TR, Honeycutt EF, Shaw LK, Al-Khatib SM, Middleton JP. Chronic kidney disease is associated with increased risk of sudden cardiac death among patients with coronary artery disease. *Kidney Int.* 2009 Sep;76(6):652–8.

[27] Deo R, Sotoodehnia N, Katz R, Sarnak MJ, Fried LF, Chonchol M, et al. Cystatin C and sudden cardiac death risk in the elderly. *Circ Cardiovasc Qual Outcomes.* 2010 Mar;3(2):159–64.

[28] Shlipak MG, Katz R, Sarnak MJ, Fried LF, Newman AB, Stehman-Breen C, et al. Cystatin C and prognosis for cardiovascular and kidney outcomes in elderly persons without chronic kidney disease. *Ann Intern Med.* 2006 Aug 15;145(4):237–46.

[29] Davis TR, Young BA, Eisenberg MS, Rea TD, Copass MK, Cobb LA. Outcome of cardiac arrests attended by emergency medical services staff at community outpatient dialysis centers. *Kidney Int.* 2008 Apr;73(8):933–9.

[30] US Renal Data System: USRDS 2006 Annual Data Report. National Institutes of Health, National Institute of Diabetes and Digestive and Kidney Diseases, Bethesda, MD. 2006;

[31] Cheung AK, Sarnak MJ, Yan G, Berkoben M, Heyka R, Kaufman A, et al. Cardiac diseases in maintenance hemodialysis patients: results of the HEMO Study. *Kidney Int.* 2004 Jun;65(6):2380–9.

[32] Wanner C, Krane V, März W, Olschewski M, Mann JFE, Ruf G, et al. Atorvastatin in patients with type 2 diabetes mellitus undergoing hemodialysis. *N Engl J Med.* 2005 Jul 21;353(3):238–48.

[33] Parekh RS, Plantinga LC, Kao WHL, Meoni LA, Jaar BG, Fink NE, et al. The association of sudden cardiac death with inflammation and other traditional risk factors. *Kidney Int.* 2008 Nov;74(10):1335–42.

[34] Jadoul M, Thumma J, Fuller DS, Tentori F, Li Y, Morgenstern H, et al. Modifiable practices associated with sudden death among hemodialysis patients in the Dialysis Outcomes and Practice Patterns Study. *Clin J Am Soc Nephrol CJASN.* 2012 May;7(5):765–74.

[35] US Renal Data System: USRDS 2011 Annual Data Report. National Institutes of Health, National Institute of Diabetes and Digestive and Kidney Diseases, Bethesda, MD. 2011;

[36] Bleyer AJ, Russell GB, Satko SG. Sudden and cardiac death rates in hemodialysis patients. *Kidney Int.* 1999 Apr;55(4):1553–9.

[37] Bleyer AJ, Hartman J, Brannon PC, Reeves-Daniel A, Satko SG, Russell G. Characteristics of sudden death in hemodialysis patients. *Kidney Int.* 2006 Jun;69(12):2268–73.

[38] Wang AY-M, Lam CW-K, Chan IH-S, Wang M, Lui S-F, Sanderson JE. Sudden cardiac death in end-stage renal disease patients: a 5-year prospective analysis. *Hypertension.* 2010 Aug;56(2):210–6.

[39] Parekh RS, Carroll CE, Wolfe RA, Port FK. Cardiovascular mortality in children and young adults with end-stage kidney disease. *J Pediatr.* 2002 Aug;141(2):191–7.

[40] Tin LL, Beevers DG, Lip GYH. Hypertension, left ventricular hypertrophy, and sudden death. *Curr Cardiol Rep.* 2002 Nov;4(6):449–57.

[41] Foley RN, Parfrey PS, Sarnak MJ. Clinical epidemiology of cardiovascular disease in chronic renal disease. *Am J Kidney Dis Off J Natl Kidney Found.* 1998 Nov;32(5 Suppl 3):S112–9.

[42] Foley RN, Parfrey PS, Kent GM, Harnett JD, Murray DC, Barre PE. Long-term evolution of cardiomyopathy in dialysis patients. *Kidney Int.* 1998 Nov;54(5):1720–5.

[43] Parfrey PS, Foley RN, Wittreich BH, Sullivan DJ, Zagari MJ, Frei D. Double-blind comparison of full and partial anemia correction in incident hemodialysis patients without symptomatic heart disease. *J Am Soc Nephrol JASN.* 2005 Jul;16(7):2180–9.

[44] Foley RN, Parfrey PS, Harnett JD, Kent GM, Murray DC, Barré PE. The prognostic importance of left ventricular geometry in uremic cardiomyopathy. *J Am Soc Nephrol JASN.* 1995 Jun;5(12):2024–31.

[45] Foley RN, Curtis BM, Randell EW, Parfrey PS. Left ventricular hypertrophy in new hemodialysis patients without symptomatic cardiac disease. *Clin J Am Soc Nephrol CJASN.* 2010 May;5(5):805–13.

[46] Kitano Y, Kasuga H, Watanabe M, Takahashi H, Ibuki K, Kawade Y, et al. Severe coronary stenosis is an important factor for induction and lengthy persistence of ventricular arrhythmias during and after hemodialysis. *Am J Kidney Dis Off J Natl Kidney Found.* 2004 Aug;44(2):328–36.

[47] London GM, Pannier B, Guerin AP, Blacher J, Marchais SJ, Darne B, et al. Alterations of left ventricular hypertrophy in and survival of patients receiving hemodialysis:

follow-up of an interventional study. *J Am Soc Nephrol JASN*. 2001 Dec;12(12):2759–67.

[48] Amann K, Kronenberg G, Gehlen F, Wessels S, Orth S, Münter K, et al. Cardiac remodelling in experimental renal failure--an immunohistochemical study. *Nephrol Dial Transplant Off Publ Eur Dial Transpl Assoc - Eur Ren Assoc*. 1998 Aug;13(8):1958–66.

[49] Haider AW, Larson MG, Benjamin EJ, Levy D. Increased left ventricular mass and hypertrophy are associated with increased risk for sudden death. *J Am Coll Cardiol*. 1998 Nov;32(5):1454–9.

[50] Reinier K, Dervan C, Singh T, Uy-Evanado A, Lai S, Gunson K, et al. Increased left ventricular mass and decreased left ventricular systolic function have independent pathways to ventricular arrhythmogenesis in coronary artery disease. *Heart Rhythm Off J Heart Rhythm Soc*. 2011 Aug;8(8):1177–82.

[51] Multicentre, cross-sectional study of ventricular arrhythmias in chronically haemodialysed patients. Gruppo Emodialisi e Patologie Cardiovasculari. *Lancet Lond Engl*. 1988 Aug 6;2(8606):305–9.

[52] Sforzini S, Latini R, Mingardi G, Vincenti A, Redaelli B. Ventricular arrhythmias and four-year mortality in haemodialysis patients. Gruppo Emodialisi e Patologie Cardiovascolari. *Lancet Lond Engl*. 1992 Jan 25;339(8787):212–3.

[53] Thygesen K, Alpert JS, Jaffe AS, Simoons ML, Chaitman BR, White HD, et al. Third universal definition of myocardial infarction. *J Am Coll Cardiol*. 2012 Oct 16;60(16):1581–98.

[54] Stacy SR, Suarez-Cuervo C, Berger Z, Wilson LM, Yeh H-C, Bass EB, et al. Role of troponin in patients with chronic kidney disease and suspected acute coronary syndrome: a systematic review. *Ann Intern Med*. 2014 Oct 7;161(7):502–12.

[55] Dierkes J, Domröse U, Westphal S, Ambrosch A, Bosselmann HP, Neumann KH, et al. Cardiac troponin T predicts mortality in patients with end-stage renal disease. *Circulation*. 2000 Oct 17;102(16):1964–9.

[56] Hojs R, Bevc S, Ekart R. Biomarkers in hemodialysis patients. *Adv Clin Chem*. 2012;57:29–56.

[57] Ikeda Y, Suehiro T, Itahara T, Inui Y, Chikazawa H, Inoue M, et al. Human serum paraoxonase concentration predicts cardiovascular mortality in hemodialysis patients. *Clin Nephrol*. 2007 Jun;67(6):358–65.

[58] Sharma R, Gaze DC, Pellerin D, Mehta RL, Gregson H, Streather CP, et al. Ischemia-modified albumin predicts mortality in ESRD. *Am J Kidney Dis Off J Natl Kidney Found*. 2006 Mar;47(3):493–502.

[59] Dirican M, Akca R, Sarandol E, Dilek K. Serum paraoxonase activity in uremic predialysis and hemodialysis patients. *J Nephrol*. 2004 Dec;17(6):813–8.

[60] Dantoine TF, Debord J, Charmes JP, Merle L, Marquet P, Lachatre G, et al. Decrease of serum paraoxonase activity in chronic renal failure. *J Am Soc Nephrol JASN*. 1998 Nov;9(11):2082–8.

[61] Gugliucci A, Mehlhaff K, Kinugasa E, Ogata H, Hermo R, Schulze J, et al. Paraoxonase-1 concentrations in end-stage renal disease patients increase after hemodialysis: correlation with low molecular AGE adduct clearance. *Clin Chim Acta Int J Clin Chem*. 2007 Feb;377(1-2):213–20.

[62] Bhagavan NV, Lai EM, Rios PA, Yang J, Ortega-Lopez AM, Shinoda H, et al. Evaluation of human serum albumin cobalt binding assay for the assessment of myocardial ischemia and myocardial infarction. *Clin Chem.* 2003 Apr;49(4):581–5.

[63] Pantazopoulos I, Papadimitriou L, Dontas I, Demestiha T, Iakovidou N, Xanthos T. Ischaemia modified albumin in the diagnosis of acute coronary syndromes. *Resuscitation.* 2009 Mar;80(3):306–10.

[64] Turedi S, Cinar O, Yavuz I, Mentese A, Gunduz A, Karahan SC, et al. Differences in ischemia-modified albumin levels between end stage renal disease patients and the normal population. *J Nephrol.* 2010 Jun;23(3):335–40.

[65] Ravani P, Tripepi G, Malberti F, Testa S, Mallamaci F, Zoccali C. Asymmetrical dimethylarginine predicts progression to dialysis and death in patients with chronic kidney disease: a competing risks modeling approach. *J Am Soc Nephrol JASN.* 2005 Aug;16(8):2449–55.

[66] Hoffman BF, Guo SD, Feinmark SJ. Arrhythmias caused by platelet activating factor. *J Cardiovasc Electrophysiol.* 1996 Feb;7(2):120–33.

[67] Hoffman BF, Feinmark SJ, Guo SD. Electrophysiologic effects of interactions between activated canine neutrophils and cardiac myocytes. *J Cardiovasc Electrophysiol.* 1997 Jun;8(6):679–87.

[68] Mallamaci F, Zoccali C, Tripepi G, Fermo I, Benedetto FA, Cataliotti A, et al. Hyperhomocysteinemia predicts cardiovascular outcomes in hemodialysis patients. *Kidney Int.* 2002 Feb;61(2):609–14.

[69] Stewart GA, Gansevoort RT, Mark PB, Rooney E, McDonagh TA, Dargie HJ, et al. Electrocardiographic abnormalities and uremic cardiomyopathy. *Kidney Int.* 2005 Jan;67(1):217–26.

[70] Pye MP, Cobbe SM. Mechanisms of ventricular arrhythmias in cardiac failure and hypertrophy. *Cardiovasc Res.* 1992 Aug;26(8):740–50.

[71] Suzuki R, Tsumura K, Inoue T, Kishimoto H, Morii H. QT interval prolongation in the patients receiving maintenance hemodialysis. *Clin Nephrol.* 1998 Apr;49(4):240–4.

[72] Covic A, Diaconita M, Gusbeth-Tatomir P, Covic M, Botezan A, Ungureanu G, et al. Haemodialysis increases QTc interval but not QTc dispersion in ESRD patients without manifest cardiac disease. *Nephrol Dial Transplant.* 2002 Dec 1;17(12):2170–7.

[73] Cupisti A, Galetta F, Morelli E, Tintori G, Sibilia G, Meola M, et al. Effect of hemodialysis on the dispersion of the QTc interval. *Nephron.* 1998;78(4):429–32.

[74] Genovesi S, Rivera R, Fabbrini P, Dossi C, Bonforte G, Mircoli L, et al. Dynamic QT interval analysis in uraemic patients receiving chronic haemodialysis. *J Hypertens.* 2003 Oct;21(10):1921–6.

[75] Redaelli B, Locatelli F, Limido D, Andrulli S, Signorini MG, Sforzini S, et al. Effect of a new model of hemodialysis potassium removal on the control of ventricular arrhythmias. *Kidney Int.* 1996 Aug;50(2):609–17.

[76] Buemi M, Aloisi E, Coppolino G, Loddo S, Crascì E, Aloisi C, et al. The effect of two different protocols of potassium haemodiafiltration on QT dispersion. *Nephrol Dial Transplant Off Publ Eur Dial Transpl Assoc - Eur Ren Assoc.* 2005 Jun;20(6):1148–54.

[77] Santoro A, Mancini E, London G, Mercadal L, Fessy H, Perrone B, et al. Patients with complex arrhythmias during and after haemodialysis suffer from different regimens of potassium removal. *Nephrol Dial Transplant Off Publ Eur Dial Transpl Assoc - Eur Ren Assoc.* 2008 Apr;23(4):1415–21.

[78] Karnik JA, Young BS, Lew NL, Herget M, Dubinsky C, Lazarus JM, et al. Cardiac arrest and sudden death in dialysis units. *Kidney Int.* 2001 Jul;60(1):350–7.
[79] Näppi SE, Virtanen VK, Saha HH, Mustonen JT, Pasternack AI. QTc dispersion increases during hemodialysis with low-calcium dialysate. *Kidney Int.* 2000 May;57(5):2117–22.
[80] Genovesi S, Dossi C, Viganò MR, Galbiati E, Prolo F, Stella A, et al. Electrolyte concentration during haemodialysis and QT interval prolongation in uraemic patients. *Eur Eur Pacing Arrhythm Card Electrophysiol J Work Groups Card Pacing Arrhythm Card Cell Electrophysiol Eur Soc Cardiol.* 2008 Jun;10(6):771–7.
[81] Beaubien ER, Pylypchuk GB, Akhtar J, Biem HJ. Value of corrected QT interval dispersion in identifying patients initiating dialysis at increased risk of total and cardiovascular mortality. *Am J Kidney Dis Off J Natl Kidney Found.* 2002 Apr;39(4):834–42.
[82] Howse M, Sastry S, Bell GM. Changes in the corrected QT interval and corrected QT dispersion during haemodialysis. *Postgrad Med J.* 2002 May;78(919):273–5.
[83] Block GA, Hulbert-Shearon TE, Levin NW, Port FK. Association of serum phosphorus and calcium x phosphate product with mortality risk in chronic hemodialysis patients: a national study. *Am J Kidney Dis Off J Natl Kidney Found.* 1998 Apr;31(4):607–17.
[84] Amann K, Ritz E. Microvascular disease--the Cinderella of uraemic heart disease. *Nephrol Dial Transplant Off Publ Eur Dial Transpl Assoc - Eur Ren Assoc.* 2000 Oct;15(10):1493–503.
[85] Ganesh SK, Stack AG, Levin NW, Hulbert-Shearon T, Port FK. Association of elevated serum PO(4), Ca x PO(4) product, and parathyroid hormone with cardiac mortality risk in chronic hemodialysis patients. *J Am Soc Nephrol JASN.* 2001 Oct;12(10):2131–8.
[86] Flythe JE, Kimmel SE, Brunelli SM. Rapid fluid removal during dialysis is associated with cardiovascular morbidity and mortality. *Kidney Int.* 2011 Jan;79(2):250–7.
[87] Saran R, Bragg-Gresham JL, Levin NW, Twardowski ZJ, Wizemann V, Saito A, et al. Longer treatment time and slower ultrafiltration in hemodialysis: associations with reduced mortality in the DOPPS. *Kidney Int.* 2006 Apr;69(7):1222–8.
[88] Movilli E, Gaggia P, Zubani R, Camerini C, Vizzardi V, Parrinello G, et al. Association between high ultrafiltration rates and mortality in uraemic patients on regular haemodialysis. A 5-year prospective observational multicentre study. *Nephrol Dial Transplant Off Publ Eur Dial Transpl Assoc - Eur Ren Assoc.* 2007 Dec;22(12):3547–52.
[89] Burton JO, Jefferies HJ, Selby NM, McIntyre CW. Hemodialysis-induced repetitive myocardial injury results in global and segmental reduction in systolic cardiac function. *Clin J Am Soc Nephrol* CJASN. 2009 Dec;4(12):1925–31.
[90] Burton JO, Jefferies HJ, Selby NM, McIntyre CW. Hemodialysis-induced cardiac injury: determinants and associated outcomes. *Clin J Am Soc Nephrol CJASN.* 2009 May;4(5):914–20.
[91] Hothi DK, Rees L, Marek J, Burton J, McIntyre CW. Pediatric myocardial stunning underscores the cardiac toxicity of conventional hemodialysis treatments. *Clin J Am Soc Nephrol* CJASN. 2009 Apr;4(4):790–7.
[92] Besarab A. Iron and cardiac disease in the end-stage renal disease setting. *Am J Kidney Dis Off J Natl Kidney Found.* 1999 Oct;34(4 Suppl 2):S18–24.

[93] Wardman P, Candeias LP. Fenton chemistry: an introduction. *Radiat Res.* 1996 May;145(5):523–31.

[94] Wu V-C, Huang J-W, Wu M-S, Chin C-Y, Chiang F-T, Liu Y-B, et al. The effect of iron stores on corrected QT dispersion in patients undergoing peritoneal dialysis. *Am J Kidney Dis Off J Natl Kidney Found.* 2004 Oct;44(4):720–8.

[95] Converse RL, Jacobsen TN, Toto RD, Jost CM, Cosentino F, Fouad-Tarazi F, et al. Sympathetic overactivity in patients with chronic renal failure. *N Engl J Med.* 1992 Dec 31;327(27):1912–8.

[96] Rump LC, Amann K, Orth S, Ritz E. Sympathetic overactivity in renal disease: a window to understand progression and cardiovascular complications of uraemia? *Nephrol Dial Transplant Off Publ Eur Dial Transpl Assoc - Eur Ren Assoc.* 2000 Nov;15(11):1735–8.

[97] Amann K, Rump LC, Simonaviciene A, Oberhauser V, Wessels S, Orth SR, et al. Effects of low dose sympathetic inhibition on glomerulosclerosis and albuminuria in subtotally nephrectomized rats. *J Am Soc Nephrol JASN.* 2000 Aug;11(8):1469–78.

[98] Johansson M, Gao SA, Friberg P, Annerstedt M, Bergström G, Carlström J, et al. Reduced baroreflex effectiveness index in hypertensive patients with chronic renal failure. *Am J Hypertens.* 2005 Jul;18(7):995–1000; discussion 1016.

[99] Johansson M, Gao SA, Friberg P, Annerstedt M, Carlström J, Ivarsson T, et al. Baroreflex effectiveness index and baroreflex sensitivity predict all-cause mortality and sudden death in hypertensive patients with chronic renal failure. *J Hypertens.* 2007 Jan;25(1):163–8.

[100] Brophy JM, Joseph L, Rouleau JL. Beta-blockers in congestive heart failure. A Bayesian meta-analysis. *Ann Intern Med.* 2001 Apr 3;134(7):550–60.

[101] Matsue Y, Suzuki M, Nagahori W, Ohno M, Matsumura A, Hashimoto Y. β-blocker prevents sudden cardiac death in patients with hemodialysis. *Int J Cardiol.* 2013 May 25;165(3):519–22.

[102] Badve SV, Roberts MA, Hawley CM, Cass A, Garg AX, Krum H, et al. Effects of beta-adrenergic antagonists in patients with chronic kidney disease: a systematic review and meta-analysis. *J Am Coll Cardiol.* 2011 Sep 6;58(11):1152–61.

[103] Myerburg RJ, Kessler KM, Mallon SM, Cox MM, deMarchena E, Interian A, et al. Life-threatening ventricular arrhythmias in patients with silent myocardial ischemia due to coronary-artery spasm. *N Engl J Med.* 1992 May 28;326(22):1451–5.

[104] Luft FC, Johnston CI. Are calcium antagonists of value in ameliorating the course of chronic renal disease? *Kidney Int Suppl.* 1992 May;36:S114–8.

[105] Tepel M, Giet MV der, Park A, Zidek W. Association of calcium channel blockers and mortality in haemodialysis patients. *Clin Sci Lond Engl* 1979. 2002 Nov;103(5):511–5.

[106] Pun PH, Lehrich RW, Smith SR, Middleton JP. Predictors of survival after cardiac arrest in outpatient hemodialysis clinics. *Clin J Am Soc Nephrol CJASN.* 2007 May;2(3):491–500.

[107] Packer M, Gheorghiade M, Young JB, Costantini PJ, Adams KF, Cody RJ, et al. Withdrawal of digoxin from patients with chronic heart failure treated with angiotensin-converting-enzyme inhibitors. RADIANCE Study. *N Engl J Med.* 1993 Jul 1;329(1):1–7.

[108] Digitalis Investigation Group. The effect of digoxin on mortality and morbidity in patients with heart failure. *N Engl J Med.* 1997 Feb 20;336(8):525–33.

[109] Chan KE, Lazarus JM, Hakim RM. Digoxin associates with mortality in ESRD. *J Am Soc Nephrol JASN*. 2010 Sep;21(9):1550–9.

[110] Piccini JP, Berger JS, O'Connor CM. Amiodarone for the prevention of sudden cardiac death: a meta-analysis of randomized controlled trials. *Eur Heart J*. 2009 May;30(10):1245–53.

[111] Domanski MJ, Exner DV, Borkowf CB, Geller NL, Rosenberg Y, Pfeffer MA. Effect of angiotensin converting enzyme inhibition on sudden cardiac death in patients following acute myocardial infarction. A meta-analysis of randomized clinical trials. *J Am Coll Cardiol*. 1999 Mar;33(3):598–604.

[112] Mann JF, Gerstein HC, Pogue J, Bosch J, Yusuf S. Renal insufficiency as a predictor of cardiovascular outcomes and the impact of ramipril: the HOPE randomized trial. *Ann Intern Med*. 2001 Apr 17;134(8):629–36.

[113] Zannad F, Kessler M, Lehert P, Grünfeld JP, Thuilliez C, Leizorovicz A, et al. Prevention of cardiovascular events in end-stage renal disease: results of a randomized trial of fosinopril and implications for future studies. *Kidney Int*. 2006 Oct;70(7):1318–24.

[114] Takahashi A, Takase H, Toriyama T, Sugiura T, Kurita Y, Ueda R, et al. Candesartan, an angiotensin II type-1 receptor blocker, reduces cardiovascular events in patients on chronic haemodialysis--a randomized study. *Nephrol Dial Transplant Off Publ Eur Dial Transpl Assoc - Eur Ren Assoc*. 2006 Sep;21(9):2507–12.

[115] Pitt B, Zannad F, Remme WJ, Cody R, Castaigne A, Perez A, et al. The effect of spironolactone on morbidity and mortality in patients with severe heart failure. Randomized Aldactone Evaluation Study Investigators. *N Engl J Med*. 1999 Sep 2;341(10):709–17.

[116] Chua D, Lo A, Lo C. Spironolactone use in heart failure patients with end-stage renal disease on hemodialysis: is it safe? *Clin Cardiol*. 2010 Oct;33(10):604–8.

[117] Green D, Ritchie JP, Kalra PA. Meta-analysis of lipid-lowering therapy in maintenance dialysis patients. *Nephron Clin Pract*. 2013;124(3-4):209–17.

[118] Sun L, Zou L, Chen M, Liu B. Meta-analysis of statin therapy in maintenance dialysis patients. *Ren Fail*. 2015 Jul 3;1–8.

[119] Palmer SC, Navaneethan SD, Craig JC, Johnson DW, Perkovic V, Nigwekar SU, et al. HMG CoA reductase inhibitors (statins) for dialysis patients. *Cochrane Database Syst Rev*. 2013;9:CD004289.

[120] Connolly SJ, Hallstrom AP, Cappato R, Schron EB, Kuck KH, Zipes DP, et al. Meta-analysis of the implantable cardioverter defibrillator secondary prevention trials. AVID, CASH and CIDS studies. Antiarrhythmics vs Implantable Defibrillator study. Cardiac Arrest Study Hamburg. Canadian Implantable Defibrillator Study. *Eur Heart J*. 2000 Dec;21(24):2071–8.

[121] Alsheikh-Ali AA, Trikalinos TA, Ruthazer R, Terrin N, Wong JB, Sarnak MJ, et al. Risk of arrhythmic and nonarrhythmic death in patients with heart failure and chronic kidney disease. *Am Heart J*. 2011 Jan;161(1):204–9.e1.

[122] Herzog CA, Li S, Weinhandl ED, Strief JW, Collins AJ, Gilbertson DT. Survival of dialysis patients after cardiac arrest and the impact of implantable cardioverter defibrillators. *Kidney Int*. 2005 Aug;68(2):818–25.

[123] Khan F, Adelstein E, Saba S. Implantable cardioverter defibrillators confer survival benefit in patients with renal insufficiency but not in dialysis-dependent patients. *J Interv Card Electrophysiol Int J Arrhythm Pacing*. 2010 Aug;28(2):117–23.

[124] Voigt A, Ezzeddine R, Barrington W, Obiaha-Ngwu O, Ganz LI, London B, et al. Utilization of implantable cardioverter-defibrillators in survivors of cardiac arrest in the United States from 1996 to 2001. *J Am Coll Cardiol*. 2004 Aug 18;44(4):855–8.

[125] de Bie MK, Lekkerkerker JC, van Dam B, Gaasbeek A, van Buren M, Putter H, et al. Prevention of sudden cardiac death: rationale and design of the Implantable Cardioverter Defibrillators in Dialysis patients (ICD2) Trial--a prospective pilot study. *Curr Med Res Opin*. 2008 Aug;24(8):2151–7.

[126] Daemen J, Boersma E, Flather M, Booth J, Stables R, Rodriguez A, et al. Long-term safety and efficacy of percutaneous coronary intervention with stenting and coronary artery bypass surgery for multivessel coronary artery disease: a meta-analysis with 5-year patient-level data from the ARTS, ERACI-II, MASS-II, and SoS trials. *Circulation*. 2008 Sep 9;118(11):1146–54.

[127] Bravata DM, Gienger AL, McDonald KM, Sundaram V, Perez MV, Varghese R, et al. Systematic review: the comparative effectiveness of percutaneous coronary interventions and coronary artery bypass graft surgery. *Ann Intern Med*. 2007 Nov 20;147(10):703–16.

[128] Castelli P, Condemi AM, Munari M. Immediate and long-term results of coronary revascularization in patients undergoing chronic hemodialysis. *Eur J Cardio-Thorac Surg Off J Eur Assoc Cardio-Thorac Surg*. 1999 Jan;15(1):51–4.

[129] Herzog CA, Ma JZ, Collins AJ. Comparative survival of dialysis patients in the United States after coronary angioplasty, coronary artery stenting, and coronary artery bypass surgery and impact of diabetes. *Circulation*. 2002 Oct 22;106(17):2207–11.

[130] Herzog CA, Ma JZ, Collins AJ. Long-term outcome of dialysis patients in the United States with coronary revascularization procedures. *Kidney Int*. 1999 Jul;56(1):324–32.

[131] Stettler C, Wandel S, Allemann S, Kastrati A, Morice MC, Schömig A, et al. Outcomes associated with drug-eluting and bare-metal stents: a collaborative network meta-analysis. *Lancet Lond Engl*. 2007 Sep 15;370(9591):937–48.

[132] Tsai TT, Messenger JC, Brennan JM, Patel UD, Dai D, Piana RN, et al. Safety and efficacy of drug-eluting stents in older patients with chronic kidney disease: a report from the linked CathPCI Registry-CMS claims database. *J Am Coll Cardiol*. 2011 Oct 25;58(18):1859–69.

[133] Abdel-Latif A, Mukherjee D, Mesgarzadeh P, Ziada KM. Drug-eluting stents in patients with end-stage renal disease: meta-analysis and systematic review of the literature. *Catheter Cardiovasc Interv Off J Soc Card Angiogr Interv*. 2010 Dec 1;76(7):942–8.

[134] Nevis IF, Mathew A, Novick RJ, Parikh CR, Devereaux PJ, Natarajan MK, et al. Optimal method of coronary revascularization in patients receiving dialysis: systematic review. *Clin J Am Soc Nephrol CJASN*. 2009 Feb;4(2):369–78.

[135] Genovesi S, Valsecchi MG, Rossi E, Pogliani D, Acquistapace I, De Cristofaro V, et al. Sudden death and associated factors in a historical cohort of chronic haemodialysis patients. *Nephrol Dial Transplant Off Publ Eur Dial Transpl Assoc - Eur Ren Assoc*. 2009 Aug;24(8):2529–36.

[136] Kovesdy CP, Regidor DL, Mehrotra R, Jing J, McAllister CJ, Greenland S, et al. Serum and dialysate potassium concentrations and survival in hemodialysis patients. *Clin J Am Soc Nephrol CJASN*. 2007 Sep;2(5):999–1007.

[137] Pun PH, Lehrich RW, Honeycutt EF, Herzog CA, Middleton JP. Modifiable risk factors associated with sudden cardiac arrest within hemodialysis clinics. *Kidney Int*. 2011 Jan;79(2):218–27.

[138] Pun PH, Horton JR, Middleton JP. Dialysate calcium concentration and the risk of sudden cardiac arrest in hemodialysis patients. *Clin J Am Soc Nephrol CJASN*. 2013 May;8(5):797–803.

[139] Ferrario M, Moissl U, Garzotto F, Cruz DN, Clementi A, Brendolan A, et al. Effects of fluid overload on heart rate variability in chronic kidney disease patients on hemodialysis. *BMC Nephrol*. 2014;15:26.

[140] Suri RS, Nesrallah GE, Mainra R, Garg AX, Lindsay RM, Greene T, et al. Daily hemodialysis: a systematic review. *Clin J Am Soc Nephrol CJASN*. 2006 Jan;1(1):33–42.

[141] Fagugli RM, Reboldi G, Quintaliani G, Pasini P, Ciao G, Cicconi B, et al. Short daily hemodialysis: blood pressure control and left ventricular mass reduction in hypertensive hemodialysis patients. *Am J Kidney Dis Off J Natl Kidney Found*. 2001 Aug;38(2):371–6.

[142] Traeger J, Galland R, Delawari E, Arkouche W, Hadden R. Six years' experience with short daily hemodialysis: do the early improvements persist in the mid and long term? *Hemodial Int Int Symp Home Hemodial*. 2004 Apr 1;8(2):151–8.

[143] FHN Trial Group, Chertow GM, Levin NW, Beck GJ, Depner TA, Eggers PW, et al. In-center hemodialysis six times per week versus three times per week. *N Engl J Med*. 2010 Dec 9;363(24):2287–300.

[144] Lacson E, Xu J, Suri RS, Nesrallah G, Lindsay R, Garg AX, et al. Survival with three-times weekly in-center nocturnal versus conventional hemodialysis. *J Am Soc Nephrol JASN*. 2012 Apr;23(4):687–95.

In: Comorbidities in Chronic Kidney Disease
Editor: Luca Di Lullo

ISBN: 978-1-63485-070-4

Chapter 8

CARDIORENAL SYNDROME

***Luca Di Lullo*[1,*] *and Claudio Ronco*[2]**

[1]Department of Nephrology and Dialysis "L. Parodi,
Delfino Hospital," Colleferro, Roma, Italy
[2]International Renal Research Institute "S. Bortolo Hospital," Vicenza, Italy

ABSTRACT

The term cardiorenal syndrome (CRS) has been used to define different clinical conditions in which heart and kidney dysfunction overlap. An effective classification of CRS has been proposed in a Consensus Conference by the Acute Dialysis Quality Group in 2008. This classification essentially divides CRS in two main groups, cardio - renal and reno - cardiac CRS, on the basis of primum movens of disease (cardiac or renal); both cardio – renal and reno – cardiac CRS are then divided into acute and chronic according to disease's onset. Type 5 of CRS integrates all cardio – renal involvement induced by systemic disease.

Pathophysiological pathways are different according to primary disease but final pathways often overlap except for type – 5 that is closely related to primary disease. Therapeutic approaches differ for acute and chronic syndromes and they are characterized both by pharmacological and non – pharmacological strategies.

Keywords: cardiorenal syndrome, acute kidney injury, heart failure, sepsis

INTRODUCTION

According to recent definition proposed by Consensus conference of Acute Dialysis Quality Initiative Group [1], the term cardiorenal syndrome (CRS) has been used to define different clinical conditions in which heart and kidney dysfunction overlap.

* Correspondence to: L. Di Lullo, Department of Nephrology and Dialysis. Colleferro County Hospital, Piazza Aldo Moro, 1 Colleferro, Rome, Italy, Tel: +39 069 722 3205; Fax: +39 069 722 3213; Email: dilulloluca69@gmail.com.

CRS complexity needs to be explained starting by its pathogenesis and epidemiology and then by analyzing diagnostic, clinical and therapeutic pathways.

Table 1. Classification of Cardio – Renal Syndrome

Type	Denomination	Description	Example
1	Acute cardiorenal	Heart failure leading to AKD	Acute coronary syndrome leading to acute heart and kidney failure
2	Chronic cardiorenal	Chronic heart failure leading to kidney failure	Chronic heart failure
3	Acute nephrocardiac	AKD leading to acute heart failure	Uremic cardiomiopathy AKD - related
4	Chronic nephrocardiac	Chronic kidney disease leading to heart failure	Left ventricular hypertrophy and diastolic heart failure due to kidney failure
5	Secondary	Systemic disease leading to heart and kidney failure	Sepsis, vasculitis, diabetes mellitus

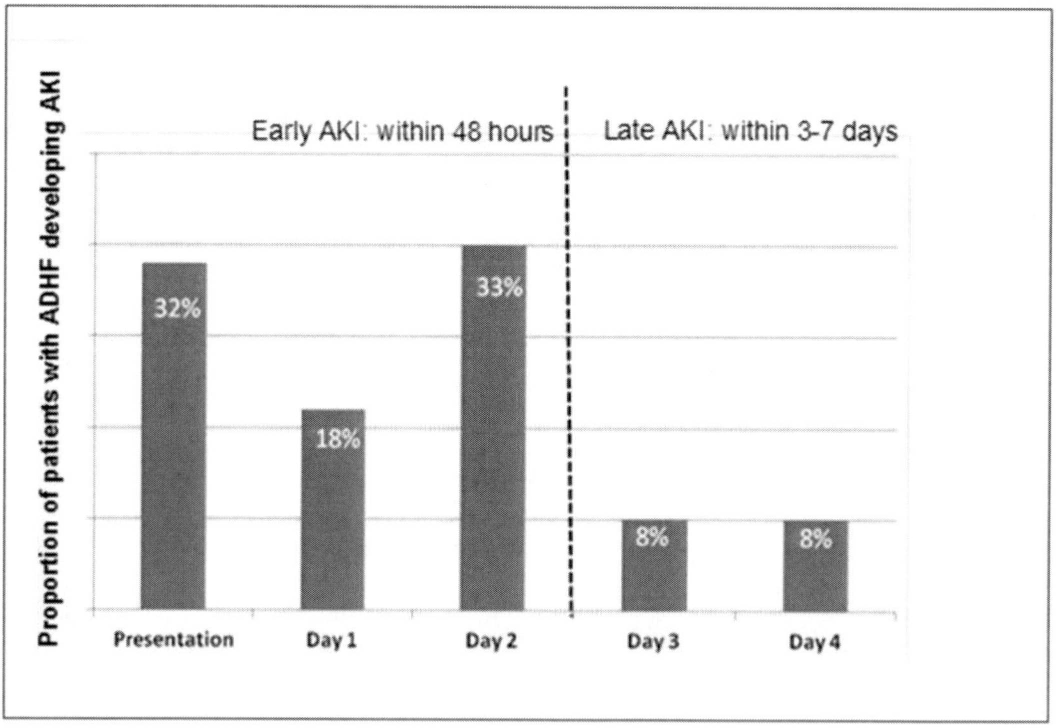

Figure 1. Timing of acute kidney injury in the setting of acute decompensated heart failure.

An effective classification of CRS has been proposed in a Consensus Conference by the Acute Dialysis Quality Group [1] in 2008 (Table 1). This classification essentially divides CRS in two main groups, cardio - renal and reno - cardiac CRS, on the basis of primum movens of disease (cardiac or renal); both cardio – renal and reno – cardiac CRS are then divided into acute and chronic according to disease's onset. Type 5 of CRS integrates all cardio – renal involvement induced by systemic disease.

1. Type – 1 Cardio – Renal Syndrome

Type – 1 occurs in about 25% of patients hospitalized for acute decompensated heart failure [2, 3]; among these patients a pre – existent chronic kidney disease is quite common and contributes to AKI in 60% of all cases studied. AKI can be considered an independent mortality risk factor in acute decompensated heart failure (ADHF) patients, including those with ST – myocardial infarction and/or reduced left ventricular ejection fraction [4].

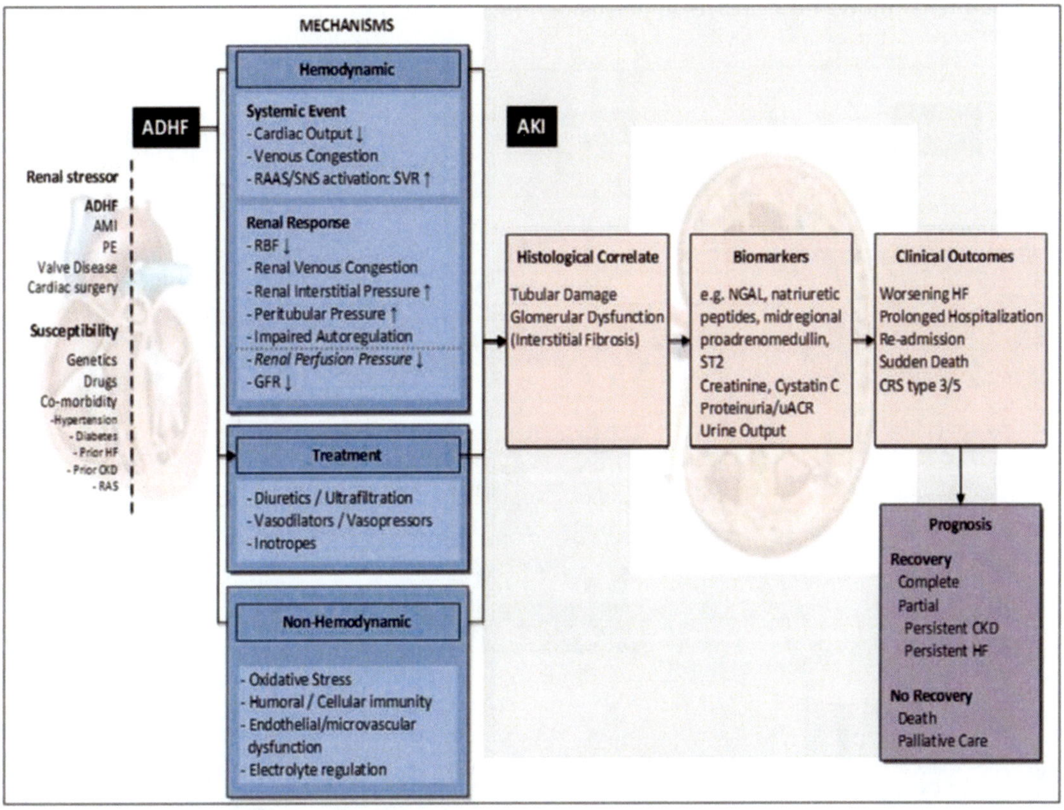

Figure 2. Overview on mechanisms, histological correlates biomarkers and outcomes in cardiorenal syndrome type 1 in the setting of acute decompensated heart failure. Reproduced with permission from ADQI [53]. ADHF, acute decompensated heart failure; AKI, acute kidney injury (the term AKI also covers the term "WRF," "worsening renal function which is usually defined as doubling in serum creatinine); AMI, acute myocardial infarction; PE, pulmonary embolism; SVR, systemic vascular resistance; HF, heart failure; CKD, chronic kidney disease; RAS, renal artery stenosis; GFR, glomerular filtration rate; NGAL; neutrophil gelatinase-associated lipocalin; IL-18, interleukin 18; KIM-1, kidney injury molecule 1; L-FABP, liver-type fatty acid binding protein; NAG, N-acetylglucosamine.

1.1. Pathophysiology

Type – 1 CRS (acute cardio – renal) is characterized by acute worsening of cardiac function leading to acute kidney injury (AKI) [5, 6] in the setting of an acute cardiac disease such as acute decompensated heart failure (ADHF) Preliminary observations point up the importance of timing in the development of AKI and its early diagnosis (Figure 1).

Hemodynamic mechanisms probably play a major role in CRS type 1 in presence of an ADHF leading to decreased renal arterial flow and consequent fall in glomerular filtration rate. Once hemodynamics has restored, renal and cardiac parameters come back to normal [7] (Figure 2). Different hemodynamic profiles have been proposed [8]: in "cold" pattern patients' reduction in ECFV (effective circulation fluid volume) represent main hemodynamic change with marked increase in CVP (central venous pressure) in "wet" pattern patients'

"Cold" patients also present renal blood flow decrease probably related to renin – angiotensin system and systemic nervous system activation causing afferent vasoconstriction, decreased renal blood flow and renal perfusion pressure falling.

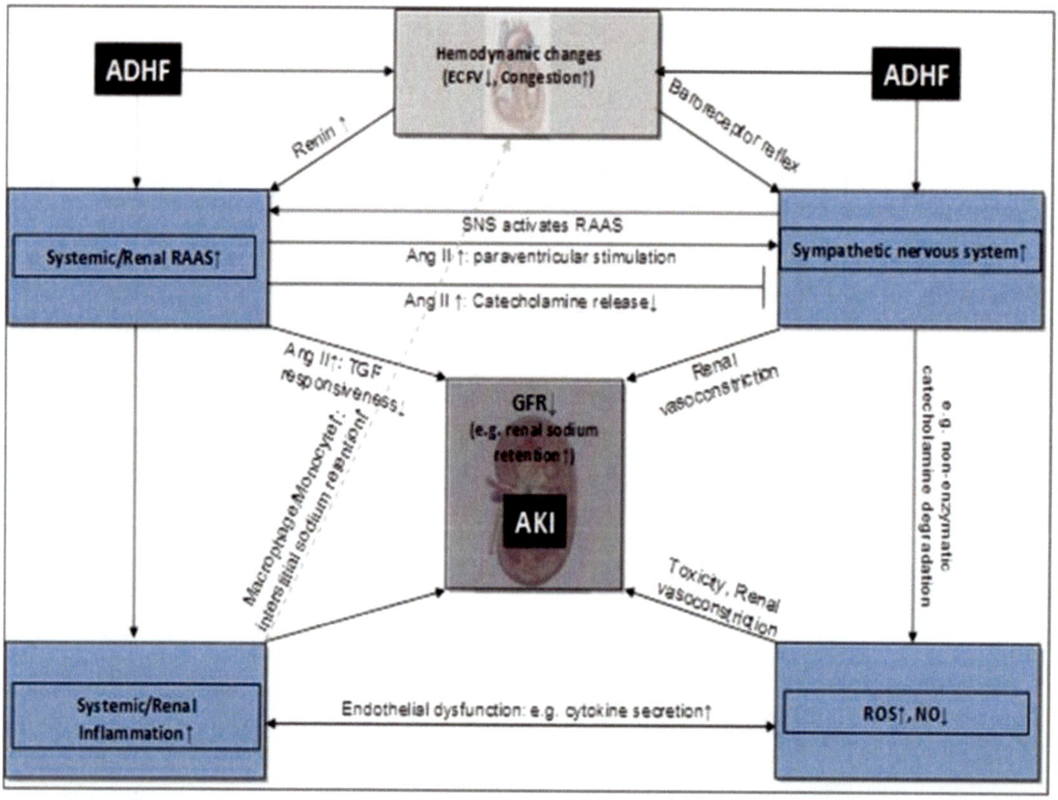

Figure 3. Non-hemodynamic network of pathophysiological interactions in CRS type 1. Note the emerging potential role of macrophages/monocytes as mediator of sodium and fluid retention. Reproduced with permission from ADQI.

Other patients present as "wet" due to increased pulmonary and/or systemic congestion; in these patients high CVP directly affects renal vein and kidney perfusion pressure [9, 10]; CVP increase also results in increased interstitial pressure with tubules' collapse and progressive lack of renal function [11].

Also "warm" profiles patients present reduction in cardiac output and ECFV but not as in "cold" patients [12].

"Warm and wet" patients represent the most occurring profile in acute and chronic advanced heart failure [13]. Mechanisms of increased CVP are quite similar to "cold" profiles patients' but renal perfusion pressure is less affected because of higher arterial blood pressures [9].

Non – hemodynamics mechanisms were also proposed as involved in type – 1 CRS, including sympathetic nervous system (SNS) and renin – angiotensin aldosterone system (RAAS) activation, chronic inflammatory status and impairment of ROS/NO production (Figure 3). Patients with ADHF show more frequent defective regulation of monocyte apoptosis and activation of inflammatory pathways in respect of healthy subjects [14, 15].

Gut under - perfusion and endotoxin release in HF patients have been proposed as pathophysiologic mechanisms in progression of heart failure and CRS [16].

1.2. Diagnosis

Since morbidity and mortality rates of type – 1 CRS are still high, an early diagnosis is required. NGAL has to be involved in cardiomyocyte apoptosis by increasing intracellular iron accumulation [19]. These findings agree with those reported in human myocarditis where NGAL was strongly induced in affected myocardiocytes, vascular wall cells, fibroblasts and neutrophils [23].

Neurohormonal involvement is underlined by incretion of natriuretic peptides, mid – regional proadrenomedullin and copeptin [24, 25, 26]. Patients with type – 1 CRS present abnormalities in cell signaling pathways: soluble ST – 2, new predictor risk factor in HF patients for risk of hospitalization and death [27, 28, 29].

ST2 is the receptor for interleukin-33, an angiohypertrophic and antifibrotic cytokine with myocardial effects [30]; soluble ST is a circulating inhibitor of the ST2 receptor, and counteracts regenerative effects of IL-33. As illustrated above it's clear how systemic cell signaling could manage negative tubuloglomerular feedback and consequent transient reduction in renal filtration [31, 32].

Cystatin C, a 25kDa glomerularly filterable protein secreted by all nucleated cells, represent valid surrogate to test renal function and it has been recognized as more predictive of long term mortality and re – hospitalization for ADHF than serum creatinine or serum BNP [33, 34].

Due to its biochemical characteristics, serum cystatin C could be helpful for earlier diagnosis of AKI in CRS type 1.

Other tubular injury biomarkers are represented by Kidney Injury Molecule 1 (KIM-1), Liver-type Fatty Acid Binding Protein (L-FABP), Interleukin 18 (IL-18), while Neutrophil Gelatinase-Associated Lipocalin (NGAL) has collected most comprehensive experimental and clinical data in ADHF patients in which it strongly correlates with renal function markers [35] and adverse cardiovascular outcomes or death [36]. Serum NGAL level was found as stronger predictor of 30-day all-cause death and ADHF readmissions than BNP [37]. On these basis, acute tubular damage in CRS type 1 is probably accountable for future development of CRS type 3. Preliminary data suggest how NGAL levels could predict AKI in patients with ADHF better than serum cystatin C and serum creatinine levels [38-40]. Other potential helpful biomarkers to be tested for early diagnosis of AKI in HF patients include osteopontin, N-acetyl-b-d-glucosaminidase, stromal cell-derived factor-1, endoglin, galectin-3 and exosomes but we have actually few data to employ them in routine diagnosis [41].

Together with laboratory diagnosis, type – 1 CRS can be diagnosed also by bioelectrical devices, especially for whom to concern fluid assessment in those patients. Several clinical studies showed an association between decreased impedance values (increased body fluid volume) and adverse events as rehospitalization and death; bioimpedance measurement also helped to distinguish cardiogenic dyspnea from noncardiogenic dyspnea [42, 43]. High sensitivity and specificity of reduced bioimpedance value were confirmed by radiographic findings consistent with pulmonary edema [44]. Bioimpedance test result may be a potential criterion for discharge readiness and testing re – hospitalization ratio [45].

Bioimpedance measurement may provide early diagnosis of ADHF, differential diagnosis of dyspnea and therapy management on CRS type 1 but need further clinical data.

Ultrasonography can provide further elements for type – 1 CRS diagnosis; echocardiographic typical findings are following: abnormal myocardial kinetics (indicating an ischemic condition) and left ventricular hypertrophy, valvular stenosis and insufficiency (particularly in case of rapid deterioration, such as valvular endocarditis or valvular rupture), pericardial effusions, normal inspiratory collapse of the inferior vena cava (excluding severe hypervolemia), aortic aneurysms or dissection [46].

Kidneys' ultrasonographic evaluation usually show normal or larger dimensions with preserved cortical – medullary ratio; color – doppler evaluation shows regular intra - parenchymal blood flow, often associated to raised resistance index (>0.8 cm/sec) [46].

1.3. Outcomes and Treatment

Renal function often improves in response to standard therapy aimed to reduce filling pressures with loop diuretics and nitrates in warm & wet ADHF patients with AKI at presentation; this observation suggests that increased renal venous congestion may be the predominate mechanisms underlying AKI

Pre-RELAX study found that drop in systolic blood pressure within the first 48 hours of vasodilator therapy was an independent predictor of AKI by day 5 [47]. These data together with clinical experience support the idea that therapy-related reduction in renal perfusion pressure and/or ECFV are the predominate mechanisms underlying AKI that develops within the first days of hospitalization.

Usually, ACE-inhibitors are slowly uptitrated during the course of hospitalization. The hemodynamic effect of ACE-inhibitors (vasodilation of the efferens glomerular vessel) and its associated drop in filtration pressure as well as "pre-renal" kidney dysfunction due to the reduction in ECFV associated with intensified therapy with loop diuretics may be the predominate mechanism underlying AKI developing late during hospitalization.

Finally, severity and duration of AKI seem to relate to long-term patient outcome; early diagnosis and treatment is quite recommended [48].

2. Type – 2 Cardio – Renal Syndrome

Cardiorenal syndrome Type 2 (CRS2) is characterized by chronic abnormalities in cardiac function leading to kidney injury or dysfunction; temporal relationship between heart and kidney disease is an epidemiological and pathophysiological aspect of the definition itself. Literature data show that chronic heart and kidney disease often coexist but large cohort studies assess the onset of one disease (e.g., chronic heart failure [HF]) subsequently describing the prevalence of the other (chronic kidney disease [CKD]) [49, 50]. It's quite difficult to establish which of two disease is primary versus secondary. CKD has been observed in 45 - 63% of CHF patients [49 - 51] but it's unclear how to classify these patients often including those ones shifting from a clinical condition of Type – 1 CRS. At the same time it's not easy to recognize these patients from Type – 4 CRS (chronic reno – cardiac syndrome) [52].

2.1. Pathophysiology

Due to definition itself, type – 2 CRS is characterized by CKD onset in HF patients, but co – existence of cardiovascular disease and CKD is not enough to propose a type – 2 CRS diagnosis. Two fundamental features are proposed for a CRS – 2 diagnosis: CHF and CKD are to be simultaneously present and CHF causally underlies CKD occurrence or progression [53]. Examples of type – 2 CRS can be provided by "cyanotic nephropathy" occurring in patients with congenital heart disease when heart disease clearly precedes kidney involvement or acute coronary syndrome leading to left ventricular dysfunction and onset/progression of co – existing CKD.

Although multiple and complex mechanisms have been proposed to explain pathophysiology of CRS – 2, neuro - hormonal activation, kidney hypoperfusion and venous congestion, inflammation, atherosclerosis and oxidative stress represent most important ones.

On the other hand recurrent episodes of acute heart and/or kidney decompensation can be associated to HF and CKD progression such as demonstrated by data showing how previous hospitalizations for HF are mortality predictors after we have controlled other HF risk factors [54]. Re – occurrence of HF admissions is independently associated with development of CKD (EPI eGFR < 60 ml/min) [55].

In HF experimental studies a reduction in glomerular plasma flow together with elevated glomerular filtration rate (efferent arteriolar constriction) is observed; if these changes persist (up to six months in experimental model) podocytes injury, focal and segmental glomerulosclerosis can occur. Many of these histologic changes can be referred to local renal increase in sympathetic nervous system and RAAS activation [56].

Kidneys of HF patients seems to release large amounts of circulating renin with consequent abnormal angiotensin II production [57] causing efferent arteriolar constriction and increase in oncotic pressure of peritubular capillaries. High venous pressure is described as an alternative worsening GFR factor in HF patients, especially in those with preserved ejection fraction. Patients with heart failure and venous congestion often present signs of RAAS activation not requiring decreased circulating volume as stimulus [58]; it has been supposed that RAAS and SNS activation contribute to CKD progression in type – 2 cardio – renal syndrome. As a consequence angiotensin II production and aldosterone release lead to distal nephron augmented sodium reabsorption and subsequent pressure and volume overload. Increased aldosterone levels can contribute to glomerular fibrosis due to up - regulation of transforming growth factor-β (TGF-β) and increased secretion of fibronectin [59, 60].

Chronic and acute inflammation could be also accountable for CKD progression in CHF patients; in presence of cardiac ischemia, myocytes can release inflammatory cytokines [61] and venous congestion itself, increasing endotoxin gut absorption, can provide to synthesis and release of inflammatory mediators, such as tumor necrosis factor (TNF)-α and large numbers of interleukins (IL) including IL-1β, IL-18 and IL-6 [62].

Table 2. Selected studies on novel renal biomarkers in chronic heart failure

Study	Study population	Specimen	Biomarker	HF vs control subjects	Biomarker correlates with (in HF patients only)			Renal outcomes
					Renal function	Clinical HF severity	Natriuretic peptides	
Tang 2008	Clinically stable CHF outpatients (n = 139)	Plasma	Cystatin C	No controls	Yes	Yes	Yes	NS
Damman 2008, 2010	Clinically stable CHF outpatients (n = 90)	Urine	NGAL	HF > controls	No	NS	No	NS
			NAG	HF > controls	Yes	NS	Yes	NS
			KIM-1	HF > controls	No	NS	Yes	NS
Jungbauer 2011	CHF (n = 173)	Urine	NGAL	HF = controls	Yes, with albuminuria No, with Cr/eGFR	No	No	No association with diuretic dose
			NAG	HF = controls	Yes	Yes	Yes	Elevated in patients on higher (vs. lower) diuretic doses
			KIM-1	HF > controls	Yes, with albuminuria No, with Cr/eGFR	Yes	Yes	Elevated in patients on higher (vs. lower) diuretic doses
Poniatowski 2009	CHF due to CAD (n = 150)	Serum	NGAL	No controls	Yes	Yes	NS	NS
			Cystatin C		Yes	NS	NS	NS
		Urine	NGAL		Yes	Yes	NS	NS
			Cystatin C		NS	NS	NS	NS
Bolignano 2009	CHF (elderly, age>65 yr) (n = 46)	Serum	NGAL	HF > controls	No	Yes	NS	NS
Yndestad 2009	CHF (n = 150)	Serum	NGAL	HF > controls	NS	Yes	Yes	NS
Shrestha 2011	CHF (LVEF ≤ 35%) (n = 130)	Plasma	NGAL	No controls	Yes	Yes	Yes	

2.2. Diagnosis

Assessment of kidney injury in HF patients has been previously limited to creatinine (and eGFR) and urinary protein excretion assay. Undoubtedly, decreased eGFR and increased urinary albumin excretion are independent predictors of prognosis and associated to higher risk of death, cardiovascular death and hospitalization in patients with preserved or reduced left ventricular ejection fraction (LVEF) as well as eGFR and albuminuria levels are prognostic for renal outcomes in CKD patients [63 – 65] but not in HF patients [66].

Recently novel kidney biomarkers (cystatin C, NGAL, KIM – 1 and NAG) has been evaluated in CHF patients [67 – 69].

In many clinical studies levels of these biomarkers are slightly elevated in CHF patients compared to control population, even in patients with normal renal function. These data suggest as biomarkers levels could have prognostic properties for whom to concern cardiovascular outcomes but not for renal outcome (Table 2).

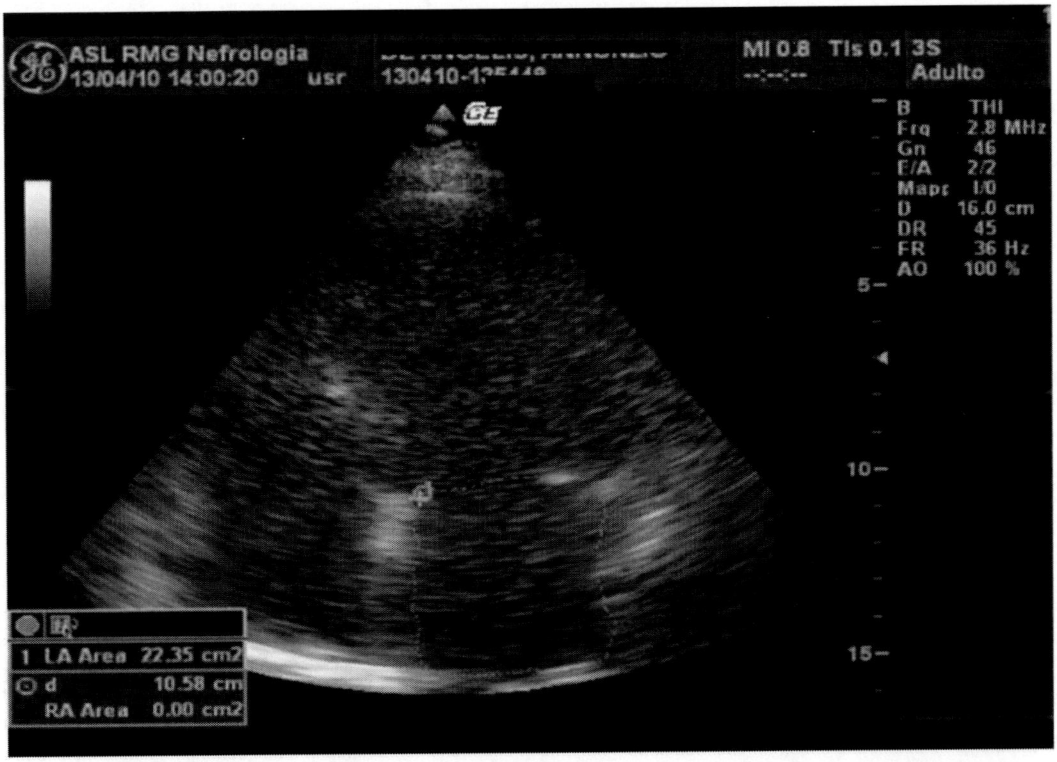

Figure 4. Left atrial dilation in Type – 2 CRS patient.

Cystatin C has been reported as independent predictor of cardiac transplantation and hospitalizations for recurrent heart failure and it correlates with pro – BNP levels and left ventricular dysfunction [68, 69].

NGAL seems to be highly expressed in myocardial cells during myocarditis and acute coronary syndrome as well as in atherosclerotic plaques; in many, but not all, clinical studies blood and urine NGAL levels both correlate with eGFR and biochemical markers of heart failure degree and associate with increased mortality and hospitalization for acute heart failure [70, 71].

Urinary KIM – 1 levels are elevated in symptomatic HF patients [72], while KIM – 1 and NAG levels correlate with severity of heart involvement and they are predictors of mortality and hospitalization for ADHF.

Ultrasound diagnosis of type – 2 CRS both involves renal and cardiac evaluation. Kidneys ultrasound pattern usually points up of classic parameters of "chronicity" such as reduction of cortical thickness, reduction of cortico – medullary ratio and increased parenchymal echogenicity.

Echocardiography shows high atrial volumes or areas as indices of volume overload (Figure 4), normal or decreased ejection fraction, right chamber dilation and decreases in estimated pulmonary arterial pressure and tricuspid annulus plane systolic excursion (TAPSE index) as parameters of congestive heart failure, pulmonary hypertension or decreased ejection fraction, pericardial effusion (Figure 5), and chronic valvular pathology, giving particular attention to valvular calcifications [46].

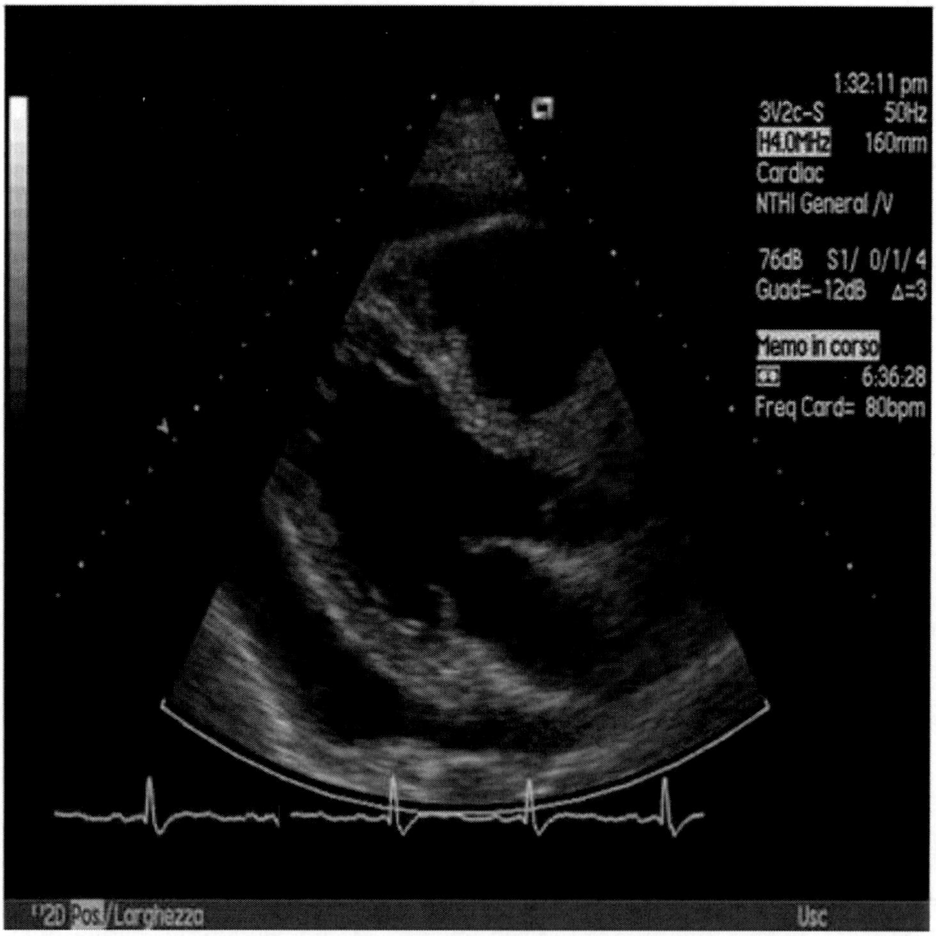

Figure 5. Pericardial effusion in CKD Stage V patient.

2.3. Outcomes and Treatment

Based on RAAS activation in CRS – 2 patients, many clinical studies have focused their attention in blocking RAAS both with angiotensin converting enzyme inhibitors (ACEIs) and angiotensin II receptor blockers (ARBs). Drugs mainly investigated have been enalapril and captopril as ACEIs and valsartan and candesartan as ARBs.

SOLVD study showed as GFR delay was slightly greater in the enalapril group compared to placebo; in the same study diabetic patients showed proteinuria reduction when treated with enalapril [73, 74]. In the CONSENSUS trial enalapril group showed medium creatinine increase of 10 – 15% [75].

VALHEFT study demonstrated slight decrease in GFR levels in valsartan patients, while proteinuria dipstick – positive was associated with increased (28%) mortality risk [76].

At present time, literature evidences are inconclusive regarding ACEIs and ARBs role in prevention of type – 2 CRS progression.

Therapy with inhibitors of aldosterone receptors in CHF patients underlines significant improvement for whom to concern survival and hospitalizations rates. RALES trial, conducted with spironolactone, showed benefits on mortality despite 17% worsening renal function in treated patients towards 7% of placebo group [77]; decrease of collagen synthesis markers was also observed in patients treated with spironolactone, suggesting a protective role against fibrosis [78].

It's crucial to point up that a slight creatinine increase (expected in patients treated with ACEIs or ARBs) does not mean a type – 2 CRS progression; it is also true that serum creatinine is an inadequate biomarker for progression of disease because of difficulty in discerning true progressive CKD from hemodynamic (and probably reversible) eGFR changes due to RAAS inhibition.

After COPERNICUS and CAPRICORN trials published data, β-blockers have become first choice treatment for heart failure; carvedilol was associated with a transient increase in serum creatinine in CKD patients [79].

Bisoprolol showed benefits in Syage III CKD patients compared to placebo group with no increase in serum creatinine levels [80], while nebivolol treatment did not modify GFR levels [81].

Since chronic inflammation has been postulated as progression risk factor in type – 2 CRS, some investigators used TNFα inhibitors in the treatment of HF; trials with infliximab or etarnecept showed decrease in CRP and IL- 6 levels but there are no reports about renal function [82].

Cardiac Resynchronization (CRT) or Left Ventricular Assist Devices (LVAD) can improve hypoperfusion in HF patients; one study showed how CRT increased GFR in a subgroup of Stage II – IIIa CKD patients [83].

3. Type – 3 Cardiorenal Syndrome

Type – 3 cardio – renal syndrome, also defined as acute reno – cardiac syndrome, occurs when acute kidney injury (AKI) contributes and/or precipitates development of acute cardiac injury. Many pathophysiological AKI causes can predispose to development of CRS Type 3 (Table 3, Table 4).

Table 3. Summary of potential contributing causes for AKI contributing to CRS Type 3

Prototypical Condition	
Contrast-induced AKI	Post-inflammatory GN
Drug-induced AKI	Rhabdomyolysis
Major surgery	Acute pyelonephritis
Cardiac surgery	Post-obstructive uropathy

Table 4. Summary of susceptibilities for CRS type 3

Risk Modifying Factors	
Age	Congestive heart failure
Sex	Pulmonary disease
Coronary artery disease	Chronic kidney disease
Hypertension	Systemic vascular disease
Hypercholesterolemia	Systemic immune disease
Diabetes mellitus	Infection/sepsis

AKI may directly or indirectly produce an acute cardiac event; many experimental data suggest that cardiac damage con be supported by inflammatory status, oxidative stress and secretion of neurohormones following AKI [84, 85].

AKI can be associated to volume overload, metabolic acidosis and electrolytes disorders such as hyperkalemia and hypocalcemia; coronary artery disease, left ventricular dysfunction and fibrosis has been also described in patients with AKI with consequent direct negative effects on cardiac performance [86].

AKI can affect cardiac function contributing to alterations in drug pharmacokinetics and dynamics.

Poor epidemiologic data are actually available about incidence and prevalence of acute cardiac events (arrhythmia, coronary artery disease, heart failure) following AKI as well as about temporal lack between AKI onset and cardiac events [87].

3.1. Pathophysiology

Direct and indirect pathophysiologic mechanisms can produce acute cardiac events and injuries during or after an AKI episode.

First of all, we focus our attention to direct mechanisms following AKI able to induce an acute cardiac event.

AKI is always characterized by non – hemodynamic events originating in the kidney with long – distance effects, including heart and cardiovascular asset [88].

Pathophysiological interactions between kidney and heart during AKI has been referred to "cardio – renal connectors" [89], like activation of immune (i.e., pro- and anti-inflammatory cytokines and chemokines release) and sympathetic nervous systems and hyperactivity of RAAS and coagulation cascade; unfortunately there are no widespread data suggesting pathophysiological role in type – 3 CRS onset.

Most of experimental available data are focused on immune cardio – renal connectors and, among them, especially on renal ischemia and reperfusion injury; animal models show as AKI encourages an immune response characterized by secretion of pro – and anti – inflammatory mediators and structural and functional changes in immune cell responsiveness; leukocytes function is also affected with alterations in adhesion. It is well known as leukocytes play an important role in cardiac dysfunction following acute coronary disease; blocking leukocyte activity can protect against myocardial damage [90].

Circulating levels of tumor necrosis factor-alpha (TNFα), interleukin-1 (IL-1) and IL-6 seems to increase immediately after renal experimental ischemia and, together with other cytokines as well as and interferon- alfa (IFN-α), they have direct cardio – depressant effects underlined by reduction in left ventricular ejection fraction and elevation of left ventricular end diastolic and systolic volumes and areas [91].

Cytokines release can affect myocardial cells directly on their contractility or by close interactions with extracellular matrix leading to negative inotropic effects; complete cellular mechanisms are still unclear but they probably involve secondary mediators such as sphingolipids, arachidonic acid and intracellular Ca^{2+} alterations [85].

In animal models, infusion of TNF-α results in decrease of left ventricular diastolic pressure with secondary coronary vasoconstriction; more infusions causes time – dependent dysfunction (regional contractility alterations) of left ventricle and its dilation lasting up to 10 days [92]. Together with left ventricular systolic dysfunction, several diastolic abnormalities are observed including slow relaxation of left ventricle and raised left atrium filling pressure to indicate an increase in left ventricle diastolic stiffness. TNF – α acute infusion directly increase oxygen consumption by myocardial cells affecting contractility, excitation and contraction coupling [93].

In presence of renal ischemia, rat hearts show increased expression of adhesion molecules such as ICAM – 1 together with myocardial apoptosis (this is not true in case of bilateral nephrectomy) to prove that systemic inflammation, and not AKI, plays an immediate role in myocardial damage and dysfunction.

Also patients with chronic heart failure show increased levels of pro – inflammatory cytokines associated with higher rates of impaired left ventricle remodelling, chronic cachexia and mortality [94].

In an AKI rat model, administration of cyclosporine A (1-5 mg/kg) attenuated development of AKI, IL – 6 expression and cellular apoptosis if compared with control population [95].

On the other hand, an incomplete or miler form of renal ischemia can provide a "protective" effect on heart; in rat model, a 15 minutes renal artery occlusion at 30°C, induced marked reductions in total infarcted areas in respect of control population; this effect can be partially referred to alterations in SNS and up – regulation of anti – inflammatory and anti - apoptotic mediators [96].

Limited data describing neuro – endocrine activation (SNS and RAAS) in type – e CRS are published. Surely, SNS activation is a key point in both developing AKI and heart failure [97].

During AKI is described an hyperactivity of SNS with abnormal secretion of norepinephrine impairing myocardial activity by several ways: direct norepinephrine effect, impairment in Ca^{2+} metabolism, increase in myocardial oxygen demand with potential evolution to myocardial ischemia, myocardial cells β1-adrenergic mediated apoptosis, stimulation of α1 receptors and, finally, activation of RAAS. β1-adrenergic stimulus on iuxta – glomerular cells simplifies renal blood flow reduction and stimulates further renin secretion by RAAS.

Abnormal and uncontrolled RAAS activation leads to angiotensin II release with consequent systemic vasoconstriction and elevation of vascular resistance; on the other hand, angiotensin II itself directly modifies myocardial structure promoting cellular hypertrophy and apoptosis [98].

In experimental model of renal ischemia, authors postulated how increased RAAS activity could be accountable for diminished coronary response to adenosine, bradykinin and L- arginine [99].

These data probably underline that AKI could directly account for impaired coronary vaso – reactivity and increased susceptibility to ischemia and other major cardiovascular events.

Other animal models allowed to discover how AKI can contribute to altered permeability of lung vessels, with resultant interstitial edema and bleeding, mediated by inflammatory mediators, altered expression of epithelial sodium channel and aquiporin – 5 expression [100].

As mentioned above, myocardial cells apoptosis and neutrophil activation greatly contribute to pathophysiologic pathways of coronary artery following AKI leading to lethal major cardiac events as can be seen in rat transgenic models [101]: in these models, kidney ischemia, not uremia, induces apoptosis in myocardial cells.

It seems that an apoptotic rate of 23 cardiomyocytes/10^5 nuclei are enough to develop a lethal dilated cardiomyopathy [102].

Best evidence for a cardio – renal link between AKI and cardiac fibrosis is beta-galactoside-binding lectin galectin-3 whose mRNA expression is up – regulated after renal ischemia; it is also implicated in the development of myocardial fibrosis and heart failure in AKI and its inhibition can delay progression of myocardial fibrosis [103].

Indirect pathophysiological mechanisms during AKI development can also affect cardiac function and outcome, such as volume overload, hypertension, acidemia, hyperkalemia, hypophosphatemia and uremic toxins.

In critical care patients volume overload is associated with poor outcomes and fluid restriction is significantly associated with improved lung function instead of liberal fluid regimen [104].

Several studies show strong association between fluid overload and less favorable outcomes in critical care patients with AKI [105]; fluid retention can also lead to fatal arrhythmias and contribute to left ventricular hypertrophy and fibrosis [106].

Hypertension is particularly prevalent in critically ill patients with AKI, probably due to AKI etiology itself (i.e., sepsis, cardiogenic shock) but also related to several mechanisms contributing to systemic and pulmonary hypertension, as elevated preload (due to volume overload), activation of SNS and RAAS. In critical care patients, these modifications lead easier to myocardial ischemia and ventricular failure [107].

Metabolic acidosis is a common feature of chronic kidney disease and AKI and it's accountable for majority of renal replacement therapy in critical care units [108]; acidemia can directly affect myocardial contractility by acting on β-receptor expression and altered intracellular calcium balance [109].

Strictly linked to acid – base impairment, hyperkalemia represent potential lethal complication in subjects presenting AKI requiring immediate renal replacement therapy and it is close linked to development of arrhythmias [110].

Chronic kidney disease and AKI are often characterized by presence of hyperphosphatemia but, once renal replacement therapy is started, hypophosphatemia often occurs leading to left systolic ventricular dysfunction [111].

Finally, uremic toxins, including beta-2-microgliobulin, and FGF-23, are associated with cardiovascular injury in CKD patients although with different pathways in respect of CKD [112]; final result is development of left ventricular hypertrophy and cardiac fibrosis [112].

All pathophysiological findings reported previously determine various effects on cardiac functions:

Electrophysiological effects: electrolytes alterations directly affect cellular membrane potentials with development of potential fatal arrhythmias. Classical ECG aspect of hyperkalemic patients is represented by tenting of T wave due to rapid and consistent changes in extracellular potassium levels leading to increased activity of potassium channel (and inactivation of sodium channel) with faster repolarization and inclination to arrhythmias.

Thus, hyperkalemia reduces resting membrane potentials (both atrial and ventricular), induces ST – T segment abnormalities (i.e., elevations in V1 and V2) simulating an ischemic pattern. In some patients, hyperkalemia can simulate a Brugada – like pattern, characterized by right bundle branch block and persistent ST – T segment elevation in at least two precordial leads.

Hypermagnesemia is often related to AV nodal and intra – ventricular conduction impairment 'till to cardiac arrest.

Hypercalcemia is accountable to short ventricular action potential duration during phase 2 and ECG shows shortening of QT interval.

Hypercalcemia can also produce ST – T segment abnormalities simulating ischemic pattern because Ca^{2+} plays central role in regulation of cardiac cycle (contraction and relaxation) [113].

Ischemic effects: Acidemia, neuro – hormonal activation and abnormal production and accumulation of uremic toxins and cytokines are linked to myocardial ischemia occuring during AKI [92]. Sympathetic activation leads to vasoconstriction and increased oxygen request by myocardial tissue; when oxygen delivery is restricted, ischemia can occur. TNF – α, endothelin and bradykinin induce coronary vasoconstriction leading to vessels stenosis.

Higher levels of oxygen demand can produce subendocardial ischemia due to oxygen redistribution; evidences demonstrate how, during AKI, coronary autoregulation is imbalanced and coronary vascular reserve and coronary vascular conductance are markedly diminished [92].

Recent data have pointed up a potential link between neutrophil gelatinase-associated lipocalin (NGAL) and cardio – renal syndromes [114]. NGAL expression rapidly increases in kidneys after acute inflammation and/or tubular injury (i.e., renal ischemia) and it has also been involved in pathophysiological pathways of heart failure, myocarditis and coronary atherosclerotic disease [115].

Kidney injury molecule (KIM) – 1, marker of kidney tubular damage, is also involved in heart failure risk during AKI acting on myocardial inflammation, modifications of atherosclerotic plaques and susceptibility to ischemic events [115].

Myocardial effects: animal models of renal ischemia showed functional changes in myocardium including left ventricular eccentric hypertrophy, increased left ventricular end – diastolic and end – systolic volumes, decreased shortening and ejection fraction. Pathophysiological pathways are ascribable to accumulation of inflammatory mediators, acute fluid retention, metabolic acidosis and accumulation of uremic toxins [85].

3.2. Diagnosis

For whom to concern laboratory findings, creatinine and GFR assessment still remains crucial points to evaluate together with electrolytes and acid – base patterns.

Other crucial biomarkers, as mentioned above, are represented by NGAL and KIM – 1, markers of kidney tubular damage able to predict heart failure in AKI patients.

Ultrasound evaluation of type – 3 CRS patients shows several pattern both on kidney and heart examination.

Kidney size and echogenicity provide primary features to discern between acute and

chronic nephropathies always remembering how kidney volume and longitudinal diameters correlate with patient height and body surface [116, 117] and that chronic renal failure does not exclude normal or enlarged kidneys (e.g., early stages of diabetic nephropathy, HIV-related glomerulonephritis or cast nephropathy).

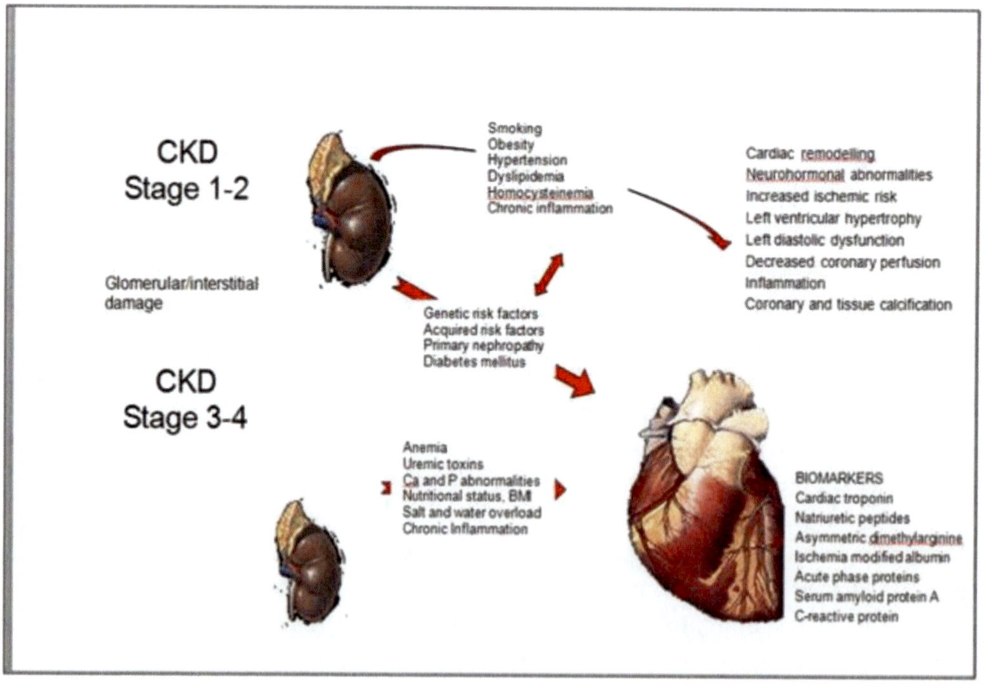

Figure 6. Pathophysiology of Type – 4 Cardio Renal Syndrome.

An hyperechogenic renal cortex with low cortico - medullary ratio is predictive of chronic nephropathy [116, 117] (Figure 4, 5). At the same time cortical hyperechogenicity can also present in acute tubular necrosis (Figure 6) or systemic lupus erythematosus nephritis [116, 117]. In these cases, enlarged renal parenchyma may suggest a condition of edema in the acute setting.

Doppler and color Doppler evaluation can be crucial in the diagnosis and prognosis in the acute setting, mainly in relation with diastolic flow evaluation in interlobulary arteries [118]. Renal ultrasound is also crucial in differential diagnosis of obstructive nephropathies.

Echocardiographic pattern is not diagnostic showing an increase in atrial volumes or areas as indices of volume overload, pleural or pericardial effusion and it's often associated to lung comets evidence on thoracic ultrasound [46].

3.3. Outcomes and Treatment

Poor data on the impact of AKI on cardiac events and outcomes are available at the moment. In cohort study association between AKI following coronary angiography (CI-AKI) and cardiovascular – related hospitalizations was evaluated [119]. Severity of CI-AKI was associated with dose – response versus risk of hospitalization for heart failure.

Other available data are from prospective evaluation of patients receiving reperfusion therapy after anterior myocardial infraction; 22% of them developed AKI in 48 hours; AKI was independently associated with higher risk of heart failure, ventricular arrhythmias and cardiac death [120].

Type – 3 CRS represent a typical scenario after cardiovascular surgery or contrast exposure. Prevention is a key point to manage this kind of cardio renal syndrome. To prevent contrast nephropathy available data and evidences indicates that isotonic fluids are the gold standard to prevent kidney injury, while contrasting data surround N- acetylcysteine [121].

More recently, a possible role for the low – osmolar, non ionic monomer iopamidol was postulated [122].

In patients affected by left ventricular dysfunction undergoing cardiovascular surgery, nesiritide employment was associated with improved post – operatory renal function compared to patients without nesiritide therapy, suggesting nephro - protective properties [123].

4. Type – 4 Cardio Renal Syndrome

Type – 4 CRS, also defined as chronic reno – cardiac, is characterized by cardiovascular involvement in patients affected by chronic kidney disease at any stage according to National Kidney Foundation (NKF) classification.

Prevalence of end stage renal disease (ESRD) is still raising and it represents worldwide epidemiological trouble [124]. Last US data estimate up to 13% population present CKD at any stage of disease.

It's well established how renal dysfunction is an independent risk factor for cardiovascular disease; CKD patients show higher mortality risk for myocardial infection and sudden death [124].

At present time pathophysiological mechanisms leading to increased cardiovascular risk in CKD patients are not completely known but we are confident in strict connections between heart and kidney.

Decline of glomerular filtration rate (GFR) leads to activation of RAAS and sympathetic nervous system and, on the other hand, it stimulates calcium – parathyroid axis; this can be due to primary diseases such as diabetes or hypertension, main causes of CKD development in western countries.

Loss of kidney function usually leads to accumulation of sodium and water with consequent stimulus to angiotensin II and aldosterone production and development of arterial hypertension. Hypertension, together with angiotensin and aldosterone, accelerates left ventricular hypertrophy and cardiac fibrosis.

4.1. Pathophysiology

To better understand pathophysiological pathways underlying type – 4 CRS (Figure 6), we have to consider various aspects of this cardio – renal syndrome from atherosclerotic damage to vascular calcifications development up to left ventricular hypertrophy development and cardiomyocites remodelling. Finally galectin – 3 and FGF-23 roles will be cleared based on last experimental evidences.

Coronary atherosclerotic heart disease: epidemiological and clinical evidences have been proved association between renal dysfunction and cardiovascular disease; it's well established that late stages of CKD are closely associated to higher cardiovascular morbidity. On the other hand it's still unclear increased incidence of cardiovascular disease at early stages of chronic kidney disease.

CKD patients present increased rates of atherosclerotic coronary disease, acute coronary syndrome, left ventricular hypertrophy and sudden death.

Cardiovascular risk for patients with eGFR less 30 mls/min/1.73/m^2 is ten fold higher in respect of patients with eGFRs above 60 ml/min/1.73/m^2.

These higher rates are in contrast with risk expected from typical risk factor present in CKD patients (hypertension, diabetes, dyslipidemia and so on); CKD is probably able to directly contribute to cardiovascular complications [125, 126].

CKD patients present, at early and late stages of disease, higher prevalence of coronary artery disease at angiographic evaluation; these patients also show multivessel disease and ECG evidence of previous silent ischemia [127].

Recent data showed that dobutamine stress echocardiography presents best accuracy for non – invasive coronary artery disease (CAD) screening in renal transplant candidates [128].

To assess CAD prevalence in early stages of CKD, an accurate review has evaluated coronary catheterization in 261 patients with eGFR between 30 and 90 ml/min; despite preserved renal function, more than half patients with eGFR >90 mls/min had a 70% stenosis in at least one coronary artery. On the other hand, more than 84% patients with late stages of CKD (eGFR < 30 ml/min) showed significant CAD with higher involvement of left coronary artery and multivessel disease [129].

Coronary calcification, myocardial calcification and aortic compliance: accelerated coronary atherosclerosis is not sufficient to completely explain higher rates of cardiovascular involvement in CKD patients.

We are now confident that osteoblastic transformation of smooth muscle cells is a key point in pathogenesis of vascular and valvular calcification during CKD.

Impaired vitamin D synthesis, secondary hyperparathyroidism and altered calcium – phosphate metabolism contribute to vascular calcification because of their direct effects on osteoblastic cells [130].

Coronary calcifications can predict major cardiac events contributing to reduced coronary reserve in CKD patients and higher risk of coronary acute syndromes [131, 132] raising with progression of renal disease.

Clinical studies conducted with high resolution multislice computed tomography (CT) demonstrated early detection of coronary calcifications since CKD stage 3 according to NKF classification; patients data showed how 83% of them presented coronary calcification did not related to CKD stage [133]. Calcifications were also extended to low limbs arteries explaining high rates of lower extremity amputation among ESRD patients presenting also greater quantity and density of calcium deposits not limited to intima, but extended to vessels' media [134]. In other studies immunostaining assay of calcified areas demonstrated presence of bone matrix proteins such as osteopontin, type I collagen and bone sialoprotein [135].

An autoptic evaluation showed how medial calcification was present in 16% of uremic patients but only in 3% of patients with normal renal function; medial calcification was also associated to presence of osteocalcin, inflammatory markers (TGF-α) and activated complement elements (C3 and C4) [136].

Increased calcium content can be accountable both reduced left ventricular compliance and prevalence of arrhythmias.

Aortic calcification is strongly associated to reduced aortic compliance and coronary artery perfusion leading to increased central pressure inducing sub – endocardial ischemia because of reduced diastolic filling [137].

Left Ventricular Hypertrophy: left ventricular hypertrophy (LVH) has been always recognized, together left ventricular systolic and diastolic dysfunction, main cardiovascular damage marker in CKD patients. LVH prevalence surely increases with declining renal function because of traditional risk factors as hypertension, diabetes and volume overload. More recent data have focused their attention of secondary hyperparathyroidism, malnutrition and even dialysis as further risk factors for development of LVH in CKD. LVH prevalence varies from 16 – 31% in patients with GFR > 30 ml/min up to 60 – 75% in ESRD and 90% prevalence in people starting renal replacement therapy [138].

Foley et al. found that 74% of ESRD patients had echocardiographic evidence of LVH and 30% presented left ventricular failure [139].

In another survey including 596 incident hemodialysis patients with no history of cardiac disease, Foley demonstrated that, after 18 months of dialysis, left ventricular mass index (LVMI) increased in 62% patients with left ventricular failure in 49% of them [140].

At present time mechanisms contributing to left ventricular dysfunction in CKD patients are unknown but many evidences suggest uremia products can directly affect cardiac structure; many of these toxins are highly protein bound and they present limited clearance by conventional dialyzers; these limitations could be accountable of dialysis effects on LVH and left heart failure [141].

Clinical conditions leading to LVH in CKD patients are similar to those observed in other clinical patterns including hypertension, atherosclerosis, pressure overload and RAAS activation. Atherosclerosis and hypertension directly promote myocites hypertrophy with consequent increased left ventricular mass, increased ventricular wall thickness, secondary myocardial fibrosis and compensatory hypertrophy [142].

In CKD patients aortic compliance is affected by accelerated atherosclerotic damage but other typical CKD variables, such as hyperphosphatemia, can affect aortic compliance [143].

In middle and end stage of CKD progression, progressive loss of nephron leads to salt and water accumulation with hypertension and volume/pressure overload; these changes up - regulate RAAS with release of pro – fibrotic factors such as galectin – 3, TGF – β and endogenous cardiac steroids [144].

As a LVH consequence, myocytes enlarge capillaries density because of increased oxygen demand; myocite diameter and interstitial volume space are increased in CKD patients compared to other patients groups: Long lasting periods of hemodynamic load promote cardiac remodeling and increase cardiac expression of interstitial myofibroblasts not ever present in normal myocardium [145].

Reduction in myocardial capillary density may explain marked CKD patients susceptibility to myocardial ischemia, LVH and myocardial fibrosis [145].

Uremia and Cardiac Fibrosis: lot of evidence now suggest that CKD patients, especially late stages, develop particular pattern of cardiac fibrosis. CKD and ESRD patients present intermyocardial fibrosis features quite different from those of hypertensive and chronic ischemic heart disease patients in which endocardial and epicardial fibrosis predominate [146].

Mechanisms leading to CKD cardiac fibrosis are still understood but recent evidences suggest that uremic toxins such as indoxyl sulfate and p – cresol can contribute to cardiac fibrosis in renal patients. In CKD patients indoxyl sulfate concentrations are 300 fold higher than control population and it directly contributes to cardiac fibrosis by synthesis of TGF – β, tissue inhibitor of metalloproteinase – 1 (TIMP-1) and alpha – 1 collagen [147, 148].

Galectin-3 and cardiac fibrosis: it's well established that diastolic dysfunction is characterized by monocytes and macrophages myocardial infiltration. Recent evidences are consistent with an up – regulation of galectin-3, member of the β-galactoside-binding lectin family synthesized by macrophages and able to interact with extracellular matrix protein like laminin, synexin and integrins.

Galectin-3 can bind to cardiac fibroblasts and increase collagen production in myocardium [149]. Lok et al. enrolled 232 patients with heart and kidney failure using NT-proBNP and eGFR as cardiac and renal function markers, demonstrating that galectin-3 levels were independent predictors of cardiovascular mortality [150].

Galecti-3 levels seems to correlate with type III amino - terminal pro - peptide of pro – collagen and TIMP – 1 suggesting that macrophage infiltration of myocardium plays a role in extracellular matrix proteins turnover of heart failure patients [151].

On the other hand, other recent studies failed in demonstrating macrophages' role in galectin-3 synthesis and consequent heart failure severity.

A Gopal et al. study reports failed in correlating galectin-3 levels and heart failure (evaluated in terms of left ventricular ejection fraction) degree, but they pointed up how galectin-3 levels were affected by kidney disease: patients with eGFR < 30 ml/min showed plasma galectin-3 levels two fold higher compared to control population [152].

Fibroblast Growth Factor 23: once verified close linkage between eGFR decline and cardiovascular structure changes, other further biomarkers have to be investigated.

One of them is represented by fibroblast growth factor – 23 (FGF-23), member of fibroblast growth factor family (implicated in regulation, growth and differentiation of cardiac myocytes) holding paracrine functions in kidneys because of its phosphaturic properties; it blocks vitamin D3 synthesis and inhibits proximal nephron reabsorption [153].

During CKD progression, accumulation of phosphate leads to increase in FGF-23 incretion, which prolonged high levels can contribute to LVH and cardiac remodeling.

New data have shown that modest reduction in GFR can stimulate FGF-23 production; echocardiographic assays demonstrated a 5% LVMI rise for every log increase in plasma FGF-23 levels. Patients included in highest tertile of FGF-23 also have a 2.4 fold higher risk for coronary artery calcifications [154].

4.2. Diagnosis

Type – 4 CRS diagnosis is based on serological and instrumental diagnosis of both chronic heart and kidney disease.

On one hand, cardiac function is more widely assessed by NT-proBNP scrum levels, while, on the other hand, eGFR represent most employed biochemical test to evaluate kidney function.

Based on recent evidence, evaluation of FGF- 23 levels can be helpful in monitoring secondary hyperparathyroidism status but it is also involved in cardiac fibrotic remodeling.

Ultrasound diagnosis of type – 4 CRS is classically based upon kidney and heart evaluation.

Kidneys ultrasound evaluation usually shows classic features of chronic nephropathy such as thin and hyperechogenic cortex with reduced cortico – medullary ratio.

It's quite frequent to observe small dilation of urinary tract and parapyelic cysts.

Echocardiographic assay allows to point out signs of volume overload, left ventricular dysfunction and right ventricular dysfunction especially in ESRD and hemodialysis patients.

At echocardiographic evaluation we can find increased atrial volumes or areas, pleural or pericardial effusion and lung comets (all signs of volume overload) [46].

Cardiac ultrasound also allow to discover presence of valvular calcifications (related to secondary hyperparathyroidism) [46] and possible right heart dysfunction features (high pulmonary artery pressure, low tricuspid annulus plane systolic excursion or right chamber dilation) [155].

4.3. Outcomes and Treatment

Since type – 4 CRS is characterized by chronic cardiovascular involvement in CKD patients, correction of traditional and non traditional cardiovascular risk factors is crucial.

Therapeutic interventions for traditional risk factors are less effective in patients with chronic kidney disease [156] also for certain kind of "therapeutic nihilism" for which treatments with antiplatelets, statins, β – blockers and ACEi in CKD patients with coronary artery disease are often denied [156].

Strategies to reduce cardiovascular risk in CKD patients have to target both traditional (hypertension, dyslipidemia, diabetes, obesity) and non traditional (anemia, chronic inflammation, secondary hyperparthyroidism, LVH, oxydative stress, RAAS and SNS hyperactivity, renal replacement therapy complications).

Specific treatment targets are quite complicated especially in hemodialysis patients in which a lot of evidences support existence of a U – shaped curve associating mortality with blood pressure levels, BMI, dyslipidemia and hyperphosphatemia [157, 158].

While it's clearly established role of secondary anemia correction [159], controversies are aroused about other risk factors corrections such as secondary hyperparathyroidism, hypertension and dyslipidemia.

For whom to concern secondary hyperparathyroidism, EVOLVE study conduced in hemodialysis patients found that cinacalcet therapy did not significantly reduce the risk of death or major cardiovascular events in patients with moderate-to-severe secondary hyperparathyroidism who were undergoing dialysis [160].

SHARP study investigated dyslipidemia treatment in CKD patients and it has been able to demonstrate a significant reduction in cardiovascular events, such as myocardial infarction, stroke, or need for coronary artery revascularization, with the use of a combination of ezetimibe plus simvastatin [161].

Pre – dialysis patients are closely recommended to maintain blood pressure levels below 130/80 mmHg, HbA1c levels below 7%, hemoglobin levels between 11 and 12 g/dl, C – LDL below 90 mg/dl. Patients should avoid nephrotoxic drugs and follow low protein diet (0.6 g/kg/day) [162, 163].

Patients on dialysis should keep their blood pressure below 140/90 before starting dialytic session and below 130/80 after dialysis session.

Special consideration have to be focused on mineral bone disorders preventing hyperphosphatemia and vascular calcifications, also in early stages of CKD [158, 164].

Treatment of arrhythmias and sudden death is still a challenge for nephrologists and cardiologists; together with prior attention to electrolytes disorders prevention (low potassium dialysate), use of β – blockers appears beneficial. ACE inhibitors and ARBs efficacy have to be proven in more prospective trials [165].

Implantation of cardiac defibrillators in dialysis patients is associated with increased risk for bleeding and infection and does not significantly affect morbidity and mortality [165].

5. Type – 5 Cardio Renal Syndrome

Type – 5 CRS is a recently defined clinical syndrome and complete epidemiological data are still missing. Type – 5 CRS occurs when heart and kidney are involved at once. Literature data underline as CRS – 5 encompasses many clinical syndromes such as sepsis, hepato - renal syndrome and drug toxicity where heart and kidney are involved secondarily to basic disease (166). Temporary sequence in which heart and kidney are involved is depending upon underlying disease.

5.1. Pathophysiology

The pathophysiology of CRS-5 depends on the underlying disease. Acute CRS-5 results from systemic processes e.g., sepsis, infections, drugs, toxins and connective tissue disorders such as lupus, Wegener's granulomatosis, and sarcoidosis. Timing from underlying condition to development of CRS is not always the same. For example, in sepsis induced acute CRS-5 there is a fulminant disease process with dramatic impact on both kidney and heart, with obvious clinical manifestations. On the other hand in cirrhotic liver disease patients, CRS-5 has a more insidious onset and the kidney and cardiac dysfunction may develop slowly until a crucial point is reached and full decompensation occurs. Several factors influence the course of CRS-5 (Table 5). Although the mechanisms invoked in acute and chronic CRS-5 are different (Figure 7, Figure 8), the nature, severity and duration of cardio – renal involvement is strictly linked to therapeutic approach (Table 5).

Acute CRS – 5 develops into four following steps and it can be hyper – acute (0 – 72 hours after diagnosis), acute (3 – 7 days), sub – acute (7 – 30 days) and chronic (over 30 days) (Figure 9, Table 6).

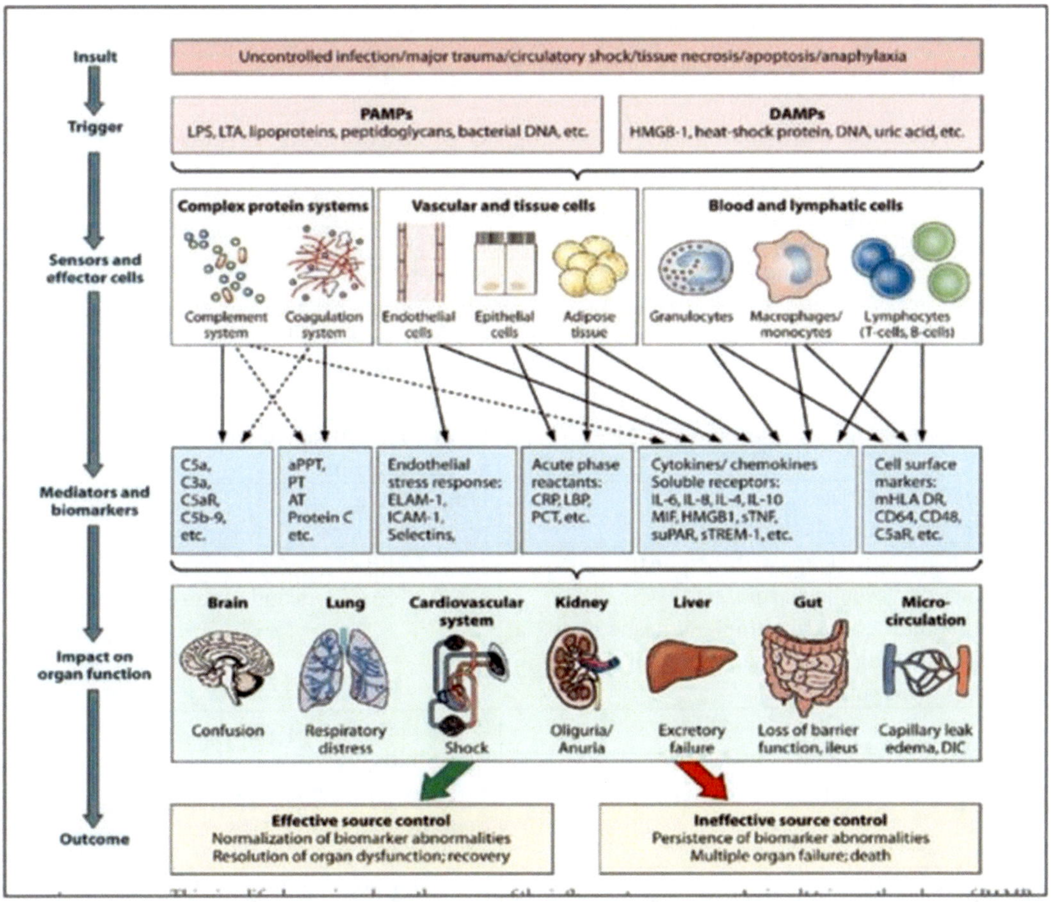

Figure 7. Pathophysiology of sepsis induced organ dysfunction.

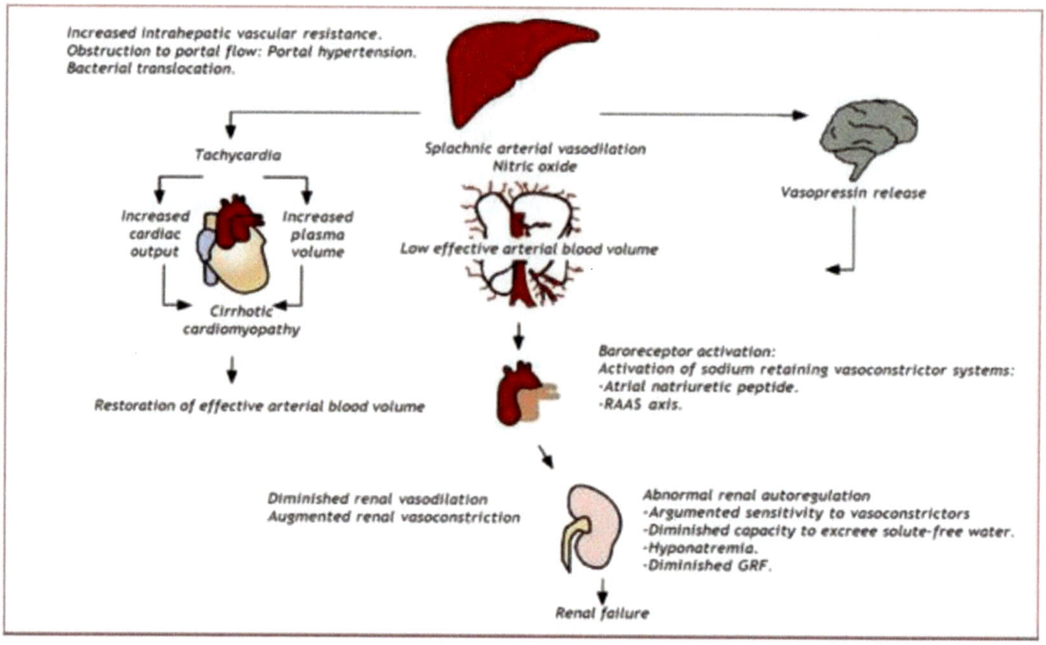

Figure 8. Pathophysiology of cirrhosis induced CRS-5.

Table 5. Predisposing and modifying factors influencing development of sepsis induced CRS-5

Patient Attributes	Process of Care
Inducing event and immunological response	Resuscitation • Volume effect on tissue edema and renal venous hypertension • Abdominal compartment syndrome • Glycocalyx
Underlying condition of heart and kidney	Search for primary focus • contrast use
Physiological responses • Peripheral vasodilatation • Compensatory Hormonal Response • Increased vascular permeability • Mitochondrial dysfunction and tissue hypoxia • Cardiac filling • Renal Hypoperfusion	Drug dosing • Antibiotics • Sedatives • Vasopressors and ionotropes
	General supportive care • Fluids • Inotropes, Pressors
	Specific Interventions • Ventilator • Surgery • RRT

Literature references are usually referred to the hyper – acute phase because most of them have focused CRS during sepsis.

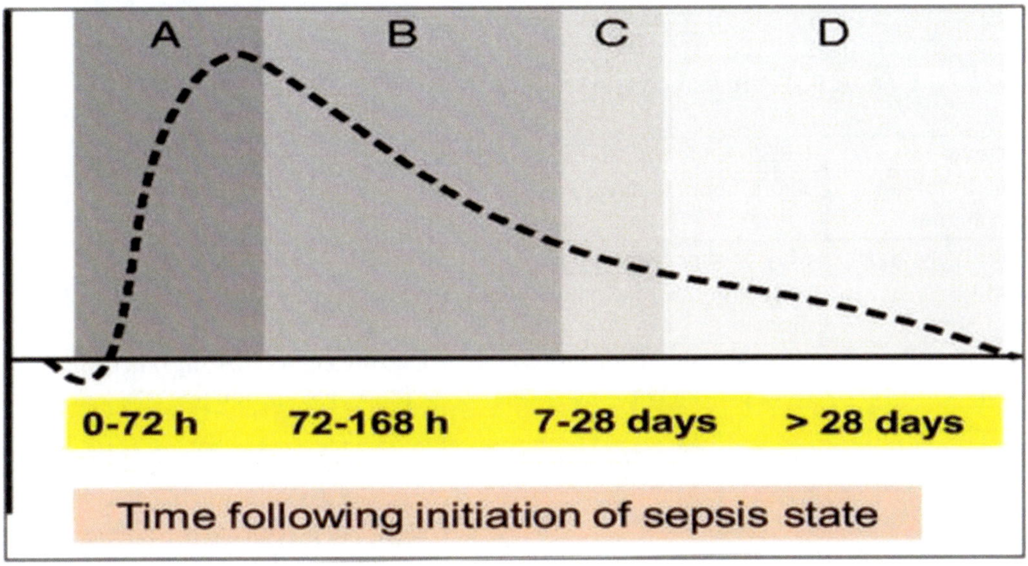

	Hyperacute	Acute	Subacute	Chronic
Systemic Hemodynamics	normal - ↑↑↑*	- ↑ or ↓*	Normal*	normal
Microcirculation	Maldistribution#	???	???	???
Autonomic Nervous system	↓ HRV# *	normal - ↓ HRV# *	???	???
RAAS	↑↑↑# *	↑ - normal# *	???	???
HPA	↓↓↓*	↓↓ - ↓*	???	???

* Clinical evidence.
# Experimental evidence.

Figure 9. Pathophysiologic Changes in sepsis induced Acute CRS-5. Organ dysfnction in sepsis can be considered in several different phases that reflect the severity of the disease. The underlying pathophysiological mechanisms are different in each phase and thus provide specific opportunties for targeted diagnostic and therapeutic strategies Phase A: 0 to 72 hours = hyperacute phase; Phase B: 72-168 hrs = Acute Phase; Phase C: 7 days – 28 days = Subacute Phase; Phase D: >28 days = Chronic.

Chronic CRS – 5 (i.e., CRS in cirrhotic patients) presents time sequence quite variable because in most cases of CRS – 5 there is an underlying condition and related precipitating event leading to attention. For instance, cirrhotic patients are subject to infections and an acute CRS – 5 can overlap a chronic process.

Pathophysiological changes in sepsis – related CRS, can depend from systemic effects of sepsis itself, from sepsis direct effect to systemic metabolic pathways or, at least, from direct cross – talk between damaged heart and kidney.

Table 6. Temporal considerations in pathophysiology of CRS-5

Attribute	CRS5 Acute (Sepsis) (Figure 1)	CRS5 Chronic (Cirrhosis) (Figure 2)
Time for organ dysfunction	Short: hours to days	Long: weeks to months
Underlying organ function	May be superimposed on underlying cardiac and kidney disease	Heart and kidney have adaptive responses that fail over time
Sequence of organ involvement	Generally simultaneous or in close proximity to each other	One organ precedes the other e.g., cardiac dysfunction precedes renal in cirrhosis
Underlying disease	Systemic event contributes to CRS5	Precipitating events can transition to an acute deterioration in CRS5 e.g., GI bleed can precipitate hepatorenal syndrome
Pathophysiology	Direct effects on organs	Failure of adaptive responses over time
Mechanisms	Determined by underlying disease	Determined by adaptive changes
Reversibility	Possible with control of sepsis and organ support	Limited unless there is replacement of diseased organ e.g., liver transplant

In early stages of sepsis microcirculation is often initially involved in contrast with normal systemic hemodynamics [167, 168] and strongly correlates with morbidity and mortality rates.

Sepsis occurring heart involvement (septic cardiomyopathy) represents one of main predictors of mortality in septic patients and it's diagnosed in almost half patients [169]. Both left and right ventricle can be injured with dilation and decreased ejection fraction often unresponsive to fluid and catecholamine therapy [170].

Septic cardiomyopathy, when severe, can mimic cardiogenic shock but it is usually reversible within 7 – 10 days [171]; myocardial blood flow and oxygen consumption do not seem involved in pathophysiology of septic cardiomyopathy [172]. On the other hand, pro – inflammatory mediators and complement factors, have been proposed as crucial actors in the development of cardiac involvement during sepsis [173, 174].

Concerning sepsis – related kidney involvement, there are clear alterations in intra – parenchymal blood flow independent by systemic hemodynamic changes linked to septic process [175, 176].

Mechanisms underlying these intra – parenchymal vascular changes are not totally understood. Recent experimental survey have compared two different sepsis models in pigs in which, irrespective of systemic hemodynamics, only pigs developing septic AKI demonstrated increased renal vascular resistance and early rises in pro – inflammatory cytokines (IL – 6) and oxidative stress markers [176].

Sepsis, therefore, is able to affect autonomic nervous system (ANS), RAAS and hypothalamus – pituitary gland – adrenal gland axis (HPA) which can impact, in several and distinctive steps, cardiac and/or renal function.

Severity of ANS dysfunction correlates with morbidity and mortality [177, 178]; autonomic dysfunction can be assessed by observing decreased heart rate variability (HRV), often associated with release of inflammatory biomarkers such as IL-6, IL.10 and C- reactive protein (CRP). Data about kidney – related ANS changes are only available in animal models in which changes in renal sympathetic activity do not affect renal blood flow [179].

Sepsis also activates RAAS as attempt to restore and maintain blood pressure; blockade of RAAS might be beneficial because RAAS activation has also been involved in endothelial dysfunction and mortality during severe sepsis [180, 181].

Experimental data suggest negative RAAS activation effects on renal function during sepsis [182]. ACE inhibitors administration improves GFR and diuresis as well as ARBs employment improves renal blood flow during experimental endotoxemia [183].

Sepsis is also involved in causing severe alteration in HPA leading to adrenal insufficiency [184] and increased production of pro – inflammatory biomarkers, free radicals, prostaglandins. Therefore inhibition of chemotaxis and expression of adhesion molecules can occur; administration of low – dose glucocorticoids can reduce vasopressors employment and critical care units hospitalization period [185].

It's not easy to determine sepsis role in heart and kidney dysfunction but some effects of heart and kidney cross –talk can be deduced by sepsis pathophysiology.

During sepsis there's reduced cardiac output leading to reduced renal perfusion further worsening sepsis – induced kidney injury; therefore, AKI is characterized by fluid overload leading to chronic heart failure in already dilated heart. At the end, metabolic acidosis due to AKI directly affects myocardial contractility, increases heart rate and encourage myocardial dysfunction. Experimental data make us confident that AKI depresses cardiac function inducing pro – inflammatory and pro – apoptotic pathophysiological mechanisms [186].

Together with hemodynamic effects of decompensated heart on renal blood flow, there are cardiac metabolic changes due to reduced fluid removal by kidneys. In experimental model AKI led to cardiac apoptosis, partially limited by anti – TNF therapy [186], hypertrophy [187] and increase in cardiac macrophages [188].

It's clear that during combined heart and kidney dysfunction, as it happens during sepsis, several cellular and molecular changes occur in both tissues.

Activation and induction of cytokines (TNF – α and IL – 6) and leukocytes (macrophages, neutrophils and lymphocytes) is well documented both in heart and kidney during sepsis.

Abnormalities in oxidative stress are also found, from mitochondrial dysfunction to alteration in anti – oxidant stress enzymes [189, 190].

Contractile heart function is mainly affected and muscle protein expression (actin and myosin) is abnormal in sepsis as well as membrane associated proteins, as dystrophin, normally regulating cell shape, mechanical strength and myocardial cells contractility.

Mean amount of dystrophin and other similar glycoproteins are reduced in septic myocardium [191].

Cardiomyocytes are connected each other at intercalated discs whose components include connexin43 and N- cadherin that are reduced during sepsis explaining electrical impairment [192].

Sepsis induces tubular damage in kidneys affected by increased secretion of lipopolysaccharide that alters HCO3 transport leading to abnormalities in urine acidification [193]. Lipopolysaccharide also modifies megalin, a glomerular protein involved in increasing albuminuria [194].

5.2. Diagnosis

For whom to concern diagnostic approach to sepsis, prototype of type – 5 CRS, initial emphasis has to be on setting of severe sepsis and septic shock, then on heart and kidney assessment and risk evaluation to star an appropriate treatment.

Systemic inflammation, like sepsis, has to be suspected when body temperature is less than 36°C (96.8°F) or greater 38°C (100.4°F), heart rate is greater than 90 beats/minute and tachypnea is already present (more than 20 breaths/minute). White blood cells count can be less than 4 x 100 cells /L or greater than 12 x 100 cells/L.

Recent review has pointed out some characteristic biomarkers whose elevation is typical during septic process: lipopolysaccharide binding protein, pro – calcitonin, C – reactive protein, pro – inflammatory cytokines (IL – 6, TGF – β) [195].

Assessment of cardiac function in type – 5 CRS is quite similar to other clinical situation in which myocardial dysfunction is present. Natriuretic peptides and troponins levels assays provide information about cardiac chambers (especially left cardiac chambers) and myocardial cells damage. Leukocytosis and C- reactive protein are not specific for myocardial injury diagnosis and imaging devices are preferred by clinicians.

Sepsis cardiomyopathy present complex clinical picture and its pathophysiology is not well understood at all. In early stages of septic process there is a low output myocardial involvement. After starting fluid therapy clinical pictures shifts to typical distributive shock characterized by increased cardiac output and systemic vasodilatation [196]. Echocardiographic assay confirm high output cardiomyopathy with abnormalities in left ventricular regional contractility together with dilation of left heart chambers [197].

Diagnosis of kidney involvement in sepsis related type 5 CRS is overlapping to other forms of AKI with acute changes in serum creatinine levels according to RIFLE, AKIN and KDIGO criteria [198, 199, 200].

At present time, several other biomarkers are proposed such as Cystatin C (only new biomarker approved in the USA), KIM-1, NGAL, NAG but RIFLE, KDIGO and AKIN criteria still recommend serum creatinine levels and urine output for diagnosis and monitoring of AKI in type 5 CRS.

5.3. Outcomes and Treatment

Once diagnosis of type 5 – CRS is made, every organ and tissue involved must be investigated to pay attention at risk prediction and protect from further and irreversible alterations in organ function.

Preliminary data (not published at present time) seem to indicate that biomarkers of cell cycle regulation may be predict patients will develop severe AKI in few days.

Regarding cardiac risk, patients who survive to septic shock showed to have lower ejection fractions and higher left ventricular end – diastolic volumes to suggest myocardial depression protective role [201].

Treatment of type – 5 CRS is mainly based on underlying disease management and on kidney and heart complications (Table 7).

First of all, maintaining hemodynamic stability and guarantee tissue perfusion are key points to prevent type – 5 CRS in hyperacute phase of sepsis together with fluid control and correct antibiotic treatment. Fluid therapy must be carefully managed to avoid fluid overload and other iatrogenic complications [202, 203].

Since inflammation and immune – disorders play an important role in the pathogenesis of sepsis, removal of cytokines and immunomodulation are two approaches based on extracorporeal techniques utilizing convection, high volume hemofiltration and high permeability membranes [204, 205, 206]. Best results were obtained with high permeability membranes and absorption [207].

Therapeutic alternative is provided by hit cellular elements accountable for apoptosis and neutrophil activation and remove them by polymyxin filters [208] or citrate anticoagulan based selective cytopheretic device [209].

Table 7. Therapeutic Interventions in Sepsis induced CRS-5

Disease Modification		Organ Support	
Removal of inflammatory mediators	- Rationale based on targeting removal of inflammatory molecules as molecular weight of most cytokines (e.g., TNF) ranges from 17-50K - Cytokine removal is variable and depends on operational characteristics - Removal can be enhanced by • Increasing permeability of membrane (High Cut Off membranes, plasma filtration) • Increasing convection (HVHF, Pulse HVHF) • Utilizing adsorption (PMMA CHDF, Polymyxin, Osiris Membrane)	Cardiac	-cardiac dysfunction contributes to shock and poor tissue perfusion -increased vascular permeability results in maldistribution of fluid in various compartments -Strategies include • Ionotropes • Vasopressors • Vasodilators
Immuno-modulation	Rationale based on targeting cellular elements of disease response • Immunoparalysis • Apoptosis • Neutrophil activation -Strategies include • Endotoxin removal by selective binding to Polymyxin • Anticoagulant based strategies (Citrate enabled selective cytophoretic device (SCD) • Plasma filtration coupled to binding to sorbents	Renal	-Renal dysfunction contributes to organ failure • Solute clearance • Fluid management • Acid Base and electrolyte homeostasis -Strategies include • Diuretics • RRT

To manage heart complications, especially in hyperacute stage, multi – pronged approach is required to maintain filling pressures with fluid therapy together with vasopressors, vasodilators and inotropes; vasopressors should be carefully employed because of depressive effects on cardiac output (increased afterload) especially with concomitant hypovolemia. Vasodilators increase cardiac output, especially in ischemic patients, while phosphodiesterase inhibitors have inotropic and vasodilatatory effects but they provide less increase of myocardial oxygen requirements.

Vasopressin increases arterial pressure but it has negative effects on cardiac output; more recently levosimendan has to be proven to provide benefits in decompensated heart failure to increase ejection fraction and diuresis [210, 211]; levosimendan efficacy is still to be proven in prevention of type – 5 CRS.

Renal support include removal of any nephrotoxic drug and media, maintenance of adeguate perfusion pressure and, if indicated, early intervention with dialysis therapy [212].

There is no role for dopamine for improving renal hemodynamics [213, 214] and there limited studies with fenoldopam [215, 216]. Norepinephrine decreases renal perfusion in normal conditions but increases systemic blood pressure in septic patients [217], while vasopressin increases diuresis and GFR in septic patients [218, 219].

Diuretics have limited role in managing heart and kidney involvement in septic patients [220] and renal replacement therapy with CRRT (continuous renal replacement therapy) should be promptly started [212]; early ultrafiltration seems to improve renal outcomes in septic shock patients but these data have to be confirmed in further clinical trials.

REFERENCES

[1] Ronco C: The cardiorenal syndrome: basis and common ground for a multidisciplinary patient-oriented therapy. *Cardiorenal Med* 2011; 1: 3–4.

[2] Bargshaw SM, Cruz DM, Aspromonte N et al. for the Acute Dialysis Quality Initiative (ADQI) Consensus Group. Epidemiology of cardio – renal syndromes: workgroup statements from from the 7th ADQI Consensus Conference. *Nephrol Dial Transplant* 2010; 25: 1406 – 16.

[3] Damman K, Navis G, Voors AA et al. Worsening renal function and prognosis in heart failure: systematic review and meta – analysis. *J Card Fail* 2007; 13: 599 – 608.

[4] McCullough PA. Cardiorenal syndromes: pathophysiology to prevention. *Int J Nephrol* 2010; 2010: 762590.

[5] Ronco C. Cardiorenal syndromes: definition and classification. *Contrib Nephrol* 2010;164:33-8.

[6] Eren Z, Ozveren O, Buvukoner E, Kaspar E, Degertekin M, Kantarci G. A Single-Centre Study of Acute Cardiorenal Syndrome: Incidence, Risk Factors and Consequences. *Cardiorenal Med* 2012;2:168-176.

[7] Hanada S, Takewa Y, Mizuno T, Tsukiyan T, Taenaka Y, Tatsumi E: Effect of the technique for assisting renal blood circulation on ischemic kidney in acute cardiorenal syndrome. *J Artif Organs* 2012;15:140-145.

[8] Stevenson LW, Perloff JK: The limited reliability of physical signs for estimating hemodynamics in chronic heart failure. *JAMA* 1989;261:884-888.

[9] Mullens W, Abrahams Z, Francis GS, Sokos G, Taylor DO, Starling RC, Young JB, Tang WH: Importance of venous congestion for worsening of renal function in advanced decompensated heart failure. *J Am Coll Cardiol* 2009;53:589-596.

[10] Uthoff H, Breidthardt T, Klima T, Aschwanden M, Arenja N, Socrates T, Heinisch C, Noveanu M, Frischknecht B, Baumann U, Jaeger KA, Mueller C: Central venous pressure and impaired renal function in patients with acute heart failure. *Eur J Heart Fail* 2011;13:432-439.

[11] Braam B, Cupples WA, Joles JA, Gaillard C: Systemic arterial and venous determinants of renal hemodynamics in congestive heart failure. *Heart Fail Rev* 2012;17:161-175.

[12] De Silva R, Loh H, Rigby AS, Nikitin NP, Witte KK, Goode K, Bhandari S, Nicholson A, Clark AL, Cleland JG: Epidemiology, associated factors, and prognostic outcomes of renal artery stenosis in chronic heart failure assessed by magnetic resonance angiography. *Am J Cardiol* 2007;100:273-279.

[13] Nohria A, Tsang SW, Fang JC, Lewis EF, Jarcho JA, Mudge GH, Stevenson LW: Clinical assessment identifies hemodynamic profiles that predict outcomes in patients admitted with heart failure. *J Am Coll Cardiol* 2003;41:1797-1804.

[14] Machnik A, Neuhofer W, Jantsch J, Dahlmann A, Tammela T, Machura K, Park JK, Beck FX, Müller DN, Derer W, Goss J, Ziomber A, Dietsch P, Wagner H, van Rooijen N, Kurtz A, Hilgers KF, Alitalo K, Eckardt KU, Luft FC, Kerjaschki D, Titze J: Macrophages regulate salt-dependent volume and blood pressure by a vascular endothelial growth factor-C-dependent buffering mechanism. *Nat Med* 2009;15:545-552.

[15] Virzì GM, Torregrossa R, Cruz DN, Chionh CY, de Cal M, Soni SS, Dominici M, Vescovo G, Rosner MH, Ronco C: Cardiorenal Syndrome Type 1 May Be Immunologically Mediated: A Pilot Evaluation of Monocyte Apoptosis. *Cardiorenal Med* 2012;2:33-42.

[16] Kraut EJ, Chen S, Hubbard NE, Erickson KI, Wisner DH. Tumor necrosis factor depresses myocardial contractility in endotoxemic swine. *J Trauma* 1999; 46: 900 – 6.

[17] Van Sloten TT, Pijpers E, Steouwer CD, Brouwers MC. Metformin – associated lactic acidosis in a patient with normal kidney function. *Diabetes Res Clinic Pract* 2012; 96x: 57 – 8.

[18] Arroio D, Melero R, Panizo M et al. Metformin – associated acute kidney injury and lactic acidosis. *Int J Nephrol*, 2011; 2011: 749 – 763.

[19] Xu G, Ahn J, Chang S, Eguchi M, Ogier A, Han S, Park Y, Shim C, Jang Y, Yang B, Xu A, Wang Y, Sweeney G: Lipocalin-2 induces cardiomyocyte apoptosis by increasing intracellular iron accumulation. *J Biol Chem* 2012;287:4808-4817.

[20] Prawle JR, Liu YI, Licari E et al. Oliguria as predictive biomarker of acute kidney injury in critically ill patients. *Crit Care* 2011; 15:R172.

[21] Mc Donagh TA, Komajda M, Maggioni AP et al. Clinical trials in acute heart failure: simpler solution to complex problems. Consensus document arising from a Euro pean Society of Cardiology cardiovascular round –table think tank on acute heart failure. *Eur J Heart Fail* 2011; 13:1253 – 60.

[22] Prowle JR, Echeverri JE, Ligabo EV, Ronco C, Bellomo R. Fluid balance and acute kidney injury. *Nat Rev Nephrol* 2010; 6: 107 – 115.

[23] Latouche C, El Moghrabi S, Messaoudi S, Nguyen Dinh Cat A, Hernandez-Diaz I, Alvarez de la Rosa D, Perret C, López Andrés N, Rossignol P, Zannad F, Farman N,

Jaisser F: Neutrophil gelatinase-associated lipocalin is a novel mineralocorticoid target in the cardiovascular system. *Hypertension* 2012;59:966-972.

[24] Maisel A, Xue Y, Shah K, Mueller C, Nowak R, Peacock WF, Ponikowski P, Mockel M, Hogan C, Wu AH, Richards M, Clopton P, Filippatos GS, Di Somma S, Anand IS, Ng L, Daniels LB, Neath SX, Christenson R, Potocki M, McCord J, Terracciano G, Kremastinos D, Hartmann O, von Haehling S, Bergmann A, Morgenthaler NG, Anker SD: Increased 90-day mortality in patients with acute heart failure with elevated copeptin: secondary results from the Biomarkers in Acute Heart Failure (BACH) study. *Circ Heart Fail* 2011;4:613-620.

[25] Shah RV, Truong QA, Gaggin HK, Pfannkuche J, Hartmann O, Januzzi JL Jr: Mid-regional pro-atrial natriuretic peptide and pro-adrenomedullin testing for the diagnostic and prognostic evaluation of patients with acute dyspnoea. *Eur Heart J* 2012;33:2197-2205.

[26] Maisel AS, Katz N, Hillege HL, Shaw A, Zanco P, Bellomo R, Anand I, Anker SD, Aspromonte N, Bagshaw SM, Berl T, Bobek I, Cruz DN, Daliento L, Davenport A, Haapio M, House AA, Mankad S, McCullough P, Mebazaa A, Palazzuoli A, Ponikowski P, Ronco F, Sheinfeld G, Soni S, Vescovo G, Zamperetti N, Ronco C; Acute Dialysis Quality Initiative consensus group: Biomarkers in kidney and heart disease. *Nephrol Dial Transplant* 2011; 26:62-74.

[27] Aldous SJ, Richards AM, Troughton R, Than M: ST2 has diagnostic and prognostic utility for all-cause mortality and heart failure in patients presenting to the emergency department with chest pain. *J Card Fail* 2012;18:304-310.

[28] Boisot S, Beede J, Isakson S, Chiu A, Clopton P, Januzzi J, Maisel AS, Fitzgerald RL: Serial sampling of ST2 predicts 90-day mortality following destabilized heart failure. *J Card Fail* 2008;14:732-738.

[29] Ky B, French B, McCloskey K, Rame JE, McIntosh E, Shahi P, Dries DL, Tang WH, Wu AH, Fang JC, Boxer R, Sweitzer NK, Levy WC, Goldberg LR, Jessup M, Cappola TP: High-sensitivity ST2 for prediction of adverse outcomes in chronic heart failure. *Circ Heart Fail* 2011;4:180-187.

[30] Dhillon OS, Narayan HK, Quinn PA, Squire IB, Davies JE, Ng LL: Interleukin 33 and ST2 in non-ST-elevation myocardial infarction: comparison with Global Registry of Acute Coronary Events Risk Scoring and NT-proBNP. *Am Heart J* 2011;161:1163-1170.

[31] Tojo A, Gross SS, Zhang L, Tisher CC, Schmidt HH, Wilcox CS, Madsen KM: Immunocytochemical localization of distinct isoforms of nitric oxide synthase in the juxtaglomerular apparatus of normal rat kidney. *J Am Soc Nephrol* 1994;4:1438-1447.

[32] Singh P, Okusa MD: The role of tubuloglomerular feedback in the pathogenesis of acute kidney injury. *Contrib Nephrol* 2011;174:12-21.

[33] Campbell CY, Clarke W, Park H, Haq N, Barone BB, Brotman DJ: Usefulness of cystatin C and prognosis following admission for acute heart failure. *Am J Cardiol* 2009;104:389-392.

[34] Lassus JP, Nieminen MS, Peuhkurinen K, Pulkki K, Siirilä-Waris K, Sund R, Harjola VP; FINN-AKVA study group: Markers of renal function and acute kidney injury in acute heart failure: definitions and impact on outcomes of the cardiorenal syndrome. *Eur Heart J* 2010;31:2791-2798.

[35] Cruz DN, Gaiao S, Maisel A, Ronco C, Devarajan P: Neutrophil gelatinase-associated lipocalin as a biomarker of cardiovascular disease: a systematic review. *Clin Chem Lab Med* 2012;50:1533-1545.

[36] Alvelos M, Lourenço P, Dias C, Amorim M, Rema J, Leite AB, Guimarães JT, Almeida P, Bettencourt P: Prognostic value of neutrophil gelatinase-associated lipocalin in acute heart failure. *Int J Cardiol* 2011 Aug 26. [Epub ahead of print].

[37] Maisel AS, Mueller C, Fitzgerald R, Brikhan R, Hiestand BC, Iqbal N, Clopton P, van Veldhuisen DJ: Prognostic utility of plasma neutrophil gelatinase-associated lipocalin in patients with acute heart failure: the NGAL EvaLuation Along with B-type NaTriuretic Peptide in acutely decompensated heart failure (GALLANT) trial. *Eur J Heart Fail* 2011;13:846-851.

[38] Alvelos M, Pimentel R, Pinho E, Gomes A, Lourenço P, Teles MJ, Almeida P, Guimarães JT, Bettencourt P: Neutrophil gelatinase-associated lipocalin in the diagnosis of type 1 cardio-renal syndrome in the general ward. *Clin J Am Soc Nephrol* 2011;6:476-481.

[39] Aghel A, Shrestha K, Mullens W, Borowski A, Tang WH: Serum neutrophil gelatinase-associated lipocalin (NGAL) in predicting worsening renal function in acute decompensated heart failure. *J Card Fail* 2010;16:49-54.

[40] Collins SP, Hart KW, Lindsell CJ, Fermann GJ, Weintraub NL, Miller KF, Roll SN, Sperling MI, Sawyer DB, Storrow AB: Elevated urinary neutrophil gelatinase-associated lipocalcin after acute heart failure treatment is associated with worsening renal function and adverse events. *Eur J Heart Fail* 2012;14:1020-1029.

[41] Valente MA, Damman K, Dunselman PH, Hillege HL, Voors AA: Urinary proteins in heart failure. *Prog Cardiovasc Dis* 2012;55:44-55.

[42] Di Somma S, De Berardinis B, Bongiovanni C, Marino R, Ferri E, Alfei B: Use of BNP and bioimpedance to drive therapy in heart failure patients. *Congest Heart Fail* 2010;16:S56-61.

[43] Parrinello G, Paterna S, Di Pasquale P, Torres D, Fatta A, Mezzero M, Scaglione R, Licata G: The usefulness of bioelectrical impedance analysis in differentiating dyspnea due to decompensated heart failure. *J Card Fail* 2008;14:676-686.

[44] Milzman D, Napoli A, Hogan C, Zlidenny A, Janchar T: Thoracic impedance vs chest radiograph to diagnose acute pulmonary edema in the ED. *Am J Emerg Med* 2009;27:770-775.

[45] Whellan DJ, Droogan CJ, Fitzpatrick J, Adams S, McCarey MM, Andrel J, Mather P, Rubin S, Bonita R, Keith S: Change in intrathoracic impedance measures during acute decompensated heart failure admission: results from the Diagnostic Data for Discharge in Heart Failure Patients (3D-HF) Pilot Study. *J Card Fail* 2012;18:107-112.

[46] Di Lullo L, Floccari F, Granata A, D'Amelio A, Rivera R, Fiorini F, Malaguti M, Timio. Ultrasonography: Ariadne's thread in the diagnosis of cardiorenal syndrome. *Cardiorenal Med* 2012; Feb; 2(1): 11 – 17 Epub 2011 Nov 30.

[47] M. Voors AA, Davison BA, Felker GM, Ponikowski P, Unemori E, Cotter G, Teerlink JR, Greenberg BH, Filippatos G, Teichman SL, Metra M; Pre-RELAX-AHF study group: Early drop in systolic blood pressure and worsening renal function in acute heart failure: renal results of Pre-RELAX-AHF. *Eur J Heart Fail* 2011;13:961-967.

[48] Shirakabe A, Hata N, Kobayashi N, Shinada T, Tomita K, Tsurumi M, Matsushita M, Okazaki H, Yamamoto Y, Yokoyama S, Asai K, Mizuno K: Prognostic Impact of

Acute Kidney Injury in Patients With Acute Decompensated Heart Failure. Circ J 2012 Dec 1. [Epub ahead of print].

[49] Heywood JT, Fonarow GC, Costanzo MR, Mathur VS, Wigneswaran JR, Wynne J: High Prevalence of Renal Dysfunction and Its Impact on Outcome in 118,465 Patients Hospitalized With Acute Decompensated Heart Failure: A Report From the ADHERE Database. *J Card Fa*il 2007, 13(6):422-430.

[50] Hebert K, Dias A, Delgado MC, Franco E, Tamariz L, Steen D, Trahan P, Major B, Arcement LM: Epidemiology and survival of the five stages of chronic kidney disease in a systolic heart failure population. *Eur J Heart Fail* 2010, 12(8):861-865.

[51] Cruz DN, Bagshaw SM: Heart-kidney interaction: epidemiology of cardiorenal syndromes. *Int J Nephrol* 2010, 2011:351291.

[52] Bagshaw SM, Cruz DN, Aspromonte N, Daliento L, Ronco F, Sheinfeld G, Anker SD, Anand I, Bellomo R, Berl T et al: Epidemiology of cardio-renal syndromes: workgroup statements from the 7th ADQI Consensus Conference. *Nephrol Dial Transplant* 2010, 25(5):1406-1416.

[53] Cruz DN, Schmidt-Ott KM, Vescovo G, House AA, Kellum JA, Ronco C, McCullough PA. Pathophysiology of Cardiorenal Syndrome Type 2 in Stable Chronic Heart Failure: Workgroup Statements from the Eleventh Consensus Conference of the Acute Dialysis Quality Initiative (ADQI). *Contrib Nephrol.* 2013;182:117-36.

[54] Setoguchi S, Stevenson LW, Schneeweiss S: Repeated hospitalizations predict mortality in the community population with heart failure. *American heart journal* 2007, 154(2):260-266.

[55] Tanaka K, Ito M, Kodama M, Maruyama H, Hoyano M, Mitsuma W, Iino N, Hirono S, Okura Y, Gejyo F et al: Longitudinal change in renal function in patients with idiopathic dilated cardiomyopathy without renal insufficiency at initial diagnosis. *Circulation journal: official journal of the Japanese Circulation Society* 2007, 71(12):1927-1931.

[56] Bongartz LG, Cramer MJ, Doevendans PA, Joles JA, Braam B: The severe cardiorenal syndrome: 'Guyton revisited.' *Eur Heart J* 2005, 26(1):11-17.

[57] Merrill AJ, Morrison JL, Branno ES: Concentration of renin in renal venous blood in patients with chronic heart failure. *The American journal of medicine* 1946, 1(5):468.

[58] Kishimoto T, Maekawa M, Abe Y, Yamamoto K: Intrarenal distribution of blood flow and renin release during renal venous pressure elevation. *Kidney Int* 1973, 4(4):259-266.

[59] Remuzzi G, Cattaneo D, Perico N: The aggravating mechanisms of aldosterone on kidney fibrosis. *J Am Soc Nephrol* 2008, 19(8):1459-1462.

[60] Onozato ML, Tojo A, Kobayashi N, Goto A, Matsuoka H, Fujita T: Dual blockade of aldosterone and angiotensin II additively suppresses TGF-beta and NADPH.

[61] Colombo PC, Ganda A, Lin J, Onat D, Harxhi A, Iyasere JE, Uriel N, Cotter G: Inflammatory activation: cardiac, renal, and cardio-renal interactions in patients with the cardiorenal syndrome. *Heart Fail Rev* 2012, 17(2):177-190.

[62] Colombo PC, Onat D, Sabbah HN: Acute heart failure as "acute endothelitis"--Interaction of fluid overload and endothelial dysfunction. *Eur J Heart Fail* 2008, 10(2):170-175.

[63] Hillege HL, Nitsch D, Pfeffer MA, Swedberg K, McMurray JJ, Yusuf S, Granger CB, Michelson EL, Ostergren J, Cornel JH et al: Renal function as a predictor of outcome in a broad spectrum of patients with heart failure. *Circulation* 2006, 113(5):671-678.

[64] Halbesma N, Jansen DF, Heymans MW, Stolk RP, de Jong PE, Gansevoort RT: Development and validation of a general population renal risk score. *Clinical journal of the American Society of Nephrology*: CJASN 2011, 6(7):1731-1738.

[65] Tangri N, Stevens LA, Griffith J, Tighiouart H, Djurdjev O, Naimark D, Levin A, Levey AS: A predictive model for progression of chronic kidney disease to kidney failure. *JAMA: the journal of the American Medical Association* 2011, 305(15):1553-1559.

[66] Khan NA, Ma I, Thompson CR, Humphries K, Salem DN, Sarnak MJ, Levin A: Kidney function and mortality among patients with left ventricular systolic dysfunction. *J Am Soc Nephrol* 2006, 17(1):244-253.

[67] Cruz DN, Fard A, Clementi A, Ronco C, Maisel A: Role of biomarkers in the diagnosis and management of cardio-renal syndromes. *Semin Nephrol* 2012, 32(1):79-92.

[68] Tang WH, Van Lente F, Shrestha K, Troughton RW, Francis GS, Tong W, Martin MG, Borowski AG, Jasper S, Starling RC et al: Impact of myocardial function on cystatin C measurements in chronic systolic heart failure. *J Card Fail* 2008, 14(5):394-399.

[69] Damman K, van Veldhuisen DJ, Navis G, Voors AA, Hillege HL: Urinary neutrophil gelatinase associated lipocalin (NGAL), a marker of tubular damage, is increased in patients with chronic heart failure. *Eur J Heart Fail* 2008, 10(10):997-1000.

[70] Bolignano D, Basile G, Parisi P, Coppolino G, Nicocia G, Buemi M: Increased plasma neutrophil gelatinase-associated lipocalin levels predict mortality in elderly patients with chronic heart failure. *Rejuvenation Res* 2009, 12(1):7-14.

[71] Shrestha K, Borowski AG, Troughton RW, Thomas JD, Klein AL, Tang WH: Renal dysfunction is a stronger determinant of systemic neutrophil gelatinase-associated lipocalin levels than myocardial dysfunction in systolic heart failure. *J Card Fail* 2011, 17(6):472-478.

[72] Jungbauer CG, Birner C, Jung B, Buchner S, Lubnow M, von Bary C, Endemann D, Banas B, Mack M, Boger CA et al: Kidney injury molecule-1 and N-acetyl-beta-D-glucosaminidase in chronic heart failure: possible biomarkers of cardiorenal syndrome. *Eur J Heart Fail* 2011, 13(10):1104-1110.

[73] Testani JM, Kimmel SE, Dries DL, Coca SG: Prognostic importance of early worsening renal function after initiation of angiotensin-converting enzyme inhibitor therapy in patients with cardiac dysfunction. *Circulation Heart failure* 2011, 4(6):685-691.

[74] Capes SE, Gerstein HC, Negassa A, Yusuf S: Enalapril prevents clinical proteinuria in diabetic patients with low ejection fraction. *Diabetes care* 2000, 23(3):377-380.

[75] Ljungman S, Kjekshus J, Swedberg K: Renal function in severe congestive heart failure during treatment with enalapril (the Cooperative North Scandinavian Enalapril Survival Study [CONSENSUS] Trial). *The American journal of cardiology* 1992, 70(4):479-487.

[76] Anand IS, Bishu K, Rector TS, Ishani A, Kuskowski MA, Cohn JN: Proteinuria, chronic kidney disease, and the effect of an angiotensin receptor blocker in addition to an angiotensin-converting enzyme inhibitor in patients with moderate to severe heart failure. *Circulation* 2009, 120(16):1577-1584.

[77] Pitt B, Zannad F, Remme WJ, Cody R, Castaigne A, Perez A, Palensky J, Wittes J: The effect of spironolactone on morbidity and mortality in patients with severe heart failure. Randomized Aldactone Evaluation Study Investigators. *N Engl J Med* 1999, 341(10):709-717.

[78] Zannad F, Dousset B, Alla F: Treatment of congestive heart failure: interfering the aldosterone-cardiac extracellular matrix relationship. *Hypertension* 2001, 38(5):1227-1232.

[79] Wali RK, Iyengar M, Beck GJ, Chartyan DM, Chonchol M, Lukas MA, Cooper C, Himmelfarb J, Weir MR, Berl T et al: Efficacy and safety of carvedilol in treatment of heart failure with chronic kidney disease: a meta-analysis of randomized trials. *Circulation Heart failure* 2011, 4(1):18-26.

[80] Castagno D, Jhund PS, McMurray JJ, Lewsey JD, Erdmann E, Zannad F, Remme WJ, Lopez-Sendon JL, Lechat P, Follath F et al: Improved survival with bisoprolol in patients with heart failure and renal impairment: an analysis of the cardiac insufficiency bisoprolol study II (CIBIS-II) trial. *Eur J Heart Fail* 2010, 12(6):607-616.

[81] Cohen-Solal A, Kotecha D, van Veldhuisen DJ, Babalis D, Bohm M, Coats AJ, Roughton M, Poole-Wilson P, Tavazzi L, Flather M: Efficacy and safety of nebivolol in elderly heart failure patients with impaired renal function: insights from the SENIORS trial. *Eur J Heart Fail* 2009, 11(9):872-880.

[82] Mann DL, McMurray JJ, Packer M, Swedberg K, Borer JS, Colucci WS, Djian J, Drexler H, Feldman A, Kober L et al: Targeted anticytokine therapy in patients with chronic heart failure: results of the Randomized Etanercept Worldwide Evaluation (RENEWAL). *Circulation* 2004, 109(13):1594-1602.

[83] Boerrigter G, Costello-Boerrigter LC, Abraham WT, Sutton MG, Heublein DM, Kruger KM, Hill MR, McCullough PA, Burnett JC, Jr.: Cardiac resynchronization therapy improves renal function in human heart failure with reduced glomerular filtration rate. *J Card Fail* 2008, 14(7):539-546.

[84] Yap SC, Lee HT. Acute kidney injury and extrarenal organ dysfunction: new concepts and experimental evidence. *Anesthesiology.* May 2012;116(5):1139-1148.

[85] Prabhu SD. Cytokine-induced modulation of cardiac function. *Circ Res.* Dec 10 2004;95(12):1140-1153.

[86] Kingma JG, Jr., Vincent C, Rouleau JR, Kingma I. Influence of acute renal failure on coronary vasoregulation in dogs. *J Am Soc Nephrol.* May 2006;17(5):1316-1324.

[87] Chuasuwan A, Kellum JA. Cardio-renal syndrome type 3: epidemiology, pathophysiology, and treatment. *Semin Nephrol.* Jan 2012;32(1):31-39.

[88] Grams ME, Rabb H. The distant organ effects of acute kidney injury. *Kidney Int.* May 2012;81(10):942-948.

[89] Bongartz LG, Cramer MJ, Doevendans PA, Joles JA, Braam B. The severe cardiorenal syndrome: 'Guyton revisited.' *Eur Heart J.* Jan 2005;26(1):11-17.

[90] Ma XL, Lefer DJ, Lefer AM, Rothlein R. Coronary endothelial and cardiac protective effects of a monoclonal antibody to intercellular adhesion molecule-1 in myocardial ischemia and reperfusion. *Circulation.* Sep 1992;86(3):937-946.

[91] Blake P, Hasegawa Y, Khosla MC, Fouad-Tarazi F, Sakura N, Paganini EP. Isolation of "myocardial depressant factor(s)" from the ultrafiltrate of heart failure patients with acute renal failure. *ASAIO J.* Sep-Oct 1996;42(5):M911-915.

[92] Edmunds NJ, Lal H, Woodward B. Effects of tumour necrosis factor-alpha on left ventricular function in the rat isolated perfused heart: possible mechanisms for a decline in cardiac function. *British journal of pharmacology*. Jan 1999;126(1):189-196.

[93] Miyano H, Shishido T, Kawada T, et al. Acute effect of tumor necrosis factor-alpha is minimal on mechanics but significant on energetics in blood-perfused canine left ventricles. *Critical care medicine*. Jan 1999;27(1):168-176.

[94] Rauchhaus M, Doehner W, Francis DP, et al. Plasma cytokine parameters and mortality in patients with chronic heart failure. *Circulation*. Dec 19 2000;102(25):3060-3067.

[95] Wen X, Peng Z, Li Y, et al. One dose of cyclosporine A is protective at initiation of folic acid-induced acute kidney injury in mice. *Nephrol Dial Transplant*. Aug 2012;27(8):3100-3109.

[96] Verdouw PD, Gho BC, Koning MM, Schoemaker RG, Duncker DJ. Cardioprotection by ischemic and nonischemic myocardial stress and ischemia in remote organs. Implications for the concept of ischemic preconditioning. *Ann N Y Acad Sci*. Sep 30 1996;793:27-42.

[97] Kobuchi S, Tanaka R, Shintani T, et al. Mechanisms underlying the renoprotective effect of GABA against ischemia/reperfusion-induced renal injury in rats. *J Pharmacol Exp Ther*. Sep 2011;338(3):767-774.

[98] Kajstura J, Cigola E, Malhotra A, et al. Angiotensin II induces apoptosis of adult ventricular myocytes in vitro. *J Mol Cell Cardiol*. Mar 1997;29(3):859-870.

[99] Kingma JG, Jr., Vincent C, Rouleau JR, Kingma I. Influence of acute renal failure on coronary vasoregulation in dogs. *J Am Soc Nephrol*. May 2006;17(5):1316-1324.

[100] Nath KA, Grande JP, Croatt AJ, et al. Transgenic sickle mice are markedly sensitive to renal ischemia-reperfusion injury. *Am J Pathol*. Apr 2005;166(4):963-972.

[101] Kelly KJ. Distant effects of experimental renal ischemia/reperfusion injury. *J Am Soc Nephrol*. Jun 2003;14(6):1549-1558.

[102] Wencker D, Chandra M, Nguyen K, et al. A mechanistic role for cardiac myocyte apoptosis in heart failure. *J Clin Invest*. May 2003;111(10):1497-1504.

[103] Liu YH, D'Ambrosio M, Liao TD, et al. N-acetyl-seryl-aspartyl-lysyl-proline prevents cardiac remodeling and dysfunction induced by galectin-3, a mammalian adhesion/growth-regulatory lectin. American journal of physiology. *Heart and circulatory physiology*. Feb 2009;296(2):H404-412.

[104] Wiedemann HP, Wheeler AP, Bernard GR, et al. Comparison of two fluid-management strategies in acute lung injury. *N Engl J Med*. Jun 15 2006;354(24):2564-2575.

[105] Payen D, de Pont AC, Sakr Y, Spies C, Reinhart K, Vincent JL. A positive fluid balance is associated with a worse outcome in patients with acute renal failure. *Crit Care*. 2008;12(3):R74.

[106] Davis KL, Laine GA, Geissler HJ. Effects of Myocardial Edema on the Development of Myocardial Interstitial Fibrosis. *Microcirculation*. 2000;7:269-280.

[107] Nazar A, Guevara M, Sitges M, et al. LEFT ventricular function assessed by echocardiography in cirrhosis: Relationship to systemic hemodynamics and renal dysfunction. *J Hepatol*. Jan 2013;58(1):51-57.

[108] Legrand M, Darmon M, Joannidis M, Payen D. Management of renal replacement therapy in ICU patients: an international survey. *Intensive care medicine*. Jan 2013;39(1):101-108.

[109] Nimmo AJ, Than N, Orchard CH, Whitaker EM. The effect of acidosis on beta-adrenergic receptors in ferret cardiac muscle. *Exp Physiol.* Jan 1993;78(1):95-103.
[110] Bagshaw SM, Wald R, Barton J, et al. Clinical factors associated with initiation of renal replacement therapy in critically ill patients with acute kidney injury-a prospective multicenter observational study. *J Crit Care.* Jun 2012;27(3):268-275.
[111] Schwenger V, Weigand MA, Hoffmann O, et al. Sustained low efficiency dialysis using a single-pass batch system in acute kidney injury - a randomized interventional trial: the REnal Replacement Therapy Study in Intensive Care Unit PatiEnts. *Crit Care.* Jul 27 2012;16(4):R140.
[112] Neirynck N, Vanholder R, Schepers E, Eloot S, Pletinck A, Glorieux G. An update on uremic toxins. *Int Urol Nephrol.* Aug 15 2012.
[113] Shannon TR, Pogwizd SM, Bers DM. Elevated sarcoplasmic reticulum Ca2+ leak in intact ventricular myocytes from rabbits in heart failure. *Circulation research.* Oct 3 2003;93(7):592-594.
[114] Ronco C, Cruz D, Noland BW. Neutrophil gelatinase-associated lipocalin curve and neutrophil gelatinase-associated lipocalin extended-range assay: a new biomarker approach in the early diagnosis of acute kidney injury and cardio-renal syndrome. *Seminars in nephrology.* Jan 2012;32(1):121-128.
[115] Carlsson AC, Larsson A, Helmersson-Karlqvist J, et al. Urinary kidney injury molecule 1 and incidence of heart failure in elderly men. *Eur J Heart Fail.* Dec 7 2012.
[116] Licurse A, Kim MC, Dziura J, Forman HP, Formica RN, Makarov DV, Parikh CR, Gross CP: Renal ultrasonography in the evaluation of acute kidney injury: developing a risk stratification framework. *Arch Intern Med* 2010; 170: 1900–1907.
[117] Ozmen CA, Akin D, Bilek SU, Bayrak AH, Senturk S, Nazaroglu H: Ultrasound as a diagnostic tool to differentiate acute from chronic renal failure. *Clin Nephrol* 2010; 74: 46–52.
[118] Darmon M, Schortgen F, Vargas F, Liazydi A, Schlemmer B, Brun-Buisson C, Brochard L: Diagnostic accuracy of Doppler renal resistive index for reversibility of acute kidney injury in critically ill patients. *Intensive Care Med* 2011.
[119] James MT, Ghali WA, Knudtson ML, et al. Associations between acute kidney injury and cardiovascular and renal outcomes after coronary angiography. *Circulation.* Feb 1 2011;123(4):409-416.
[120] Selby NM, Kolhe NV, McIntyre CW, et al. Defining the cause of death in hospitalised patients with acute kidney injury. *PLoS One.* 2012;7(11):e48580.
[121] Jasuja D, Mor MK, Hartwig KC, Palevsky PM, Fine MJ, Weisbord SD. Provider knowledge of contrast-induced acute kidney injury. *Am J Med Sci.* 2009;338:280–286.
[122] Solomon RJ, Mehran R, Natarajan MK, Doucet S, Katholi RE, Staniloae CS, Sharma SK, Labinaz M, Gelormini JL, Barrett BJ. Contrast-induced nephropathy and long-term adverse events: cause and effect? *Clin J Am Soc Nephrol.* 2009;4:1162–1169.
[123] Mentzer RM, Jr, Oz MC, Sladen RN, Graeve AH, Hebeler RF, Jr, Luber JM, Jr, et al. Effects of perioperative nesiritide in patients with left ventricular dysfunction undergoing cardiac surgery:the NAPA Trial. *J Am Coll Cardiol.* 2007;49:716–726.
[124] Redo´na J, Cea-Calvob L, Lozanoc JV, Ferna´ndez-Pe´rezd C, Navarroe J, Bonete A and Estebanb JG: Kidney function and cardiovascular disease in the hypertensive population: the ERIC-HTA study. *Journal of Hypertension* 2006; 24:663–669.

[125] Anavekar NS, McMurray JJV. Velazquez EJ, Solomon SD, Kober L, Rouleau JL: Relation between renal dysfunction and cardiovascular outcomes after myocardial infarction. *New Eng. J Med* 2004; 351:1285– 1295.
[126] Rostand SG, Kirk KA, Rutsky EA: Dialysis-associated ischemic heart disease: Insights from coronary angiography. *Kidney International* 1984; 25, 653–659.
[127] Joki N, Hase H, Nakamura R: Onset of coronary artery disease prior to initiation of hemodialysis in patients with end-stage renal disease. *Nephrol Dial Transplant* 1997; 12: 718–723.
[128] Whalley GA, Marwick TH, Doughty RN, Cooper BA, Johnson DW, Pilmore A, Harris DC, Pollock CA, Collins JF: IDEAL Effect of Early Initiation of Dialysis on Cardiac Structure and Function: Results From the Echo Substudy of the IDEAL Trial. *Am J Kidney Dis*. 2012 Nov 13.
[129] Chonchol M, Whittle J, Desbien: Chronic kidney disease is associated with angiographic coronary artery disease. *Am. J. Nephrol.* 2008; 28: 354–360.
[130] McCullough PA, Agrawal V, Danielewicz E, Abela GS: Accelerated Atherosclerotic Calcification and Mo¨nckeberg's Sclerosis: A Continuum of Advanced Vascular Pathology in Chronic Kidney Disease. *Clin J Am Soc Nephrol*; 2008 3: 1585–1598.
[131] Gross ML, Meyer HP, Ziebart H, Rieger P, Wenzel U, Amann K, Berger I, Adamczak M, Schirmacher P, Ritz E: Calcification of Coronary Intima and Media: *Clin J Am Soc Nephrol*; 2007 2: 121–134.
[132] Ragosta M, Samady H, MD, Isaacs RB, Lawrence B, Gimple W, Sarembock AJ, Powers ER: Coronary flow reserve abnormalities in patients with diabetes mellitus who have end-stage renal disease and normal epicardial coronary arteries *Am. Heart J.;*2004 147:1017–23.
[133] Garland JS, Holden RM, Groome PA, Lam M, Nolan RL, Ross Morton R, William Pickett W: Prevalence and Associations of Coronary Artery Calcification in Patients With Stages 3 to 5 CKD Without Cardiovascular Disease *Am. J. Kidney Dis.*;2008 52:849-858.
[134] Adragao T, Pires A, Branco P, Castro R, Oliveira A, Nogueira C, Bordalo J, Curto JD, Prata MM: Ankle-brachial index, vascular calcifications and mortality in dialysis patients. *Nephrol Dial Transplant*; 2012 27: 318–325.
[135] Moe SM, O'Neill KD, Duan D, Ahmed S, Chen NX, Leapman SB, Fineberg N, Kopecky K: Medial artery calcification in ESRD patients is associated with deposition of bone matrix proteins. *Kidney Int.*; 2002 61: 638–647.
[136] Campean V, Nonnast-Daniel B, Garlichs C, Gross ML, Amann K, CD40-CD154 expression in calcified and non-calcified coronary lesions of patients with chronic renal failure. *Atherosclerosis*; 2007; 190: 156-66.
[137] Laurent S, Cockcroft J, Van Bortel L, Boutouyrie P, Giannattasio C, Hayoz D, Pannier B, Vlachopoulos C, Wilkinson I, Struijker-Boudier H. Expert consensus document on arterial stiffness: methodological issues and clinical applications. *Eur. Heart J.* 2006; 27; 2588 –2605).
[138] McGregor E, Jardine AG, Murray LS, Dargie HJ, Rodger RS, Junor BJ: Preoperative echocardiographic abnormalities and adverse outcome following renal transplantation. *Nephrol Dial Transplant*. 1998; 13: 1499-505.

[139] Foley RN, Parfey PS, Harneyf JD, Kent GM, Martin GJ, Murray DC, Barre PEP Clinical and echocardiographic disease in patients starting end-stage renal disease therapy *Kidney International.* 1995;47:186-1 92.

[140] Foley RN, Curtis BM, Randell EW, Parfey PS: Left Ventricular Hypertrophy in New Hemodialysis Patients without Symptomatic Cardiac Disease *Clin J. Am. Soc. Nephrol.* 2010; 5: 805–813.

[141] McIntyre CW, Burton JO, Selby NM, Leccisotti L, Korsheed S, Baker CSR, Camici PG: Hemodialysis-Induced Cardiac Dysfunction Is Associated with an Acute Reduction in Global and Segmental Myocardial Blood Flow *Clin J Am Soc Nephrol* 2008; 3; 19–26.

[142] Parfey PS, Harnett JD, Foley RN. Heart failure and ischemic heart disease in chronic uremia: *Curr. Opin. Nephrol. Hypertens.* 1995; 4: 105-10, 1995.

[143] Blancher J, Safar ME, Guerin AP, B. Pannier, Sylvain J, Marchais, SJ, London GM: Aortic pulse wave velocity index and mortality in end-stage renal disease. *Kidney International*, 2003;63:852–1860.

[144] Bogrov AY, Shapiro JI: Endogenous digitalis: pathophysiologic roles and therapeutic applications. *Nature Clinical Practice Nephrology* 2008; 4378-392.

[145] Amann K. Breitbach M, Ritz E, Mall G.: Myocyte/Capillary Mismatch in the Heart of Uremic Patients. *J. Am Soc Nephrol* 1998 9: 1018-1022.

[146] Mall G, Huther W, Schneider J, Lundin P, Ritz E,: Diffuse Intermyocardiocytic Fibrosis in Uraemic Patients *Nephrol Dial Transplant* 1990: 5: 39-44.4.

[147] Meert N, Schepers E, De Smet R, Argiles A, Cohen G, Deppisch R, Drueke T, Massy Z, Spasovski G, Stegmayr B, Zidek W, Jankowski J, Vanholder R: Inconsistency of reported uremic toxin concentrations. *Artif. Organs* 2007; 31:600–611.

[148] Miyazaki T, Ise M, Seo H, Niwa T: Indoxyl sulfate increases the gene expressions of TGF-beta 1, TIMP-1 and pro-alpha 1(I) collagen in uremic rat kidneys. *Kidney Int. Suppl.* 1997; 62:S15–S22.

[149] Sharma UC, Pokharel S, van Brakel TJ: Galectin-3 marks activated macrophages in failure-prone hypertrophied hearts and contribute to cardiac dysfunction. *Circulation* 2004; 110; 3121–8.

[150] Lok DJA, Van Der Meer P, Bruggink-Andre´ de la Porte PW, Lipsic E, Van Wijngaarden J, Hillege HL, van Veldhuisen DJ: Prognostic value of galectin-3, a novel marker of fibrosis, in patients with chronic heart failure: data from the DEAL-HF study. *Clin Res Cardiol* 2010; 99:323–328.

[151] Yen-Hung Lin, Lian-YuLin, Yen-WenWu, Kuo-Liong Chien, Chi-MingLee, Ron-BinHsu, Chia-LunChao, Shoei -ShenWang, Yenh-Chen Hsein, Lin-Chu Liaof, Yi-Lwun Hoa, d, Chena MF,: The relationship between serum galectin-3 and serum markers of cardiac extracellular matrix turnover in heart failure patients *Clinica Chimica Acta* 2009 409;96–99.

[152] Gopal DM, Kommineni M, Ayalon N, Koelbl C, Ayalon R, Biolo A, Dember LM, Downing J, Siwik DA, Liang CS, Colucci WS: Relationship of Plasma Galectin-3 to Renal Function in Patients With Heart Failure: Effects of Clinical Status, Pathophysiology of Heart Failure, and Presence or Absence of Heart Failure *J. Am. Heart Assoc.*; 2012 1: 1-7.

[153] Faul, C, Amaral AP, Oskouei B, Hu MC, Sloan A, Isakova T, Gutiérrez OM, Aguillon-Prada R, Lincoln J, Hare JM, Mundel P, Morales A, Scialla J, Fischer M, Soliman EZ,

Chen J, Go AS, Rosas SE, Nessel L, Townsend RR, Feldman HI, St. John Sutton M, Ojo A, Gadegbeku C, Di Marco SG, Reuter S, Kentrup D, Tiemann K, Brand M, Hill JA, Moe OW, Kuro-o M, Kusek JW, Keane MG, Wolf M:FGF23 induces left ventricular hypertrophy *J Clin Invest.*; 2011; 121;4393–4408.

[154] Gutiérrez OM, Januzzi JL, Isakova T, Laliberte K, Smith K, Collerone G, Sarwar AS, Hoffmann U, Coglianese E, Christenson R, Wang TJ, deFilippi C, Wolf M:Fibroblast Growth Factor 23 and Left Ventricular Hypertrophy in Chronic Kidney Disease Circulation 2009;119; 2545-2552.

[155] Di Lullo L, Floccari F, Polito P: Right ventricular diastolic function in dialysis patients could be affected by vascular access. *Nephron Clin Pract* 2011; 118:c258–c262.

[156] P. A. McCullough, "Why is chronic kidney disease the "spoiler" for cardiovascular outcomes?" *Journal of the American College of Cardiology,* vol. 41, no. 5, pp. 725–728, 2003.

[157] K. Kalantar-Zadeh, G. Block, M. H. Humphreys, and J. D. Kopple, "Reverse epidemiology of cardiovascular risk factors in maintenance dialysis patients," *Kidney International*, vol. 63, no. 3, pp. 793–808, 2003.

[158] Di Lullo L, Floccari F, Santoboni A, Barbera V, Rivera RF, Granata A, Morrone L, Russo D. Progression of cardiac valve calcification and decline of renal function in CKD patients. *J Nephrol.* 2013 Jun 28:0. doi: 10.5301/jn.5000290. In press.

[159] Dmitrieva O, de Lusignan S, Macdougall IC, Gallagher H, Tomson C, Harris K, Desombre T, Goldsmith D. Association of anaemia in primary care patients with chronic kidney disease: cross sectional study of quality improvement in chronic kidney disease (QICKD) trial data. *BMC Nephrol.* 2013 Jan 25;14:24.

[160] EVOLVE Trial Investigators, Chertow GM, Block GA, Correa-Rotter R, Drüeke TB, Floege J, Goodman WG, Herzog CA, Kubo Y, London GM, Mahaffey KW, Mix TC, Moe SM, Trotman ML, Wheeler DC, Parfrey PS. Effect of cinacalcet on cardiovascular disease in patients undergoing dialysis. *N Engl J Med.* 2012 Dec 27;367(26):2482-94.

[161] Baigent C, Landray MJ, Reith C, Emberson J, Wheeler DC, Tomson C, Wanner C, Krane V, Cass A, Craig J, Neal B, Jiang L, Hooi LS, Levin A, Agodoa L, Gaziano M, Kasiske B, Walker R, Massy ZA, Feldt-Rasmussen B, Krairittichai U, Ophascharoensuk V, Fellström B, Holdaas H, Tesar V, Wiecek A, Grobbee D, de Zeeuw D, Grönhagen-Riska C, Dasgupta T, Lewis D, Herrington W, Mafham M, Majoni W, Wallendszus K, Grimm R, Pedersen T, Tobert J, Armitage J, Baxter A, Bray C, Chen Y, Chen Z, Hill M, Knott C, Parish S, Simpson D, Sleight P, Young A, Collins R; SHARP Investigators. The effects of lowering LDL cholesterol with simvastatin plus ezetimibe in patients with chronic kidney disease (Study of Heart and Renal Protection): a randomised placebo-controlled trial. *Lancet.* 2011 Jun 25;377(9784):2181-92.

[162] Kidney Disease Outcomes Quality Initiative (K/DOQI), "Clinical practice guidelines on hypertension and antihypertensive agents in chronic kidney disease," *American Journal of Kidney Diseases*, vol. 43, no. 5, supplement 1, pp. S1–S290, 2004.

[163] Kidney Disease Outcomes Quality Initiative (K/DOQI), "Clinical practice guidelines and clinical practice recommendations for diabetes and chronic kidney disease," *American Journal of Kidney Diseases*, vol. 49, no. 2, supplement 2, pp. S12–S154, 2007.

[164] Kidney Disease Improving Global Outcomes (KDIGO), Clinical Practice Guideline for the Diagnosis, Evaluation, Prevention, and Treatment of Chronic Kidney Disease—Mineral and Bone Disorder (CKD—MBD), "Treatment of CKD-MBD targeted at lowering high serum phosphorus and maintaining serum calcium," *Kidney International*, vol. 76, supplement 113, pp. S50–S69, 2009.

[165] C. A. Herzog, J. M. Mangrum, and R. Passman, "Sudden cardiac death and dialysis patients," *Seminars in Dialysis*, vol. 21, no. 4, pp. 300–307, 2008.

[166] Ronco C, McCullough PA, Anker SD, Anand I, Aspromonte N, Bagshaw SM, Bellomo R, Berl T, Bobek I, Cruz DN, Daliento L, Davenport A, Haapio M, Hillege H, House A, Katz NM, Maisel A, Mankad S, Zanco P, Mebazaa A, Palazzuoli A, Ronco F, Shaw A, Sheinfeld G, Soni S, Vescovo G, Zamperetti N, Ponikowski P; Acute Dialysis Quality Initiative (ADQI) consensus group. Cardiorenal syndromes: an executive summary from the consensus conference of the Acute Dialysis Quality Initiative (ADQI). *Contrib Nephrol.* 2010;165:54-67.

[167] Lundy, D. J. and S. Trzeciak, Microcirculatory dysfunction in sepsis. *Crit Care Clin*, 2009. 25(4): p. 721-31

[168] Trzeciak, S., et al., Early microcirculatory perfusion derangements in patients with severe sepsis and septic shock: relationship to hemodynamics, oxygen transport, and survival. *Ann Emerg Med*, 2007. 49(1): p. 88-98, 98 e1-2.

[169] Jardin, F., et al., Sepsis-related cardiogenic shock. *Crit Care Med*, 1990. 18(10): p. 1055-60.

[170] Lambermont, B., et al., Effects of endotoxic shock on right ventricular systolic function and mechanical efficiency. *Cardiovasc Res,* 2003. 59(2): p. 412-8.

[171] Parker, M. M., et al., Profound but reversible myocardial depression in patients with septic shock. *Ann Intern Med*, 1984. 100(4): p. 483-90.

[172] Dhainaut, J. F., et al., Coronary hemodynamics and myocardial metabolism of lactate, free fatty acids, glucose, and ketones in patients with septic shock. *Circulation,* 1987. 75(3): p. 533-41.

[173] Kumar, A., et al., Tumor necrosis factor alpha and interleukin 1beta are responsible for in vitro myocardial cell depression induced by human septic shock serum. *J Exp Med*, 1996. 183(3): p. 949-58.

[174] Torre-Amione, G., et al., Proinflammatory cytokine levels in patients with depressed left ventricular ejection fraction: a report from the Studies of Left Ventricular Dysfunction (SOLVD). *J Am Coll Cardiol,* 1996. 27(5): p. 1201-6.

[175] Benes, J., et al., Searching for mechanisms that matter in early septic acute kidney injury: an experimental study. *Crit Care*, 2011. 15(5): p. R256.

[176] Bougle, A. and J. Duranteau, Pathophysiology of sepsis-induced acute kidney injury: the role of global renal blood flow and renal vascular resistance. *Contrib Nephrol*, 2011. 174: p. 89-97.

[177] Schmidt, H., et al., Autonomic dysfunction predicts both 1- and 2-month mortality in middle-aged patients with multiple organ dysfunction syndrome. *Crit Care Med*, 2008. 36(3): p. 967-70.

[178] Tateishi, Y., et al., Depressed heart rate variability is associated with high IL-6 blood level and decline in the blood pressure in septic patients. *Shock,* 2007. 28(5): p. 549-53.

[179] Ramchandra, R., et al., Septic shock induces distinct changes in sympathetic nerve activity to the heart and kidney in conscious sheep. *Am J Physiol Regul Integr Comp Physiol*, 2009. 297(5): p. R1247-53.
[180] Doerschug, K. C., et al., Renin-angiotensin system activation correlates with microvascular dysfunction in a prospective cohort study of clinical sepsis. *Crit Care*, 2010. 14(1): p. R24.
[181] Shen, L., et al., Losartan prevents sepsis-induced acute lung injury and decreases activation of nuclear factor kappaB and mitogen-activated protein kinases. *Shock,* 2009. 31(5): p. 500-6.
[182] Hagiwara, S., et al., Effects of an angiotensin-converting enzyme inhibitor on the inflammatory response in in vivo and in vitro models. *Crit Care Med*, 2009. 37(2): p. 626-33.
[183] Mortensen, E. M., et al., Impact of previous statin and angiotensin II receptor blocker use on mortality in patients hospitalized with sepsis. *Pharmacotherapy,* 2007. 27(12): p. 1619-26.
[184] Soni, A., et al., Adrenal insufficiency occurring during septic shock: incidence, outcome, and relationship to peripheral cytokine levels. *Am J Med*, 1995. 98(3): p. 266-71.
[185] Sligl, W. I., et al., Safety and efficacy of corticosteroids for the treatment of septic shock: A systematic review and meta-analysis. *Clin Infect Dis,* 2009. 49(1): p. 93-101.
[186] Kelly, K. J., Distant effects of experimental renal ischemia/reperfusion injury. *J Am Soc Nephrol*, 2003. 14(6): p. 1549-58.
[187] Burchill, L., et al., Acute kidney injury in the rat causes cardiac remodelling and increases angiotensin-converting enzyme 2 expression. *Exp Physiol*, 2008. 93(5): p. 622-30.
[188] Tokuyama, H., et al., Macrophage infiltration and cellular proliferation in the non-ischemic kidney and heart following prolonged unilateral renal ischemia. *Nephron Physiol*, 2007. 106(3): p. p54-62.
[189] Chopra, M., et al., Modulation of myocardial mitochondrial mechanisms during severe polymicrobial sepsis in the rat. *PLoS One*, 2011. 6(6): p. e21285.
[190] Liu, M., et al., Transcription factor Nrf2 is protective during ischemic and nephrotoxic acute kidney injury in mice. *Kidney Int,* 2009. 76(3): p. 277-85.
[191] Celes, M. R., C. M. Prado, and M. A. Rossi, Sepsis: going to the heart of the matter. *Pathobiology*, 2013. 80(2): p. 70-86.
[192] Stengl, M., et al., Reduced L-type calcium current in ventricular myocytes from pigs with hyperdynamic septic shock. *Crit Care Med,* 2010. 38(2): p. 579-87.
[193] Good, D. W., T. George, and B.A. Watts, 3rd, Toll-like receptor 2 mediates inhibition of HCO(3)(-) absorption by bacterial lipoprotein in medullary thick ascending limb. *Am J Physiol Renal Physiol*, 2010. 299(3): p. F536-44.
[194] Schreiber, A., et al., Acute endotoxemia in mice induces downregulation of megalin and cubilin in the kidney. *Kidney Int*, 2012. 82(1): p. 53-9.
[195] Reinhart, K., et al., New approaches to sepsis: molecular diagnostics and biomarkers. *Clin Microbiol Rev*, 2012. 25(4): p. 609-34.
[196] Dellinger, R. P., et al., Surviving Sepsis Campaign: international guidelines for management of severe sepsis and septic shock: 2008. *Crit Care Med*, 2008. 36(1): p. 296-327.

[197] Vignon, P., et al., Hand-held echocardiography with Doppler capability for the assessment of critically-ill patients: is it reliable? *Intensive Care Med,* 2004. 30(4): p. 718-23.

[198] Bellomo, R., et al., Acute renal failure - definition, outcome measures, animal models, fluid therapy and information technology needs: the Second International Consensus Conference of the Acute Dialysis Quality Initiative (ADQI) Group. *Crit Care*, 2004. 8(4): p. R204-12.

[199] Mehta, R. L., et al., Acute Kidney Injury Network: report of an initiative to improve outcomes in acute kidney injury. *Crit Care*, 2007. 11(2): p. R31.

[200] KDIGO Clinical Practice Guideline for Acute Kidney Injury: Summary of Recommendation Statements. *Kidney international*, 2012. Suppl. 2(1): p. 8-12.

[201] Calvin, J. E., A. A. Driedger, and W. J. Sibbald, An assessment of myocardial function in human sepsis utilizing ECG gated cardiac scintigraphy. *Chest*, 1981. 80(5): p. 579-86.

[202] Liu, K. D., et al., Acute kidney injury in patients with acute lung injury: impact of fluid accumulation on classification of acute kidney injury and associated outcomes. *Crit Care Med*, 2011. 39(12): p. 2665-71.

[203] Bellomo, R., et al., Fluid management in septic acute kidney injury and cardiorenal syndromes. *Contrib Nephrol*, 2010. 165: p. 206-18.

[204] De Vriese, A. S., et al., Cytokine removal during continuous hemofiltration in septic patients. *J Am Soc Nephrol,* 1999. 10(4): p. 846-53.

[205] Tapia, P., et al., Effectiveness of short-term 6-hour high-volume hemofiltration during refractory severe septic shock. *J Trauma Acute Care Surg*, 2012. 72(5): p. 1228-37; discussion 1237-8.

[206] Matson, J., A. Zydney, and P.M. Honore, Blood filtration: new opportunities and the implications of systems biology. *Crit Care Resusc,* 2004. 6(3): p. 209-17.

[207] Nakamura, M., et al., Treatment of severe sepsis and septic shock by CHDF using a PMMA membrane hemofilter as a cytokine modulator. *Contrib Nephrol*, 2010. 166: p. 73-82.

[208] Cruz, D. N., et al., Early use of polymyxin B hemoperfusion in abdominal septic shock: the EUPHAS randomized controlled trial. *JAMA,* 2009. 301(23): p. 2445-52.

[209] Humes, H. D., et al., A selective cytopheretic inhibitory device to treat the immunological dysregulation of acute and chronic renal failure. *Blood Purif*, 2010. 29(2): p. 183-90.

[210] Hou, Z. Q., et al., Effect of Levosimendan on Estimated Glomerular Filtration Rate in Hospitalized Patients with Decompensated Heart Failure and Renal Dysfunction. *Cardiovasc Ther*, 2012.

[211] Ristikankare, A., et al., Effects of levosimendan on renal function in patients undergoing coronary artery surgery. *J Cardiothorac Vasc Anesth*, 2012. 26(4): p. 591-5.

[212] Chou, Y. H., et al., Impact of timing of renal replacement therapy initiation on outcome of septic acute kidney injury. *Crit Care*, 2011. 15(3): p. R134.

[213] Bellomo, R., L. Wan, and C. May, Vasoactive drugs and acute kidney injury. *Crit Care Med*, 2008. 36(4 Suppl): p. S179-86.

[214] Schmoelz, M., et al., Comparison of systemic and renal effects of dopexamine and dopamine in norepinephrine-treated septic shock. *J Cardiothorac Vasc Anesth*, 2006. 20(2): p. 173-8.

[215] Cobas, M., et al., Fenoldopam in critically ill patients with early renal dysfunction. A crossover study. *Cardiovasc Ther,* 2011. 29(4): p. 280-4.

[216] Landoni, G., et al., Fenoldopam in cardiac surgery-associated acute kidney injury. *Int J Artif Organs*, 2008. 31(6): p. 561.

[217] Redfors, B., et al., Effects of norepinephrine on renal perfusion, filtration and oxygenation in vasodilatory shock and acute kidney injury. *Intensive Care Med*, 2011. 37(1): p. 60-7.

[218] Guzman, J. A., A. E. Rosado, and J. A. Kruse, Vasopressin vs norepinephrine in endotoxic shock: systemic, renal, and splanchnic hemodynamic and oxygen transport effects. *J Appl Physiol*, 2003. 95(2): p. 803-9.

[219] Gordon, A. C., et al., The effects of vasopressin on acute kidney injury in septic shock. *Intensive Care Med*, 2010. 36(1): p. 83-91.

[220] Nigwekar, S. U. and S. S. Waikar, Diuretics in acute kidney injury. *Semin Nephrol*, 2011. 31(6): p. 523-34.

In: Comorbidities in Chronic Kidney Disease
Editor: Luca Di Lullo
ISBN: 978-1-63485-070-4

Chapter 9

THE HEPATO – RENAL SYNDROME

Luca Di Lullo*, Francesca Santoboni and Alberto Santoboni

Department of Nephrology and Dialysis – L. Parodi – Delfino Hospital, Colleferro (Rome), Italy

ABSTRACT

Hepatic and kidney failure are often closely linked (Hepato-Renal Sindrome – HRS). Acute kidney injury (AKI) represents a well – known complication of liver or biliary tract disease. Pathophysiology of HRS is still not completely clear. At this stage, we know the biological pathways of several kidney abnormalities in end stage liver disease patients. At the same time, a patient's prognosis is poor with bad results despite the reversible nature of the kidneys' involvement. Liver transplantation represents the ultimate treatment for HRS patients.

Keywords: liver failure, renal failure, liver transplantation, dialysis

BACKGROUND

Hepatic and kidney failure are often closely linked (Hepato-Renal Sindrome – HRS). Acute kidney injury (AKI) represents a well – known complication of liver or biliary tract disease [1].

Since the late 1800s, oliguria was reported in patients with end stage liver disease (i.e., ascites and advanced cirrhosis) without any renal histological features of primary or secondary kidney involvement [2].

In 1957, Sheila Sherlock reported rapid and progressive decline in renal function in cirrhotic patients characterized by an oligo; anuria and creatinin increase; her work also

* Correspondence to: Luca Di Lullo, Department of Nephrology and Dialysis. Colleferro County Hospital, Piazza Aldo Moro, 1 Colleferro, Rome, Italy, Tel: +39 069 722 3205; Fax: +39 069 722 3213; Email: dilulloluca69@gmail.com.

demonstrated renal function recovery (both clinical and histological) once hepatic function was restored [3].

Further observations confirmed the work done by Sheila Sherlock that the kidneys transplanted from HRS patients did not show any glomerular and/or interstitial structural damage [4].

The pathophysiology of HRS is still not completely. At this stage we know the biological pathways of several kidney abnormalities in end stage liver disease patients. At the same time, a patient's prognosis is poor with bad results despite the reversible nature of the kidneys' involvement [5].

Liver transplant represents the final treatment of HRS, and unfortunately a majority of patients die before receiving a liver transplant.

Hepato – Renal Syndrome: Definition

The first definition of HRS was developed in 1996 and revised in 2007 [6, 7]; the definition criteria demonstrates close pathophysiological links between hepatic and renal dysfunction.

HRS shows itself in two distinct clinical pictures [8]: HRS types – 1 and 2.

Type – 1 has an acute form and leads to progressive renal failure in a short time, and it usually develops as a consequence of gastrointestinal bleeding, large volume paracentesis, acute alcoholic hepatitis and bacterial peritonitis [9, 10]. It is often complicated by an impairment of the heart, brain, liver and adrenal glands.

Type – 2 HRS is a chronic form and is characterized by a slow progression towards renal failure associated with diuretic resistant ascites [11].

Despite the above described classification, HRS usually moves toward progressive renal impairment and type – 2 HRS easily turns into type – 1.

Pathogenesis of Hepato – Renal Syndrome

Pathogenesis of HRS is not completely known presently, but it has been stated that a reduction in glomerular filtration rate (GFR) represents the main pathophysiological feature.

The main steps in HRS pathophysiology are summarized in figure 1 and figure 2.

Fall in GFR is strictly linked to a reduction of effective blood volume due to splanchnic vasodilation with related renin – angiotensin – aldosterone system (RAAS) and sympathetic nervous system activation. At the same time a release of antidiuretic hormone (ADH) occurs leading to renal afferent artery vasoconstriction [12 – 14].

Patients with HRS present low urinary sodium excretion due to decreased filtered and increased reabsorption of sodium; furosemide and spironolactone are both ineffective because of a decreased delivery and the low amount of sodium at the effector site (Henle's loop and distal tubule).

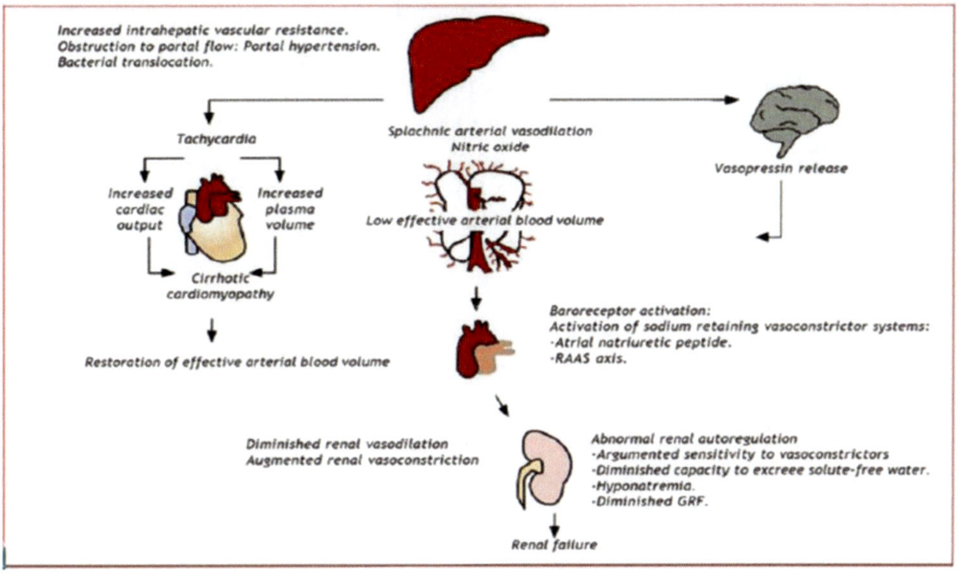

Figure 1. Pathophysiology of cirrhosis induced acute kidney injury (HRS: hepato – renal syndrome).

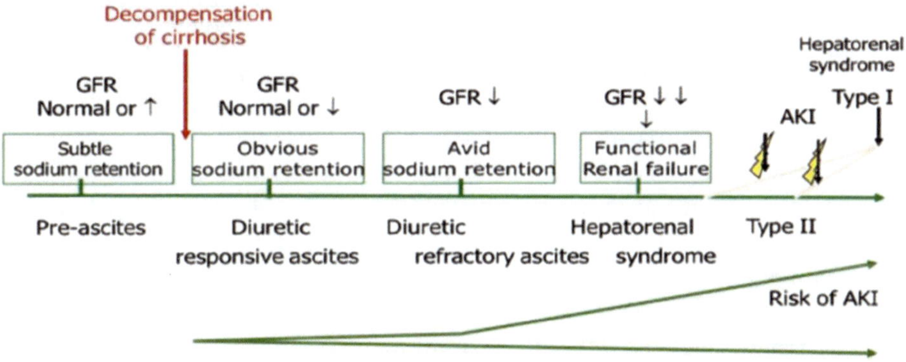

	Compensated cirrhosis	Diuretic-responsive ascites	Diuretic-resistant ascites	HRS
Splanchnic/systemic arterial vasodilation	Normal/+	+	++	+++
Effective circulating volume	Normal	-	--	---
Renin, aldosterone, vasopressin, norepinephrine	Normal	+	++	+++
Renal sodium retention/plasma volume	+	++	+++	++++
Renal vasoconstriction	Normal	Normal	++	++++

Figure 2. Hemodynamic changes during different stages of cirrhosis.

Small amounts of filtered water are absorbed at distal tubules in response to high ADH levels leading to oligo – anuria [15, 16].

Splanchnic vasodilation represents a cornerstone in HRS pathophysiology that is widely accepted in scientific literature. In early cirrhosis hepatocyte inflammation promotes the secretion of collagen into hepatic sinusoids increasing portal venous resistance and the consequent progression of liver damage.

As a consequence of the shear stress on the portal and splanchnic venous system, we observe a massive secretion of nitric oxide (NO) and other vasodilators from endothelial cells [17].

An increasing shear stress also supports the formation of collateral vessels both by opening pre-existing vessels or angiogenesis due to up – regulation of endothelial growth factor (EGF) and platelet derived growth factor (PDGF) [18, 19].

Bacterial translocation from intestinal flora to portal circulation seems to be involved in HRS pathogenesis, through the activation of immune system and massive production of cytokines as tumor necrosis factor alpha (TNF-α) and interleukin – 6 (IL – 6) [21, 22], as commonly observed in cirrhotic patients with portal hypertension [20].

TNF-α, IL - 6 and bacterial endotoxins increase NO production from endothelial cells leading to splanchnic vasodilation [23].

The splanchnic vasodilation is not a sufficient explanation for the development of HRS.

First of all, auto – regulation of renal blood flow in cirrhotic patients is right – shifted due to the activation of renal sympathetic nervous system and other vasoconstrictors agents [24].

With the progress of liver disease, the renal blood flow becomes more dependent on systemic arterial blood pressure; in advanced cirrhosis patients, mild changes in arterial blood pressure will result in a significant increase in renal blood flow. At the same time the left ventricular function can be damaged, as in the well known "cirrhotic cardiomyopathy"; the cardiac output is not adequate to balance the effective blood volume leading to impairment of renal perfusion pressure [25, 26].

The hypo – perfusion can also affect the adrenal glands with subsequent glucocorticoid insufficiency and an impaired response to vasoconstrictors agents [27].

Although splanchnic vasodilation is the most plausible pathophysiological mechanism in HRS development, progressive renal function impairment is probably related to other liver injuries such as trauma and toxic drugs abuse [28, 29].

The systemic inflammatory response to liver injury could be considered for many other pathophysiological and clinical aspects of HRS. After liver ischemia, Kuppfer cells release pro – inflammatory cytokines such as TNF-α, IL - 1α and IL – 6 promoting inflammatory changes in several organs including the lungs, heart and kidneys [30, 31].

Damaged hepatocytes release other intracellular molecules such as Damage Associated Molecular Pattern molecules (DAMPs) that are responsible for exacerbating an inflammatory response [32, 33].

Other inflammatory agents, including circulating bile acids, uric acid and circulating immune-complexes, may further lead to the development of acute kidney injury (AKI) [66].

This hypothesis has been further strengthened by recent findings showing vascular endothelial cell damage in patients with end stage liver disease [34].

Pro – inflammatory cytokines directly affect the kidney's endothelial cells leading to the loss of their ability to regulate leukocyte recruitment [35, 36].

Recent findings point out the gut's involvement in inflammatory pathway by releasing IL – 17A. High levels of IL – 17A are mainly stored in the Paneth cells, located at the base of intestinal crypts, usually secreting "defensins" (cationic proteins able to protect the gut from bacterial infections).

Because of liver or kidney ischemia, Paneth cells release great amounts of IL – 17A, that are responsible for the widespread inflammation [37].

Diagnosis and Biomarkers of HRS

The lack of universally acceptable criteria makes for a difficult diagnosis of HRS. Current ascites club criteria cannot be employ because of a high percentage of oligo – anuric patients [38].

Among available biomarkers, cystatin C (Cys-C) is actually under investigation for clinical use in HRS patients.

Cys-C crosses through glomerular membranes and is metabolized in the proximal tubular cells [39]; Cys – C levels are independent of muscle mass, age, sex and they are not influenced by inflammation or neoplasia [39].

Another biomarker, in addition to creatinine and Cys – C, is urinary NGAL (neutrophil gelatinase-associated lipocalin-2), expressed by damaged tubular cells and secreted within two hours of kidney's injury (40). We can use the urinary NGAL dosage to distinguish HRS from other secondary kidney disease; in fact, in AKI the NGAL level is highest, during HRS it has an intermediate levels and in chronic kidney disease (CKD) patients is lowest.

Other urinary biomarkers investigated include gamma – glutamyl transpeptidase, transaminase, IL – 18 and hepatitis A virus cellular receptor – 1, but these biomarkers need further investigations in cirrhotic patients.

Markers of afferent renal artery vasoconstriction have been suggested for HRS diagnosis such as plasma noradrenaline level (to test sympathetic nervous system activity) and plasma renin activity (to assess renin – angiotensin – aldosterone system activity) [40].

Management Strategies

a) Pharmacological Approach

Treatment options for HRS patients are quite limited and mainly serve to prolong the patients' life until a liver transplant is possible; furthermore, supportive therapies have to prevent and treat all precipitating factors for HRS development:

1) Paracentesis for large amounts of ascites
2) Antibiotics for peritonitis
3) Avoidance of nephrotoxic drugs and diagnostic proceedings
4) Low – salt diet and water restrictions, especially in hyponatremic patients

Few specific drugs are actually available to reduce the splanchnic vasodilation; one of these is represented by Terlipressin, a vasopressin - analog (active on vasopressin type – 1 receptors in splanchnic circulation) [41].

Terlipressin, together with albumin infusion, represents a first choice therapy in type – 1 HRS [51, 52].

Additionally, Terlipressin is effective in patients with mild liver (total bilirubin levels below 10 mg/dl) and kidney dysfunction [42].

Other vasoconstrictor agents, such as milodrine, α-adrenergic receptor agonist, and octreotide, are less effective than terlipressin.

The activation of neuro – hormonal systems leads to sodium and water retention, for this reason there is an increasing interest in drugs such as the vasopressin V2 – receptors, known as vaptans. This drug may improve circulatory and renal function in cirrhotic patients with refractory ascites and/or hyponatremia, Vasopressin (AVP) action is mediated by three receptor's subtypes: V1a, V1b and V2; V2 receptors are expressed by principal cells of renal collecting duct system and mobilize intracellular acquaporin 2 to apical plasma membrane increasing reabsorption of free water.

AVP acts on V2 receptors on the basolateral surface of principal cells leading to adenylyl cyclase and protein kinase activation; this enzymatic activation allows the water shift against osmotic gradient; the water returns to systemic circulation across basolateral membrane [43].

Active vasopressin receptor antagonists are called vaptans and cause aquaresis (i.e., excretion of solute – free urine); vaptans differ from diuretics because they promote water excretion without loss of electrolytes.

Vaptans were used both in the management of refractory ascites and especially dilutional hyponatremia.

Main therapy of hyponatremia consists in increasing solute – free water excretion, as implemented with the incoming vaptans' therapy [44, 45]. A small amount of data in research literature shows that a short period of vaptans' therapy (from 1 week to 1 month) improves solute – free water excretion leading to the increase in serum sodium levels without major side effects (i.e., reduction of renal function, natruresis, impairment of circulatory function and RAAS activity) [46 – 49].

The main side effects of vaptan therapy are represented by thirst, hypernatremia, dehydration, acute kidney failure and osmotic demyelination due to increased serum sodium levels [46 – 49].

Tolvaptan was approved in the USA and Europe for treatment of severe hypervolemic hyponatremia (< 125 mmol/L) due to SIADH and should be started with 15 mg/day titrated 'till 30 to 60 mg/day following serum sodium concentrations. It should be also be noted that the FDA (Food and Drug Administration) has forbidden tolvaptan to be used in patients with liver disease (including cirrhosis) because the ability to recover has yet to be proved [50].

Vaptan therapy should be reserved to patients with severe hypervolemic hyponatremia (< 125 mmol/L) and carefully introduced under hospitalization; patients should be discharged at home only when sodium levels become stable and no further adjustments are needed [51].

b) Non – Pharmacological Approach

Non - pharmacological approaches include renal replacement therapy, transjugular intrahepatic porto-systemic shunt (TIPS) and liver transplantation.

Renal replacement therapy is mainly indicated as a supportive therapy to contrast hyperkalemia, metabolic acidosis and volume overload [52].

TIPS can decompress portal pressure and decrease sympathetic nervous system and RAAS activities [53, 54]. TIPS itself increases cardiac output and peripheral vasodilation and it should be performed only in patients with stable liver function and as a bridge therapy waiting for liver transplant.

The ideal treatment is a liver transplant, as it best treats both liver and renal dysfunction, particularly when performed in the early stages of disease.

Liver transplantation is unfortunately limited by the availability of organs and many patients die before undergoing transplantation [55].

References

[1] Quincke, H.; Nothnagel, H. Specielle Pathologie und Therapie. Vol. xviii. Vienna: 1899. p. 63.

[2] F A. Clinical report on hydro-peritoneum, based on analysis of forty-six cases. *Am. J. Med. Sci.* 1863; 45:306–39.

[3] Hecker R, Sherlock S. Electrolyte and circulatory changes in terminal liver failure. *Lancet.* 1956; 271(6953):1121–5. [PubMed: 13377688].

[4] Koppel MH, Coburn JW, Mims MM, Goldstein H, Boyle JD, Rubini ME. Transplantation of cadaveric kidneys from patients with hepatorenal syndrome Evidence for the functionalnature of renal failure in advanced liver disease. *N. Engl. J. Med.* 1969; 280(25):1367–71. [PubMed: 4890476].

[5] Gines P, Guevara M, Arroyo V, Rodes J. Hepatorenal syndrome. *Lancet.* 2003; 362(9398): 1819–27. [PubMed: 14654322].

[6] Arroyo V, Gines P, Gerbes AL, Dudley FJ, Gentilini P, Laffi G, et al. Definition and diagnostic criteria of refractory ascites and hepatorenal syndrome in cirrhosis. International Ascites Club. *Hepatology.* 1996; 23(1):164–76. [PubMed: 8550036].

[7] Salerno F, Gerbes A, Gines P, Wong F, Arroyo V. Diagnosis, prevention and treatment of hepatorenal syndrome in cirrhosis. *Gut.* 2007; 56(9): 1310–8. [PubMed: 17389705].

[8] European Association for the Study of the L. EASL clinical practice guidelines on the management of ascites, spontaneous bacterial peritonitis, and hepatorenal syndrome in cirrhosis. *J. Hepatol.* 2010; 53(3): 397–417. [PubMed: 20633946].

[9] Gines A, Escorsell A, Gines P, Salo J, Jimenez W, Inglada L, et al. Incidence, predictive factors, and prognosis of the hepatorenal syndrome in cirrhosis with ascites. *Gastroenterology.* 1993; 105(1):229–36. [PubMed: 8514039].

[10] Follo A, Llovet JM, Navasa M, Planas R, Forns X, Francitorra A, et al. Renal impairment after spontaneous bacterial peritonitis in cirrhosis: incidence, clinical course, predictive factors and prognosis. *Hepatology.* 1994; 20(6): 1495–501. [PubMed: 7982650].

[11] Gines P, Schrier RW. Renal failure in cirrhosis. *N. Engl. J. Med.* 2009; 361(13):1279–90. [PubMed: 19776409].

[12] Moller S, Hobolth L, Winkler C, Bendtsen F, Christensen E. Determinants of the hyperdynamic circulation and central hypovolaemia in cirrhosis. *Gut.* 2011; 60(9): 1254–9. [PubMed: 21504996].

[13] Sacerdoti D, Bolognesi M, Merkel C, Angeli P, Gatta A. Renal vasoconstriction in cirrhosis evaluated by duplex Doppler ultrasonography. *Hepatology.* 1993; 17(2):219–24. [PubMed: 8428719].

[14] Maroto A, Gines A, Salo J, Claria J, Gines P, Anibarro L, et al. Diagnosis of functional kidney failure of cirrhosis with Doppler sonography: prognostic value of resistive index. *Hepatology.* 1994; 20(4 Pt 1): 839–44. [PubMed: 7927224].

[15] Linas SL, Anderson RJ, Guggenheim SJ, Robertson GL, Berl T. Role of vasopressin in impaired water excretion in conscious rats with experimental cirrhosis. Kidney Int. 1981; 20(2): 173–80. [PubMed: 7289402].

[16] Bichet DG, Van Putten VJ, Schrier RW. Potential role of increased sympathetic activity in impaired sodium and water excretion in cirrhosis. *N. Engl. J. Med.* 1982; 307(25):1552–7. [PubMed: 6755251].

[17] Schrier RW, Arroyo V, Bernardi M, Epstein M, Henriksen JH, Rodes J. Peripheral arterial vasodilation hypothesis: a proposal for the initiation of renal sodium and water retention in cirrhosis. *Hepatology*. 1988; 8(5): 1151–7. [PubMed: 2971015].

[18] Van Steenkiste C, Geerts A, Vanheule E, Van Vlierberghe H, De Vos F, Olievier K, et al. Role of placental growth factor in mesenteric neoangiogenesis in a mouse model of portal hypertension. *Gastroenterology*. 2009; 137(6):2112–24 e1-6. [PubMed: 19751735].

[19] Paternostro C, David E, Novo E, Parola M. Hypoxia, angiogenesis and liver fibrogenesis in the progression of chronic liver diseases. *World J. Gastroenterol.* 2010; 16(3):281–8. [PubMed: 20082471].

[20] Bellot P, Frances R, Such J. Pathological bacterial translocation in cirrhosis: pathophysiology, diagnosis and clinical implications. *Liver Int.* 2013; 33(1): 31–9. [PubMed: 23121656].

[21] Sugano S. Endotoxin levels in cirrhotic rats with sterile and infected ascites. *Gastroenterol. Jpn.* 1992; 27(3):348–53. [PubMed: 1624078].

[22] Heller J, Sogni P, Barriere E, Tazi KA, Chauvelot-Moachon L, Guimont MC, et al. Effects of lipopolysaccharide on TNF-alpha production, hepatic NOS2 activity, and hepatic toxicity in rats with cirrhosis. *J. Hepatol.* 2000; 33(3):376–81. [PubMed: 11019992].

[23] Wiest R, Das S, Cadelina G, Garcia-Tsao G, Milstien S, Groszmann RJ. Bacterial translocation in cirrhotic rats stimulates eNOS-derived NO production and impairs mesenteric vascular contractility. *J. Clin. Invest.* 1999; 104(9):1223–33. [PubMed: 10545521].

[24] Stadlbauer V, Wright GA, Banaji M, Mukhopadhya A, Mookerjee RP, Moore K, et al. Relationship between activation of the sympathetic nervous system and renal blood flow autoregulation in cirrhosis. *Gastroenterology*. 2008; 134(1): 111–9. [PubMed: 18166350].

[25] Ruiz-del-Arbol L, Urman J, Fernandez J, Gonzalez M, Navasa M, Monescillo A, et al. Systemic, renal, and hepatic hemodynamic derangement in cirrhotic patients with spontaneous bacterial peritonitis. *Hepatology*. 2003; 38(5): 1210–8. [PubMed: 14578859].

[26] Ruiz-del-Arbol L, Monescillo A, Arocena C, Valer P, Gines P, Moreira V, et al. Circulatory function and hepatorenal syndrome in cirrhosis. *Hepatology*. 2005; 42(2): 439–47. [PubMed: 15977202].

[27] Cooper MS, Stewart PM. Corticosteroid insufficiency in acutely ill patients. *N. Engl. J. Med.* 2003; 348(8): 727–34. [PubMed: 12594318].

[28] Helwig F, Schutz C. A further contribution to the liver-kidney syndrome. *J. Lab. and Clin. Med.* 1935; 21:264.

[29] Wilensky A. Occurrence, Distribution and Pathogenesis of So-Called Liver Death and/or the Hepatorenal Syndrome. *Arch. Surg.* 1939; 38:625.

[30] Tsung A, Hoffman RA, Izuishi K, Critchlow ND, Nakao A, Chan MH, et al. Hepatic ischemia/reperfusion injury involves functional TLR4 signaling in nonparenchymal cells. *J. Immunol.* 2005; 175(11):7661–8. [PubMed: 16301676].

[31] Tanaka Y, Maher JM, Chen C, Klaassen CD. Hepatic ischemia-reperfusion induces renal heme oxygenase-1 via NF-E2-related factor 2 in rats and mice. *Mol. Pharmacol.* 2007; 71(3):817–25. [PubMed: 17151289].

[32] Wang H, Bloom O, Zhang M, Vishnubhakat JM, Ombrellino M, Che J, et al. HMG-1 as a late mediator of endotoxin lethality in mice. *Science.* 1999; 285(5425): 248–51. [PubMed: 10398600].

[33] Andersson U, Wang H, Palmblad K, Aveberger AC, Bloom O, Erlandsson-Harris H, et al. High mobility group 1 protein (HMG-1) stimulates proinflammatory cytokine synthesis in human monocytes. *J. Exp. Med.* 2000; 192(4):565–70. [PubMed: 10952726].

[34] Lee HT, Park SW, Kim M, D'Agati VD. Acute kidney injury after hepatic ischemia and reperfusion injury in mice. *Lab. Invest.* 2009; 89(2): 196–208. [PubMed: 19079326].

[35] Teoh NC, Farrell GC. Hepatic ischemia reperfusion injury: pathogenic mechanisms and basis for hepatoprotection. *J. Gastroenterol. Hepatol.* 2003; 18(8):891–902. [PubMed: 12859717].

[36] Sutton TA, Mang HE, Campos SB, Sandoval RM, Yoder MC, Molitoris BA. Injury of the renal microvascular endothelium alters barrier function after ischemia. *Am. J. Physiol. Renal Physiol.* 2003; 285(2):F191–8. [PubMed: 12684225].

[37] Park SW, Kim M, Brown KM, D'Agati VD, Lee HT. Paneth cell-derived interleukin-17A causes multiorgan dysfunction after hepatic ischemia and reperfusion injury. *Hepatology*. 2011; 53(5): 1662–75. [PubMed: 21360570].

[38] Wong F, Nadim MK, Kellum JA, Salerno F, Bellomo R, Gerbes A, et al. Working Party proposal for a revised classification system of renal dysfunction in patients with cirrhosis. *Gut.* 2011; 60(5): 702–9. [PubMed: 21325171].

[39] Randers E, Erlandsen EJ. Serum cystatin C as an endogenous marker of the renal function--a review. *Clin. Chem. Lab. Med.* 1999; 37(4): 389–95. [PubMed: 10369108].

[40] Verna EC, Brown RS, Farrand E, Pichardo EM, Forster CS, Sola-Del Valle DA, et al. Urinary neutrophil gelatinase-associated lipocalin predicts mortality and identifies acute kidney injury in cirrhosis. *Dig. Dis. Sci.* 2012; 57(9): 2362–70. [PubMed: 22562534].

[41] Cooper MS, Stewart PM. Corticosteroid insufficiency in acutely ill patients. *N. Engl. J. Med.* 2003; 348(8):727–34. [PubMed: 12594318].

[42] Tsai MH, Peng YS, Chen YC, Liu NJ, Ho YP, Fang JT, et al. Adrenal insufficiency in patients with cirrhosis, severe sepsis and septic shock. *Hepatology*. 2006; 43(4):673–81. [PubMed: 16557538].

[43] Kumar P, Clark M, editors. Kumar and Clark's Clinical Medicine. 7 ed. Edinburgh: *Saunders Elsevier;* 2009.pp.649–663.

[44] Quittnat F, Gross P. Vaptans and the treatment of water-retaining disorders. *Semin. Nephrol.* 2006; 26: 234-243.

[45] Ginès P. Vaptans: a promising therapy in the management of advanced cirrhosis. *J. Hepatol.* 2007;46: 1150-1152.

[46] Schrier RW, Gross P, Gheorghiade M, Berl T, Verbalis JG, Czerwiec FS, Orlandi C. Tolvaptan, a selective oral vasopressin V2-receptor antagonist, for hyponatremia. *N. Engl. J. Med.* 2006;355:2099-2112.

[47] O'Leary JG, Davis GL. Conivaptan increases serum sodium in hyponatremic patients with end-stage liver disease. *Liver Transpl.* 2009; 15:1325-1329.

[48] Gerbes AL, Gülberg V, Ginès P, Decaux G, Gross P, Gandjini H, Djian J. Therapy of hyponatremia in cirrhosis with a vasopressin receptor antagonist: a randomized double-blind multicenter trial. *Gastroenterology.* 2003; 124:933-939.

[49] Wong F, Blei AT, Blendis LM, Thuluvath PJ. A vasopressin receptor antagonist (VPA-985) improves serum sodium concentration in patients with hyponatremia: a multicenter, randomized, placebo-controlled trial. *Hepatology.* 2003; 37: 182-191.

[50] Available from: http://www.fda.gov/Drugs/DrugSafety/ucm350062.htm.

[51] European Association for the Study of the Liver. EASL clinical practice guidelines on the management of ascites, spontaneous bacterial peritonitis, and hepatorenal syndrome in cirrhosis. *J. Hepatol.* 2010; 53:397-417.

[52] Wadei HM. Hepatorenal syndrome: a critical update. *Semin. Respir. Crit. Care Med.* 2012; 33(1): 55–69. [PubMed: 22447261].

[53] Somberg KA, Lake JR, Tomlanovich SJ, LaBerge JM, Feldstein V, Bass NM. Transjugular intrahepatic portosystemic shunts for refractory ascites: assessment of clinical and hormonal response and renal function. *Hepatology.* 1995; 21(3):709–16. [PubMed: 7875668].

[54] Quiroga J, Sangro B, Nunez M, Bilbao I, Longo J, Garcia-Villarreal L, et al. Transjugular intrahepatic portal-systemic shunt in the treatment of refractory ascites: effect on clinical, renal, humoral, and hemodynamic parameters. *Hepatology.* 1995; 21(4): 986–94. [PubMed: 7705810].

[55] Ng CK, Chan MH, Tai MH, Lam CW. Hepatorenal syndrome. *Clin. Biochem. Rev.* 2007; 28(1): 11– 7. [PubMed: 17603637].

In: Comorbidities in Chronic Kidney Disease
Editor: Luca Di Lullo
ISBN: 978-1-63485-070-4

Chapter 10

Contrast-Induced Acute Kidney Injury

Vincenzo Barbera* and Antonio Gorini
Department of Nephrology and Dialysis,
Colleferro County Hospital, Colleferro, Rome, Italy

Abstract

Contrast-Induced Acute Kidney Injury (CI-AKI) represents a relevant cause of mortality and morbidity in patients after diagnostic and interventional procedures. CI-AKI is the third cause of renal failure acquired during hospitalization, after surgery and hypotension. Formerly the definition of AKI wasn't well defined due to poor knowledge of risk factors, pathogenesis and prevention strategies to reduce clinical manifestations especially in presence of predisposing conditions. The aforementioned items we'll describe based on the most recent knowledge and the last KDIGO guidelines.

Keywords: CI-AKI, Low Osmolal Contrast Media (LOCM), High Osmolal Contrast Media (HOCM), diabetes

Introduction

As a result of Multiple Detector Computed Tomography (MDCT) availability in clinical routine, it has been observed in last decade a progressive growing of contrastographic examinations: in USA these ones reached the number of 30 million per years. The increasing use of contrastographic procedures (e.g., angiography) for high risk patients made CI-AKI an important cause of morbidity and mortality in the short and long term. Formerly contrast induced nephropathy (CIN) was identified as ≥25% increase of serum creatinine (sCr) level *vs* basal level or ≥0.5 mg/dL (44 μmol/L) within 48 hours from contrast infusion, in absence of other known causes [1]; currently, CIN is best defined as CI-AKI. According to KDIGO

* Correspondence to: V. Barbera, Department of Nephrology and Dialysis. Colleferro County Hospital, Piazza Aldo Moro, 1 Colleferro, Rome, Italy, Tel: +39 069 722 3205; Fax: +39 069 722 3213; Email: vincenzo.barbera@aslromag.it.

guidelines [2] we can define Acute Kidney Injury (AKI) the condition showing an increase in sCr ≥0.3 mg/dL in 48 hours, or an increase in sCr ≥50% from baseline over a period of seven days [2]. In addition to the biochemical criteria, KDIGO also recognized a reduction in urinary output <0.5 ml/kg/hr for at least 6 hours as a marker of AKI [2]. Therefore, we define CI-AKI as the AKI onset within 48 hours after intravenous administration of radiographic contrast medium and not given by other causes.

EPIDEMIOLOGY

CI-AKI epidemiology is very difficult to define in detail due to different employed diagnostic criteria, various radiological procedures and different contrast agents used, the presence of risk factors and length of follow up.

In 1985 Misson and Cutler gathered the data of seven retrospective studies and eight prospective ones, for a total of 1216 patients and 1256, respectively [3]. In the first group CI-AKI incidence ranged between 5% and 17%, while in the latter it was between 0 and 22%. An overall incidence of 14.5% is reported by McCullough et al. in a large study defining CI-AKI as an increase in sCr of at least 25% from baseline in the five days following exposure to contrast [4]. The incidence was located in a range between zero and 90% depending on the presence or absence of certain risk factors, especially chronic kidney disease (CKD), diabetes mellitus and the amount of contrast used. On the other hand, CI-AKI incidence in the general population is estimated to be less than 2% [5]. In hospitalized patients with impaired renal function CI-AKI incidence may not be directly related to the administration of contrast medium (e.g., ateroembolism during angiography). On this regard Newhouse et al. [6] conducted a retrospective study of 32,161 patients not been submitted to contrastographic examaminations in the ten days before and carrying serial sCr assays for five consecutive days. More than 50% of the patients showed a variation in sCr of at least 25% while an increase of at least 0.4 mg/dL was observed in 2/5 of them. A recent meta-analysis including 1,489 studies has demonstrated a similar rate of AKI, need for dialysis and mortality in the group receiving contrastographic procedures compared to controls where no contrast agent was administered [7]. More in detail, AKI risk was independent of the type of contrast agent, the diagnostic criteria used to define the renal damage and the presence or absence of diabetes mellitus and CKD. Despite these conflicting results, CI-AKI is universally recognized as an important cause of morbidity and mortality, the third largest (about 10%) among the causes of AKI acquired during a hospitalization and being responsible for about 5% of the hospitalizations [8]. The overall mortality rate remains high floating around 30% of the cases [9]; in patients undergoing coronary angiography this value is significantly higher (35.7%) with a 2-year survival of approximately 18.8% [4]. Similar results have been obtained by Levy et al. [10] in a cohort of about 16,000 patients undergoing various contrastographic procedures (CT, coronary and peripheral angiography). In this study the Authors showed a mortality increase in the group developing CI-AKI, while the one not showing such complication it did not appear (34% vs 7%), leading to the conclusion that this condition was an independent risk factor for death. However, this concept seems to be still under discussion. Recently, McDonald in a retrospective analysis including 21,346 patients (10,673 underwent contrastographic examinations and 10,673 contrast-free) concludes that exposure to contrast medium was not associated with an excessive risk of AKI, dialysis or death even among high risk patients [11].

Risk Factors

Several factors seem to cause CI-AKI onset (Figure 1) but only a few have been proven to be independent risk factors [12]. Since the overall CI-AKI risk raises by increasing the number of risk factors, it is appropriate to evaluate each factor in order to reduce its effect, if possible. All studies comparing patients with and without CKD show that the presence of renal failure significantly increases the risk of developing acute renal failure caused by contrast media [13, 14]. In a prospective trial including 1144 patients undergoing cardiac catheterization Davidson and coworkers showed that the CI-AKI risk begins to increase for values of sCr greater than 1.2 mg/dL, growing exponentially with the rise of the sCr (increase of about 20% for values of sCr of 2.0 mg/dL) [15]. In absence of renal impairment, CI-AKI is infrequent, appearing in less than 10% of patients.

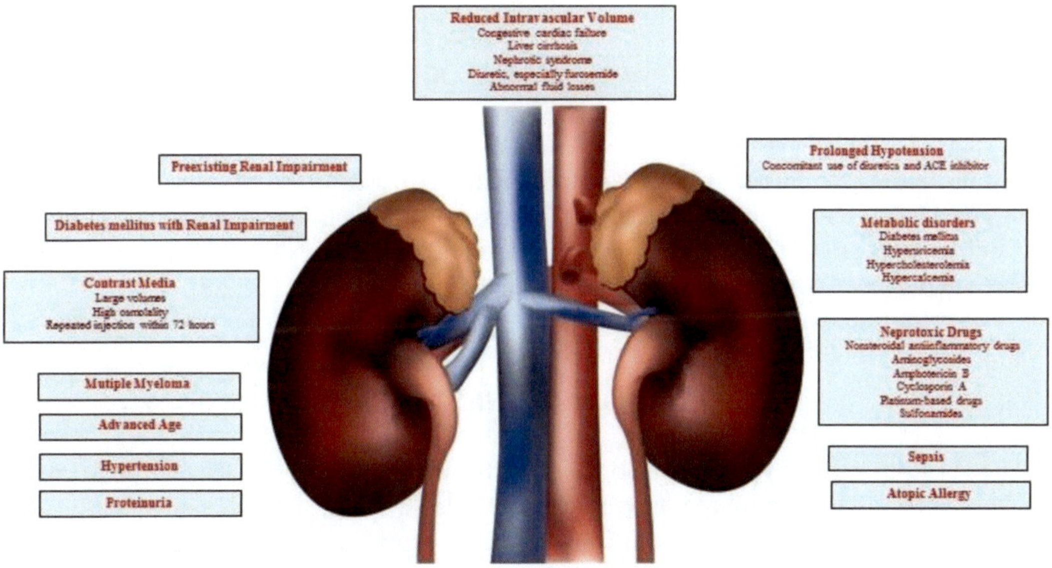

Figure 1. Risk Factors for Contrast-Induced Nephropathy.

Diabetes mellitus is an important independent risk factor for development of CI-AKI. Diabetic patients without renal impairment show a risk comparable to non-diabetics with kidney failure [14]; however, the association of the two diseases leads to doubling the risk compared to that expected for the single kidney failure [13]. Such synergy is apparently due to the endothelial and vascular damage common in diabetes patients and involving the renal plasma flow.

Even the reduction of the effective circulating volume occurring during heart failure (HF) conditions has been reported as risk factor for the CI-AKI, although not all Authors agree with this statement [15, 16]. Several patients with HF assume diuretics or RAAS (Renin

Angiotensin Aldosterone System) inhibitors drugs, which may increase AKI risk by decreasing the blood volume and by activating renal vasoconstriction.

Frequently, patients with multiple myeloma are considered at higher risk of CI-AKI [17, 18]. The pathogenetic hypothesis is linked to the intratubular contrast precipitation along with some proteins – e.g., Tamm-Horsfall protein - and cell debris coming from the tubules ischemic damage. Furthermore it should be considered the direct toxic damage of the contrast media as well as the altered integrins function [19]. However, the low CI-AKI incidence (0.6-1.25%) reported in a number of studies suggests that myeloma itself can not be an independent risk factor. Other associated conditions, such as hyperuricemia, hypercalcemia, amyloidosis, volume depletion, toxicity to light chains predispose to CI-AKI. A recent retrospective study on 476 multiple myeloma patients is not able to show an increase of CI-AKI in such patients [20].

Increasing the amount and/or frequency of the contrast medium rises CI-AKI risk. However, safe levels are not known, volumes of low osmolality contrast media (LOCM) – e.g., iohexol or iopamidol - above 30 mL were associated with a significantly higher rate of kidney injury, which increased by about 65% every time you added 5 mL in volume [21]. In addition, the administration route plays an important role. The nephrotoxicity is greater by intra arterial route as compared to intravenous route [15]: this is likely due to the much higher contrast media intrarenal peaks.

Finally, some studies showed that the use of LOCM reduces CI-AKI occurrence at a greater extent as compared to HOCM (High Osmolality Contrast Media) [22-26]. However, this advantage is only observed in patients with preexisting renal damage and in which the contrast medium is administered by intra-arterial route.

In conclusion, renal failure and the possible association with diabetes mellitus seem the only independent risk factors definitely assessed. Therefore, all necessary preventive measures to prevent CI-AKI should be implemented in these subjects [27, 28].

Pathogenesis

The exact underlying CI-AKI pathogenic mechanisms are not yet fully clarified (Figure 2). Likely both vascular and direct tubular damages play a role in CI-AKI pathogenesis. We use the following classification: intrinsic (renal) and extrinsic (pre-renal) causes. Intrinsic causes include: (1) increase of intra-renal vasoconstriction; (2) reduction of vasodilation mediated by prostaglandins (PGs) and nitric oxide (NO); (3) a direct toxic effect on renal tubular cells by reactive oxygen species (ROS); (4) increased oxygen demand; (5) increased intratubular pressure related to osmotic diuresis induced by the contrast agent; (6) increasing of urinary viscosity; (7) intratubular obstruction. All above causes may contribute to renal ischemia [29-31].

The extrinsic causes are essentially represented by dehydration and reduction of circulating volume.

Experimental models seem to confirm the hypothesis that damage from the contrast agent occurs more readily when pre-existing intra-renal hemodynamics alteration occurs. Under normal conditions there is in a delicate balance between vasoconstrictor and vasodilator factors (PGs, NO, endothelin). It is known that the infusion of contrast medium in experimental animals is accompanied by a diphasic hemodynamic response: vasodilation lasting a few seconds, followed by a vasoconstriction of variable duration leading to a fall in renal plasma flow (RPF) and a prolonged GFR reduction. In humans the hemodynamic response appears to be similar. Therefore, CI-AKI occurrence is most commonly seen in patients with a greater reduction in the RPF. A condition of good hydration can, therefore, prevent the onset of disease. Due to the osmotic load provided by the contrast medium [32], we observe: (1) increasing quantity of filtered sodium and chlorine which reaches the thin segment of the ascending limb of Henle's loop and, above all, (2) an increase in O_2 consumption. However, the fall of the medullary interstitial pO_2 is greater than one would expect only from its increased use. The reduced blood circulation as a result of a pre-existing RPF reduction likely has a role in such dynamic. Thus, under such conditions, an imbalance between vasoconstriction and vasodilation factors of the intra-renal vascular system occurs.

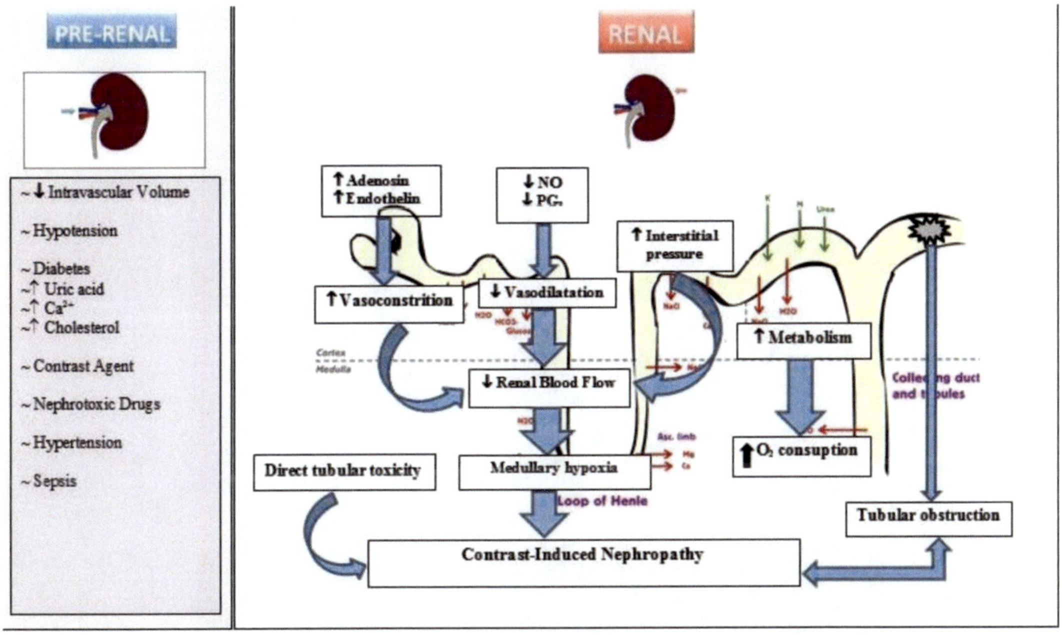

Figure 2. Proposed pathogenetic mechanisms for contrast-induced nephropathy.

A large number of potential vasoconstrictor factors, such as angiotensin, endothelin, adenosine, thromboxane, was implicated in the CI-AKI pathogenesis.

Regarding the renin angiotensin system, the blocking angiotensin II receptors partially reduces the response of vasoconstriction to the contrast agent in animals; likewise, the infusion of angiotensin II enhances kidney damage in rats.

Unfortunately no human trials have tested the effectiveness of RAAS block. A small prospective study [33] conducted in CKD patients showed that a single captopril dose administered about 20 minutes before exposure to the contrast decreases by about 20% the GFR and RPF decrease after 120 minutes. In this study it wasn't reported the incidence of CI-AKI.

Endothelins (ETs), vasoactive peptides composed of 21 amino acids, are known as ET1, ET2, ET3 and ET4. ETs bind to a specific receptor existing in at least two types: ETα (on smooth muscle cells) and ETβ (on smooth muscle cells and endothelial cells).

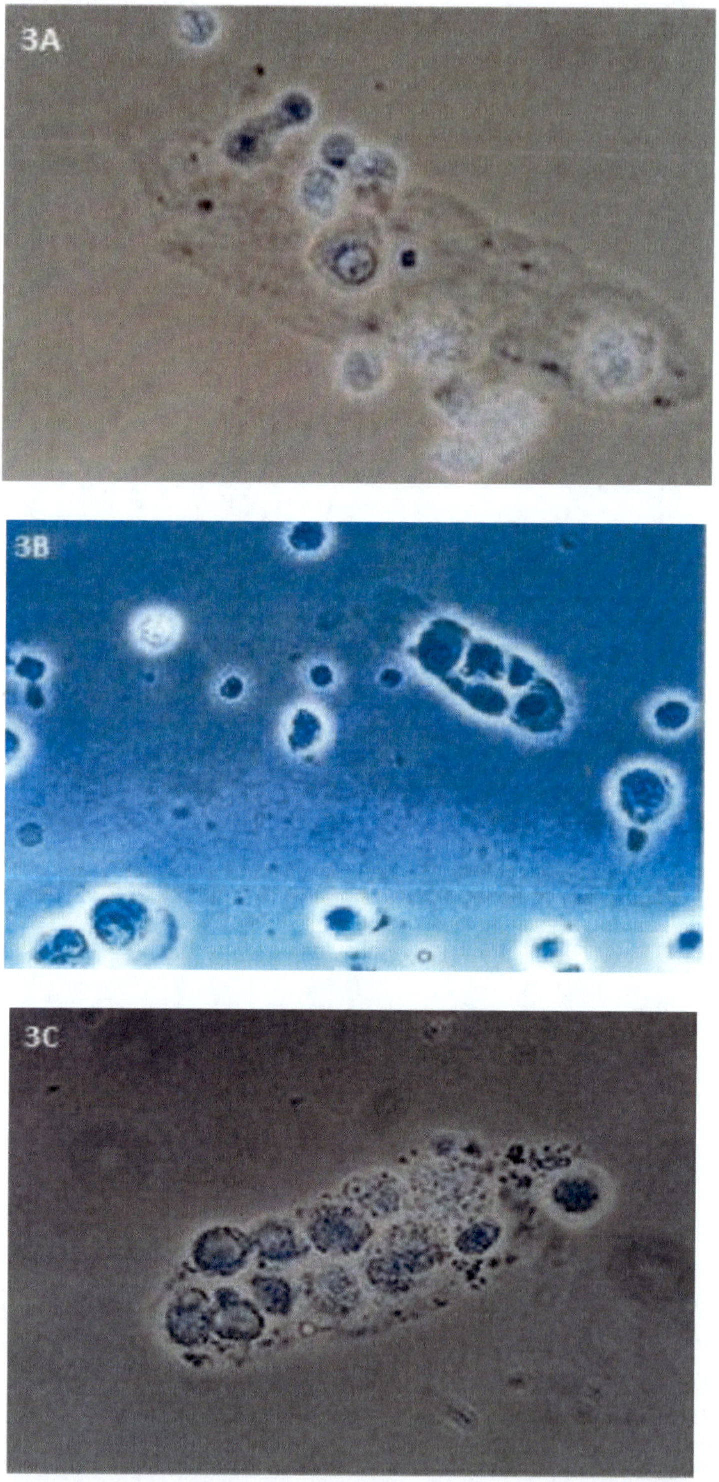

Figure 3. A. An ovoidal tubular cells within the matrix of a cast (phase contrast, x 400). B. A cast containing tubular cells; other similar cells are free in the urine (phase contract, x 400). C. An epithelial cast containing tubular cells with their typical large central nucleus (phase contrast, x 400).

ETs, produced by endothelial cells of the kidney and mesangial cells, act locally producing an intense and long-lasting vasoconstriction. Experimental *in vitro* and *in vivo* data [34] show a role of ETs in CI-AKI. In fact, administering an ETs antagonist before the contrast agent can prevent the decline of the RPF. Some systemic mediators, such as atrial natriuretic factor (ANP) and the antidiuretic hormone, may play a role in CI-AKI pathogenesis, but at the moment there are no reliable data. The final outcome of the mechanisms described above is a renal hypoxia due to osmotic stress [35, 36]: this one is poorly tolerated if the renal circulation is compromised, such as in patients with diabetes mellitus and renal failure.

The contrast medium in the renal tubule increases ATP hydrolysis resulting in increased adenosine concentrations. Such nucleoside increases the vasoconstrictor effects [37]; also the inhibition of PG synthesis as well as the sodium depletion increase the renal effects of adenosine. In animal models a renal protection by phosphodiesterase inhibitors (aminophylline and/or theophylline) has been demonstrated in respect of CI-AKI, supporting these findings [38-41]. ROS also contribute to the pathogenesis of acute renal failure from contrast media [42]. It has been shown an increase in the renal production of free radicals after contrast medium administration [43-45] while the preventive treatment with superossidodesmutasi and allopurinol has been able to reduce it [46]. Following we describe the nephrotoxic differences between contrast agents. In humans the HOCM determines a RPF reduction greater than LOCM. The reduction in renal excretion of PAI demonstrated after administration of contrast medium is certainly suggestive of tubular damage. The direct toxic effect on tubular cells is shown by a reduced sodium proximal reabsorption and with the increase in urinary excretion of lysosomal enzymes and brush border components. The contrast medium tends to accumulate in intracellular vacuoles [47-49]: this gradually leads to cell lysis resulting to tubular necrosis. In vitro, the contrast agents also exert a toxic effect on the cells of the distal tubule, detectable with the increased of potassium and adenosine triphosphate urinary excretion [50-53].

In conclusion, the evidence described so far emphasizes the central role of medullary ischemia in CI-AKI pathophysiology.

The altered balance between vasoconstrictor/vasodilators factors could be the onset of a deviation of the blood flow to the cortex, especially in the presence of pre-existing renal impairment, such as diabetes mellitus and/or renal failure.

Clinical Description

Following the use of iodinated contrast media cellular debris and epithelial cylinders can be observed in the urinary sediment (Figure 3A, 3B, 3C). Tubular cells contained in the cylinders are generally round or ovoidal, with central or peripheral nucleus. However, when cellular degeneration occurs, due to the collapse of the cytoplasmic organelles around the nucleus, these aspects may be absent. In this case, it is almost impossible to distinguish them from the leukocyte cylinders, even with the phase contrast microscope. The presence of leukocytes or tubular cells may aid in differentiating the leukocyte from epithelial cylinders. These findings are, however, non-specific and not predictive of CI-AKI. Sometimes there may be crystals of calcium oxalate and urate amorphous. Formerly, a reduction in the fraction of sodium excretion (<1%) was reported as a distinctive element of AKI by contrast medium [22, 54], but more recently this index was highly variable [55]. In some studies the persistence of nephrographic effect after 24-48 hours after the contrast medium injection, has been shown as a hallmark of CI-AKI. Sensitivity, specificity and clinical relevance of this finding have not yet been clarified [56-58]. Despite researchers look for early kidney injury biomarkers, currently the easiest, more sensitive and inexpensive method for CI-AKI diagnosis is repetitive sCr measurement. Although the CI-AKI is usually not oliguric, sometimes it may begin in the oliguric form, especially if pre-existing kidney damage occurs. Creatinine serum concentrations usually begin to rise within 24 hours of exposure to the contrast medium, reaching a peak after 3-5 days. These patients must be treated in the same way as for other AKI forms, namely:

- monitoring serum electrolytes to identify hyperkalemia;
- controlling the fluid balance and body weight for the prevention of hypo/hyper-blood volume;
- providing adequate nutritional support.

Generally, sCr levels tend to return to baseline within 7-10 days after onset, however, if a more severe kidney damage occurs, replacement therapy may be required. Fortunately, CI-AKI in most cases tend to self-restraint and resolve.

Prevention Strategies

The limited availability of treatment options make CI-AKI prophylaxis a very important strategy in clinical practice, perhaps the only one. Prevention is based on: knowledge of pathophysiological mechanisms previously considered, assessment of risk factors, choice of more appropriate contrast medium (or at doses as low as possible) and use of alternative imaging techniques (without contrast), if possible.

At the moment only a good hydration and avoiding potentially nephrotoxic drugs (e.g., NSAIDs, aminoglycosides, cisplatin, cyclosporin A, amphotericin B) at least 24 hours before the examination have been useful in reducing the incidence of CI-AKI.

Hydration. Although dehydration is not universally recognized as an independent risk factor for the onset of CI-AKI, nevertheless the hydration seems to represent the easiest and most effective method to protect kidney function against iodinated contrast medium injury.

In high-risk patients the following protocol may be used: saline solution 1 ml/kg body weight/hour IV, taking into account the cardiovascular and hydration status. This protocol can begin 6-12 hours before the contrastographic examination and should continue for the next 12-24 hours if diuresis is preserved. In a retrospective study on 158 patients with renal impairment (sCr >1.9 mg/dL) Brown et al. revealed that 76 subjects with CI-AKI had a lower blood pressure and were less hydrated than 82 control subjects [59]. Solomon et al. conducted a prospective randomized trial in 78 patients with renal impairment (sCr: 2.1 ± 0.6 mg/dL; 50% diabetics) candidates for cardiac catheterization. All patients were treated with saline solution 0.45%: 1 ml/kg/min in the 12 hours before and after exposure to contrast medium; 80 mg of furosemide were administered to a third of them and further 50 g of mannitol to 26 patients, 30 and 60 minutes before the procedure, respectively. The overall incidence of CI-AKI was 26%, comparable to that observed in previous studies. However, the group treated only with hypotonic solution showed 11% incidence compared to 26% of the group with mannitol and 46% of the furosemide group. The Authors concluded that hydration with hypotonic solution alone provides a better protection towards the onset of CI-AKI [60]. Almost all trials in which the hydration is used in patients undergoing angiography confirmed a lower frequency of CI-AKI. More recently a single-center, prospective, randomized trial of 119 patients suggested that hydration with sodium bicarbonate showed some superiority over the simple saline solution [61]. In sodium bicarbonate-treated patients, the CI-AKI incidence observed was 1.7% *vs* 13.6%. Merten et al. concluded that hydration with sodium bicarbonate was more effective than saline alone in preventing CI-AKI [61]. The higher efficacy of sodium bicarbonate may be due to extracellular environment alkalinization, which reduces ROS levels. Further study will be needed to further clarify this aspect. Meantime, we can use the administration of sodium bicarbonate solution as an effective prevention strategy of CI-AKI.

N-Acetylcysteine. The many evidences in favor of the pathogenic role of ROS in the CI-AKI represent the rationale of using N-acetylcysteine (NAC) for the prophylaxis of CI-AKI. NAC is considered an antioxidant that can increase cellular oxide-reductive capacity. Furthermore, NAC may produce the S-nitrosothiol (a potent vasodilator) through combination with the NO, thus improving the PRF [61].

In animal models, NAC has proved able to reduce ischemia-reperfusion injury in several parts of the body, including the kidney. Recent studies have focused on vasodilator properties of NAC [62, 63], demonstrating its ability to block VCAM-1 (Vascular Cell Adhesion Molecule-1) expression and nuclear mesangial factor-κβ activation [64]. Tepel et al. observed a smaller reduction of renal function in all patients with pre-existing CKD (sCr: 2.4 ± 1.3 mg/dL; GFR <50 mL/min), by administering NAC orally at 600 mg dose every 12 hours, the day before and the day of the examination with contrast medium [65]. However, this study has some limitations: (1) small sample size (n = 83); (2) lack of follow-up; (3) broad enrollment criteria so to allow inclusion of patients with normal renal function.

The APART study (Acetylcysteine to Prevent Angiography-Related Renal Tissue Injury) confirms that NAC reduces the risk of CI-AKI post-cardiac catheterization in CKD patients and suggests the use of this drug in preventing CI-AKI. There are plenty of studies that cast doubt on the protective effect of NAC. Durham et al. say that NAC is not effective in preventing CI-AKI in CKD patients undergoing cardiac catheterization [66]. The same Authors, however, highlight many differences between their study and Tepel's study, namely: in the first study higher LOCM doses (81.6 vs 75 mL) are used for intra-arterial route (IV in the second study). Even the timing of NAC intake differed in the two trials: Durham used an initial dose of 1200 mg administered 60 minutes before the diagnostic procedure and a second after 180 minutes. Since NAC after a single dose oral administration reaches a peak serum in about an hour and has a half-life of 120 minutes, it is very unlikely that this intake timing may have influenced the two studies. However, the Authors speculate that some other acetylcysteine metabolite with antioxidant properties might be responsible for the benefits observed in the Tepel's study.

The available studies, the safety and the low cost of NAC, have widely adopted this drug in preventing CI-AKI, especially in high-risk patients. The NAC dosage regimen most widely used includes the oral administration of 600 mg every 12 hours twenty-four hours before and the day of the contrastographic procedure. In patients unable to take it orally, the drug can be administered IV at a dose of 150 mg/kg half hour before or 50 mg/kg approximately four hours after contrastographic procedure [67].

Contrast media. According to their chemical and pharmacological characteristics the contrast media can be classified into ionic or non-ionic and monomeric or dimeric.

The osmotic properties have a central role in the onset of CI-AKI and are defined by the ratio between the number of iodine atoms in the molecules of contrast medium compared to the total number of dissolved particles: the higher ratio and the better X-rays attenuation.

1.5:1 ratio characterizes the HOCM, while the LOCM are characterized by a ratio of 3:1 [54]; more recently, agents so-called iso-osmolar (IOCM) with a ratio of 6:1 have been introduced [54].

It has been shown [68] that patients receiving HOCM (diatrizoate) had a 3.3 times greater risk of developing CI-AKI compared to those administered with LOCM (iohexol). Subsequently, a meta-analysis of 31 trials concluded that LOCM use in patients with preexisting renal disease was associated with a lower CI-AKI incidence compared to HOCM [69].

LOCM, while being more expensive, are better tolerated and cause fewer allergic reactions and/or adverse events to the cardiovascular apparatus compared to HOCM. Their use is strongly recommended in case of increased CI-AKI risk, while in patients with normal renal function they do not have substantial advantages compared to HOCM [69].

An interesting promise seems to be the iodixanol, IOCM, non-ionic, dimeric. Clinical studies show a lower CI-AKI incidence (odds ratio 11 times lower) with the use of iodixanol *vs* iohexol in high risk patients [69].

Mannitol and Furosemide. Some Authors suggest that the use of mannitol may prevent acute kidney injury by contrast media, in high-risk patients [70]. This suggestion comes mainly from pre-clinical experimental observations showing that mannitol is able to prevent ischemic renal failure in dogs and preserve the GFR during renal hypoperfusion in rats [71, 72]. However, the effect of nephroprotection was not reproducible in CI-AKI animal models; furthermore, the osmotic load that reaches the renal tubules increases the medullar O_2 consumption leading to a severe hypoxia. Clinical trials aimed at demonstrating the protective effect of mannitol against CI-AKI did not provide convincing results. The most often mentioned study supporting mannitol use is Anto et al. [55], in which 37 CKD patients were hydrated before and after urographic examination and submitted to infusion of 20%-mannitol one hour after exposure to the contrast medium; these subjects were compared with 40 others who received only hydration. CI-AKI incidence was 22% in the treatment group *vs* 70% of the control. However, the study has been criticized since the hydration protocol differed in the study group compared to controls. The un-effect of mannitol was later confirmed by Solomon and colleagues mentioned above [60].

Even the use of furosemide in preventing CI-AKI appears controversial. Heyman et al. observed a minor impairment of the GFR in rats by administering furosemide before exposure to contrast medium [73] However, few controlled trials support the prophylactic use of loop diuretics. On the other hand, Weinstein et al. [74] suggest a harmful effect of furosemide: in this study the renal function underwent a significant deterioration in patients with pre-existing CKD treated with furosemide and hydration before the contrastographic exam. According to the Authors, furosemide contributes to kidney damage causing a negative water balance. Solomon reaches the same conclusions [60], assuming that the adverse effect has to be found in the intra-renal blood flow reduction induced by the diuretic, worsening hypoxia induced by the contrast.

Vasodilators drugs. Many substances have been used as vasodilators in preventing CI-AKI. However, this approach does not seem entirely free from side effects; in fact reduction of systemic blood pressure and/or reduction of resistance of the renal cortex may further compromise the medullary circulation (especially in diabetic subjects).

Intra-arterial infusion of ANP (atrial natriuretic peptide) has succeeded in preventing the fall of GFR after 24 and 36 hours of exposure to the contrast medium [75]. However, a prospective randomized trial with ANP IV in 207 high-risk patients (sCr ~ 2.1 mg/dL) did not provide the expected positive results in terms of CI-AKI reduction. Similarly, the Auriculin Anaritide Acute Renal Failure Study Group, multicenter, randomized, double-blind study failed to demonstrate the superiority of anaritide (synthetic analog of ANP) over placebo in terms of dialysis-free survival in patients with acute renal failure oliguric from acute tubular necrosis [76]. Kurnik et al. observed in 247 high-risk patients (CKD and diabetes mellitus) as the CI-AKI frequency was higher in the group treated with anaritide (23-25%) compared to placebo (19%); moreover, there was no evidence of greater benefit in the group with diabetes [77]. Likewise Weisberg et al. did not obtain any benefit from ANP administration compared to hydration alone [78]. Therefore, there are currently no indications to the use of ANP in CI-AKI prophylaxis.

Dopamine is a potent renal vasodilator. Two prospective trials, one of which randomized controlled trial, have shown that dopamine administration of 2.5-3.0 μg/kg/min before and after 12- 24 hours of exposure to the contrast medium is able to prevent CI-AKI in patients with renal failure [79]. More recent studies have not confirmed these findings, noting that dopamine - when compared with hydration - worsens kidney failure, prolonging the course of the CI-AKI [80]. This results were confirmed by Weisberg [78], who observed that, similarly to diuretics, dopamine worsened kidney function in diabetic patients. Dopamine agonists (e.g., Fenoldopam) don't seem to have more advantages than the dopamine or hydration alone. For these reasons, the use of these substances is not recommended in the prevention of acute kidney injury by contrast medium.

The nitrendipine was one of the first calcium antagonists to be used in preventing CI-AKI. In a randomized double-blind trial, its use in patients undergoing urography and renal arteriography was able to slow GFR decline following the administration of contrast medium with return to baseline levels within 48 hours [81]. Similar results were obtained in a subsequent study despite a follow-up of only two hours [82], while Solomon was unable to prove a protective effect of a single dose of a calcium channel blocker before angiography on 78 patients [60].

Likewise, Khoury et al. [83] in a prospective randomized trial with nifedipine failed to reach statistical significance in 42 patients treated with 10 mg of the drug compared to the placebo group.

This led these authors to conclude that prophylaxis with nifedipine is not accompanied with any clinical benefit and therefore should not be used routinely to prevent CI-AKI.

In a more recent trial 27 patients (including 15 diabetics) with normal or only slightly reduced renal function, underwent angiography with LOCM (iohexol) and preventive hydration [84]. The Authors were unable to demonstrate a greater protective effect of felodipine (10 mg orally 3-4 hours before the exam) in 14 treated patients compared to controls ($p < 0.05$). Despite these disappointing results, Duan et al. [85] reported that amlodipine seems to prevent kidney damage by diatrizoate in rats, while the diltiazem (10 mg/kg intraperitoneally 30 minutes before exposure to the contrast medium) prevents the increase of the creatinine observed with the injection of 6 mL of diatrizoate in 5 rat models [86]. In humans lack of unequivocal results advise against the use of such drugs in CI-AKI prophylaxis.

In different experimental models of acute renal failure adenosine receptor antagonists have been shown to have a nephroprotection effect, while two clinical trials confirmed these benefits in humans. In the first, Erley [87] evaluated the effect of theophylline IV *vs* placebo in 45 patients. Inulin clearance and creatinine clearance were significantly reduced in the placebo group but were stable or only slightly declined in the treatment group. This nephroprotection occurred both in patients with or without pre-existing CKD. Similar results were obtained from Katholi et al. [37], enrolling 93 patients with baseline sCr <2.0 mg/dL to receive oral theophylline or placebo before exposure to iopamidol (LOCM) or diatrizoate (HOCM). The reduction in creatinine clearance was significantly attenuated by theophylline.

Other studies, however, do not agree with such results. Abizaid et al. [88] in a trial including 60 patients undergoing coronary angioplasty randomized to receive saline, dopamine or aminophylline failed to show significant differences between the various groups. The study by Gandhi et al. [89] similarly showed no clinical benefit from theophylline.

In the absence of a definitive prospective multicenter trial, considering the potential side effects of theophylline (arrhythmias, seizures), as well as its narrow therapeutic index, currently adenosine receptor antagonists are not recommended for routine CI-AKI prophylaxis in the clinical practice.

In some experimental models, *bosentan*, an endothelin receptor antagonist, has been able to protect kidney from acute damage induced by contrast medium.

By contrast, a recent multicenter randomized prospective trial reports such drugs led to a deterioration of nephrotoxicity. Wang et al. [43] evaluated 158 patients with CKD (sCr: 2.7 mg/dL ± 1.0 mg/dL) undergoing coronary angiography and randomized to receive a mix of A and B endothelin antagonists or placebo; they show an increase in average values sCr (>0.5 mg/dL or 25% from baseline within 48 hours of infusion of contrast) in the treated group compared with placebo. This increase occurred in patients with diabetes as well as non-diabetics.

Two pilot studies aimed at verifying the effectiveness of PGE1 (alprostadil), on 117 [90] and in 130 patients respectively [91], demonstrated the protective role in the CI-AKI. Despite the promising results, these studies are limited by the small number of subjects, the lack of control of the state of hydration, the type of contrast medium used and its mode of administration and the volume used. In addition, six patients presented significant side effects that required prostaglandins discontinuation; an undetermined number of patients complained nausea, vomiting, fatigue and skin disorders; others had a significant reduction in blood pressure. Authors did not discuss these important issues and concluded that PGE1 can be used successfully and safely in the prevention of acute renal failure from contrast media in patients with prior renal impairment. Further trials are needed to determine the safety and applicability in clinical practice.

Hemodialysis and Hemofiltration. Removing by dialysis the contrast medium in patients with pre-existing renal impairment has no effect on CI-AKI prevention and is not routinely applicable in the clinical practice.

In a randomized trial Vogt et al. evaluated the effectiveness of CI-AKI prevention by hemodialysis (HD) in CKD patients [92]. The results showed no benefit over hydration alone. Marenzi et al. evaluated the effectiveness of hemofiltration (HF) *vs* hydration in CI-AKI prevention in patients with renal failure undergoing percutaneous coronary angiography. One hundred fourteen CKD patients (sCr >2.0 mg/dL) were randomized to HF or to hydration with isotonic saline solution. sCr increase was found (>25% from baseline) lower in the HF group compared with the control (5% vs. 50%; $p < 0.001$); only 3% of HF patients underwent temporary hemodialysis (25% in control group). Adverse events during hospitalization (HF: 9% *vs* 52%; $p < 0.001$), mortality rate (HF: 2% *vs* 14%; $p = 0.02$) and cumulative mortality at 1 year (HF: 10% *vs* 30%; $p = 0.01$) were overall higher in the control group. Although the Authors confer to HF these benefits, they also acknowledge the fundamental role of intensive care received in ICU and that infusion of heparin during HF can show some advantages. The superiority of the convective method compared to hemodialysis was attributed to the greater hemodynamic stability and to prevention of renal hypoperfusion. By contrast, hypovolemia induced from HD could worsen the ischemic kidney damage and require additional substitution treatment.

A recent systematic review considered 11 studies enrolling 1,010 patients overall [94]: in 8 studies the conventional HD has been used and in 3 studies the HF or hemodiafiltration (HDF). Despite the effective removal of contrast medium, a significant reduction in the CI-AKI incidence was not observed, as compared to normal medical therapy (relative risk 1.2).

Moreover, in the HD group, there was an increased incidence of CI-AKI as compared with control patients (relative risk 1.61), while in HF or HDF groups there was a significant reduction in the use of HD (RR 0:22) and a decrease of CI-AKI (RR 0:46). Further randomized controlled trials will be required to assess the effectiveness of substitution treatment in advanced stage of renal failure.

The US Food and Drug Administration issued a “warning cautioning” with regard to the use of contrast media in patients taking metformin. Metformin is completely eliminated by renal secretion. In the presence of renal failure, increased serum levels can cause lactic acidosis that sometimes is associated with CI-AKI. Drug suspension is therefore recommended at least 48 hours before exposure to contrast medium.

The recommendations provided by the KDIGO guidelines [2] for the prevention of CI-AKI are the following:

1. volume expansion with isotonic saline or sodium bicarbonate in patients at increased risk is recommended (1A);
2. using oral fluids in patients at increased risk is not recommended (1C);
3. the use of oral N-acetylcysteine along with the use of intravenous isotonic crystalloid in patients at increased risk (2D) is recommended;
4. It is suggested not to use theophylline (2C) or the fenoldopam (1B);
5. It is suggested not to use hemodialysis or hemofiltration with preventive purposes.

Prevention strategies described so far are predominantly oriented to the patient’s preparation and treatment. The crucial factors for CI-AKI development are the type of procedure, the nephrotoxicity of the contrast medium related to its chemical-physical characteristics and the chosen route of administration.

REFERENCES

[1] Barrett BJ, Parfrey PS: Prevention of nephrotoxicity induced by radiocontrast agents. *N Engl J Med* 1994; 331:1449-1450.
[2] KDIGO Clinical Practice Guideline for Acute Kidney Injury Kidney Int 2012; Suppl. 2. (Section 4: Contrast-induced AKI: 69-88). http://www. nature.com/kisup/journal/v2/n1/ index.html.
[3] Misson R, Cutler R: Radiocontrast-induced renal failure. *West J Med* 1985; 142:657-664.
[4] McCullough PA, Wolyn R, Rocher LL, Levin RN, O'Neill WW: Acute renal failure after coronary intervention: incidence, risk factors and relationship to mortality. *Am J Med* 1997; 103:368-374.
[5] Berg KJ: nephrotoxicity related to contrast media. *Scand J Urol Nephrol* 2000; 34:317-322.
[6] Newhouse JH, Kho D, Rao QA, Starren J: Frequency of serum creatinine changes in the absence of iodinated contrast material: implications for studies of contrast nephrotoxicity. *Am J Roentgenol* 2008; 191:376-382.
[7] McDonald JS, McDonald RJ, Comin J, Williamson EE, Katzberg RW et al: Frequency of acute kidney injury following intravenous contrast medium administration: a systematic review and meta-analysis. *Radiology* 2013; 267: 119-128.
[8] Hou SH, Bushinsky DA, Wish JB, Cohen JJ, Harrington JT: Hospital-acquired renal insufficiency: a prospective study. *Am J Med* 1983; 74:243-248.
[9] Brady RB, Singer GG: Acute Renal Failure. *Lancet* 1995; 346:1533-1540.
[10] Levy EM, Viscoli CM, Horwitz RI: The effect of acute renal failure on mortality: a cohort analysis. *JAMA* 1996; 275:1489-1494.
[11] McDonald RJ, McDonald JS, Carter RE, Hartman RP, Katzberg RW et al: Intravenous contrast material exposure is not an independent risk factor for dialysis or mortality. *Radiology* 2014; 273: 714-725.
[12] Solomon R: Contrast medium induced acute renal failure. *Kidney Int* 1998; 53:230-242.
[13] Tervel JL, Marcer R, Onaindia JM, Serrano A, Quereda C et al: Renal function impairment caused by intravenous urography. *Arch Int Med* 1981; 141:1271-1274.
[14] Parfrey PS, Griffiths SM, Barret BJ, Paul MD, Genge M et al: Contrast material-induced renal failure in patients with diabetes mellitus, renal insufficiency or both: A prospective controlled study. *N Engl J Med* 1989; 320:143-149.
[15] Davidson CJ, Hlatky M, Morris KG, Pieper K, Skelton TN et al: Cardiovascular and renal toxicity of a nonionic radiographic contrast agents after cardiac catheterization. A prospective trial. *Ann Intern Med* 1989; 110:119-124.
[16] Mason RA, Arbett LA, Giron F: Renal disfunction after arteriography. *JAMA* 1985;253(7):727-732.
[17] Vix VA: Intravenous pielography in multiple myeloma; *Radiology* 1966;87:896-902.
[18] Myers GH, Witten DM: Acute renal failure after excretory urography in multiple myeloma. *Am J Roentgenol Rod Ther Nucl Med* 1971;113:583-588.
[19] Simon EE: Potential role of integrins in acute renal failure. *Nephrol Dial Transplant* 1994; 9(Suppl. 4): 26-33.

[20] McCarthy CS, Becker JA: Multiple myeloma and contrast media. *Radiology* 1992;183:519-521.

[21] Manske CL, Sprafka JM, Strony JT, Wang Y: Contrast nephropathy in azotemic diabetic patients undergoing coronary angiography. *Am J Med* 1990; 89:615-620.

[22] Fang L, Sirota R, Ebert T, Lichtenstein N: Low fractional excretion of sodium with contrast media-induced acute renal failure. *Arch Intern Med* 1980;140:531-533.

[23] Anderson RJ, Linas SL, Berns AS, Henrich WL, Miller TL, et al: Non-oliguric acute renal failure. *N Engl J Med* 1977; 296: 1134-1138.

[24] Taliercia CP, Vlietstra RE, Ilstrup DM, Burnett JC, Menke KK, et al: A randomized comparison of the nephrotoxicity of iopamidolo and diatrizoate in High-risk patients undergoing cardiac angiography. *J Am Coll Cardiol* 1991; 17:384-390.

[25] Barrett BJ: Contrast nephrotoxicity. *J Am Soc Nephrol* 1994; 5:125-137.

[26] Barrett BJ, Carlisle EJ: Metaanalysis of the relative nephrotoxicity of high- and low-osmolality iodinated contrast media. *Radiology* 1993; 188:171-178.

[27] Lepor NE, Mathur VS: Radiocontrast nephropathy. *Curr Intern Cardiol Rep* 2000; 2:335-341.

[28] Thomsen HS: Contrast-medium-induced nephrotoxicity: are all answers in for Acetylcysteine? *Eur Radiol* 2001; 11:2351-2353.

[29] Weisberg LS, Kurnik PB, Kurnik BR: Radiocontrast-induced nephropathy in humans: role of renal vasoconstriction. *Kidney Int* 1992; 41:1408-1415.

[30] Prasad PV, Priatna A, Spokes K, Epstein FH: Changes in intra-renal oxygenation as evaluated by BOLD MRI in a rat kidney model for radiocontrast nephropathy. *J Magn Reson Imaging* 2000; 13:744-747.

[31] Bakris GI, Lass N, Gaber AO, Jones JD, Burnett JC Jr: Radiocontrast medium induces declines in renal function: a role for oxygen free radicals. *Am J Physiol* 1990; 258(1 Pt 2):F115-120.

[32] Murphy ME, Tublin ME, Li S: Influence of contrast media on the response of rat renal arteries to endothelin and nitric oxide: influence of contrast media. *Invest Radiol* 1998; 33:356-365.

[33] Russo D, Minutolo R, Cianciaruso B,, Mernoli B, Conte G et al: Early effects of contrast media on renal hemodynamics and tubular function in chronic renal failure. *J Am Soc Nephrol* 1995; 6:1451-1458.

[34] Oldroyd SD, Haylor JL, Morcos SK: The acute effect of ioversol on kidney function: role of endothelin. *Eur J Radiol* 1995; 19:91-95.

[35] Weinbroum AA, Reduck V, Ben-Abraham R, Karchevsky E: N-acetylcysteine ameliorates ischemic renal failure. *Am J Physiol* 1997; 272:F292-298.

[36] Heyman SN, Rosen S, Brezis M: Radiocontrast nephropathy: a paradigm for the synergism between toxic and hypoxic insults in the kidney. *Exp Nephrol* 1994; 2:153-157.

[37] Katholi RE, Taylor GJ, McCann WP, Woods WT Jr, Womack KA, et al: Nephrotoxicity from contrast media: attenuation with theophylline. *Radiology* 1995; 195:17-22.

[38] Gouyon JB, Guignard JP: Theophylline prevents the hypoxemia-induced renal hemodynamic changes in rabbits. *Kidney Int* 1988; 33:1078-1083.

[39] Deray G, Martinez F, Cacoub P, Baumelou B, Baumelou A, et al: A role for adenosine, calcium and ischemia in radiocontrast-induced intrarenale vasoconstriction. *Am J Nephrol* 1990; 10:316-322.

[40] Rossi N, Ellis V, Kontry T, Gunther S, Churchill P, et al: The role of adenosine in HgC12-induced acute renal failure in rats. *Am J Physiol* 1990; 258:F1554-F1560.

[41] Lin JJ, Churchill PC, Bidani AK: Effect of theophylline on the initiation phase of postischemic acute renal failure in rats. *J Lab Clin Med* 1986; 108:150-154.

[42] Battenfeld R, Khater AR, Drommer W, Guenzel P, Kaup F-J: Ioxaglate-induced light and electron microscopic alterations in the renal proximal tubular epithelium of rats. *Invest Radiol* 1991; 26:35-39.

[43] Wang A, Holcslaw T, Bashore TM, Freed MI, Miller D, et al: Exacerbation of radiocontrast nephrotoxicity by endothelin receptor antagonism. *Kidney Int* 2000; 57:1675-1680.

[44] Yoshioka T, Fogo A, Beckman JK: Reduced activity of antioxidant enzymes underlies contrast media-induced renal injury in volume depletion. *Kidney Int* 1992; 41:1008-1015.

[45] Baliga R, Ueda N, Walker PD, Shah SV: Oxidant mechanisms in toxic acute renal failure. *Am J Kidney Dis* 1997; 29:465-477.

[46] Safirstein R, Andrade L, Vieria JM. Acetylcysteine and nephrotoxic effects of radiographics contrast agents: a new use for an old drug. *N Engl J Med* 2000; 343:210-212.

[47] Dobrota M, Powell C, Holtz E, Wallin A, Vik H: Biochemical and morphological effects of contrast media on the kidney. *Acta Radiol* 1995; 399(Suppl):196-203.

[48] Tervahartiala P, Kivisaari L, Kivisaari R, Virtanen I, Standerskjold-Nordenstam C: Contrast media-induced renal tubular vacuolization: a light and electron microscopy study on rat kidneys. *Invest Radiol* 1991; 26:882-887.

[49] Tervahartiala P: Contrast media-induced tubular vacuolization after dehydratation: a light and electron microscopy study in rats. *Invest Radiol* 1992; 27:114-118.

[50] Andersen K, Vik H, Eikesdal H, Christensen E: Effects of contrast media on renal epithelial cells in culture. *Acta Radiol* 1995; 399[Suppl]:213-218.

[51] Anderson K-J, Christensen E, Vik H: Effects of iodinated x-ray contrast media on renal epithelial cells in culture. *Invest Radiol* 1994; 29:955-962.

[52] Messana J, Cieslinski D, Nguyen V, Humes H: Comparison of the toxicity of the radiocontrast agents, iopamidolo and diatrizoate, to rabbit renal proximal tubule cells in vitro. *J Pharmacol Exp Ther* 1988; 244:1139-1144.

[53] Humes H, Hunt D, White M: Direct toxic effect of the radiocontrast agent diatrizoato on renal proximal tubule cells. *Am J Physiol* 1987; 252[Suppl 2, part 2]F:246-F255.

[54] Katzberg R: Urography into the 21st century: new contrast media handling, imaging characteristics, and nephrotoxicity. *Radiology* 1997; 204:297-312.

[55] Anto H, Chou S-Y, Porush J, Shapiro W: Infusion intravenous pyelography and renl function: effects of hypertonc mannitol in patients with chronic renal insufficiency. *Arch Intern Med* 1981; 141:1652-1656.

[56] Jacobsen J, Lundby B, Kristoffersen D, Borch K, Hald J, et al: Evaluation of renal function with delayed CT after injection of nonionic monomeric dimeric contrast media in healthy volunteers. *Radiology* 1992; 182:419-424.

[57] Love L, Lind J Jr, Olson M: Persistent CT nephrogram: significance in the diagnosis of contrast nephropathy. *Radiology* 1989; 172:125-129.

[58] Love L, Johnson M, Bresler M: The persistent computed tomography nephrogram: its significance in the diagnosis of contrast-associated nephrotoxicity. *Br J Radiol* 1994; 67:951-957.

[59] Brown SB, Ransil B, Clark BA: Prehydratation protects against contrast nephropathy in high-risk patients undergoing cardiac catheterization (abstract). *J Am Soc Nephrol* 1990; 1:330A.

[60] Solomon R, Werner C, Mann D, D'Elia J, Silva P: Effect of saline, mannitol, and furosemide on acute decreases in renal function induced by radiocontrast agents. *N Engl J Med* 1994; 331:1416-1420.

[61] Merten GJ, Burgess WP, Gray LV, Holleman JH, Roush TS, et al: Prevention of contrast-induced nephropathy with sodium bicarbonate: a randomized controlled trial. *JAMA* 2004; 291:2328-2334.

[62] Arstall MA, Yang J, Stafford I, Betts WH, Horowitz JD: N-acetylcysteine in combination with nitroglycerin and streptokinase for treatment of evolving acute myocardial infarction: safety and biochemical effects. *Circulation* 1995; 92:2855-2862.

[63] Weinbroum AA, Rudick V, Ben-Abraham R, Karchevsky E: N-acetyl-L-cysteine for preventing lung perfusion injury after liver ischemia-reperfusion: a possible dual protective mechanism in a dose-response study. *Transplantation* 2000; 69:853-859.

[64] Khachigian LM, Collins T, Fries JW: N-acetyl-cysteine blocks mesangial VCAM-1 and NF-kappa b expression in vivo. *Am J Pathol* 1997; 151:1225-1229.

[65] Tepel M, Van der Giet M, Schwarzfeld C, Laufer U, Liermann D, et al: Prevention of radiographic-contrast-agent-induced reduction in renal function by Acetylcysteine. *N Engl J Med* 2000; 343:180-184.

[66] Durham JD, Caputo C, Dokko J, Zaharakis T, Mohsen P, et al: A randomized controlled trial of N-acetylcysteine to prevent contrast nephropathy in cardiac angiography. *Kidney Int 2002*; 62:2202-2207.

[67] Baker C, Wragg A, Kumar S: A rapid protocol for the prevention of contrast-induced renal dysfunction: the RAPID study. *J Am Coll Cardiol* 2003; 41:2114-2118.

[68] Rudnick M, Berns J, Cohen R, Goldfarb S: Nephrotoxic risks of renal angiography: contrast media-associated nephrotoxicity and atheroembolism. A critical review. *Am J Kidney Dis* 1994; 24:713-727.

[69] Aspelin P, Aubry P, Fransson SG, Strasser R, Willembrock R, et al: Nephrotoxic effects in high-risk patients undergoing angiography. *N Engl J Med* 2003; 348:491-498.

[70] Berns A: Nephrotoxicity of contrast media. *Kidney Int* 1989; 36:730-740.

[71] Cronin R, Erickson A, De Torrente A, McDonald K, Chrier R: Norepinephrine-induced acute renal failure: a reversible ischemic model of acute renal failure. *Kidney Int* 1978; 14:187-193.

[72] Morris C. Alexander E, Bruns F, levinsky N: Restoration and manteinance of glomerular filtration by mannitol during hypoperfusion of the kidney. *J Clin Invest* 1972; 51:1555-1564.

[73] Heyman S, Brezis M, Greenfield Z, Rosen S: Protective role of furosemide and saline in radiocontrast-induced acute renal failure in the rat. *Am J Kidney Dis* 1989; 14:377-385.

[74] Weinstein JM; Heyman S, Brezis M: Potential deleterious effect of furosemide in radiocontrast nephropathy. *Nephron* 1992; 62:413-415.

[75] Margulies KB, McKinley LJ, Allgren RL, Stanson AW, Burnett JCJ: Intra-arterial atrial natriuretic factor (ANF) attenuates radiocontrast-induced nephropathy in humans (abstract): *J Am Soc Nephrol* 1991, 2(3):666.

[76] Allgren RL, Marbury TC, Rahman SN, Weisberg LS, Fenves AZ, et al. for the Auriculin Anaritide Acute Renal failure Study Group: Anaritide in acute tubular necrosis. *N Engl J Med* 1997; 336:828-834.

[77] Kurnic BRC, Allgren RL, Genter FC; Solomon RJ, Bates ER, et al: Prospective study of atrial natriuretic peptide for the prevention of radiocontrast-induced nephropathy. *Am J Kidney Dis* 1998; 31:674-680.

[78] Weisberg LS, Kurnik PB, Kurnik BR: Risk of radiocontrast nephropathy in patients with and without diabetes mellitus. *Kidney Int* 1994; 45: 259-265.

[79] Hans B, Hans SS, Mittal VK, Khan TA, Patec N: Renal functional response to dopamine during and after arteriography in patients with chronic renal insufficiency. *Radiology* 1990; 176:651-654.

[80] Shammas NW, Kapalis MJ, Harris M, McKinney D, Coyne EP: Aminophylline does not pretect against radiocontrast nephropathy in patients undergoing percutenous angiographic procedures. *J Invasive Cardiol* 2001; 13:738-740.

[81] Neumayer HH, Junge W, Kufner A, Wenning A: Prevention of radiocontrast media-induced nephrotoxicity by the calcium channel blocker nitrendipina: a prospective randomized clinical trial. *Nephrol Dial Transplant* 1989; 55:254-257.

[82] Russo D, Testa A, Della Volpe L, Sansone G: Ranomized prospective study on renal effects of two different contrast media in humans: protective role of a calcium blocker. *Nephron* 1990; 55:254-257.

[83] Khoury Z, Schlicht JE, Como J, Karschner JK, Shapiro AP, et al: The effect of prophylactic nifedipina on renal function in patients administered contrast media. *Pharmacotherapy* 1995; 15:59-65.

[84] Spangberg-Viklund B, Berglund J, Nikonoff T, Nyberg P, Skau T, et al: Does prophylactic treatment with felodipina, a calcium antagonist, prevent low-osmolar contrast-induced renal dysfunction in hydrated diabetic and non diabetic patients with normal or moderately reduced renal function? *Scand J Urol Nephrol* 1996; 30:63-68.

[85] Duan SB, Liu FY, Luo JA, Wu HW, Liu RH, et al: Nephrotoxicity of high and low-osmolar contrast media: the protective role of amlodipine in a rat model. *Acta Radiol* 2000; 41:503-507.

[86] Wang Y-XJ, Jia Y-F, Chen K-M, Morcos SK: Radiographics contrast media induced nephropathy: experimental observations and the protective effect of calcium channel blockers. *Br J Radiol* 2001; 74: 1103-1108.

[87] Erley CM, Duda SH, Dchlepckow S, Koehler J, Strohmaier WL, et al: Adenosine antagonist theophylline prevents the reduction of glomerular filtration rate after contrast media application. *Kidney Int* 1994; 45:1425-1431.

[88] Abizaid AS, Clark CE, Mintz GS, Dosa S: Effects of dopamine and aminophylline on contrast-induced acute renal failure after coronary angioplasty in patients with preexisting renal insufficiency. *Am J Cardiol* 1999; 83:260-263.

[89] Gandhi MR, Brown P, Romanowsky CAJ, Morcos K, Campbell S, et al: The use of theophylline: an adenosine antagonist in the prevention of contrast medium-induced nephrotoxicity (letter). *Br J Radiol* 1992; 65:838.

[90] Brinker JA, Sketch M, Kock JA, Bernink P: PGE_1 prophylaxis against contrast-induced nephropathy in patients with preexisting renal compromise: results of a randomized, controlled pilot trial (abstract). *Circulation* 1998; 98:707A.

[91] Koch JA, Plum J, Grabensee B, Modder U: Prostaglandine E_1: a new agent for the prevention of renal dysfunction in high-risk patients by radiocontrast media – the PGE_1 study group. *Nephrol Dial Transplant* 2000; 15:43-49.

[92] Vogt B, Ferrari P, Schonholzer C, Marti HP, Mohaupt M, et al: Prophylactic hemodialysis after radiocontrast media in patients with renal insufficiency is potentially harmful. Am J Med 2001; 111:692-698.

[93] Marenzi G, Marana I, Lauri G, Assanelli E, Grazi M, et al: The prevention of radiocontrast-agent-induced nephropathy by hemofiltration. *N Engl J Med* 2003; 349:1333-1340.

[94] Cruz DN, Goh CY, Marenzi G, Corradi V, Ronco C, et al: Renal Replacement Therapies for Prevention of Radiocontrast-induced nephropathy: a systematic review. *Am J Med* 2012; 125:66-78.e3.

[95] Sirtori CF, Pasik C: Re-evaluation of biguanide, metformin: mechanism of action and tolerability. *Pharmacol Res* 1994;30:187-228.

About the Editor

Dr. Luca Di Lullo, MD, PhD
Department of Nephrology and Dialysis
L. Parodi Delfino Hospital
Piazza Aldo Moro, 1 – 00034 Colleferro (Roma) – ITALY
Phone +39 349 4203258
dilullo.luca@inwind.it

INDEX

L

M

N

O

P

Q

R

S

T

V